Lecture Notes in Networks and Systems

The series "Lecture Notes in Networks and Systems" publishes the latest developments in Networks and Systems—quickly, informally and with high quality. Original research reported in proceedings and post-proceedings represents the core of LNNS.

Volumes published in LNNS embrace all aspects and subfields of, as well as new challenges in, Networks and Systems.

The series contains proceedings and edited volumes in systems and networks, spanning the areas of Cyber-Physical Systems, Autonomous Systems, Sensor Networks, Control Systems, Energy Systems, Automotive Systems, Biological Systems, Vehicular Networking and Connected Vehicles, Aerospace Systems, Automation, Manufacturing, Smart Grids, Nonlinear Systems, Power Systems, Robotics, Social Systems, Economic Systems and other. Of particular value to both the contributors and the readership are the short publication timeframe and the world-wide distribution and exposure which enable both a wide and rapid dissemination of research output.

The series covers the theory, applications, and perspectives on the state of the art and future developments relevant to systems and networks, decision making, control, complex processes and related areas, as embedded in the fields of interdisciplinary and applied sciences, engineering, computer science, physics, economics, social, and life sciences, as well as the paradigms and methodologies behind them.

Indexed by SCOPUS, INSPEC, WTI Frankfurt eG, zbMATH, SCImago.

All books published in the series are submitted for consideration in Web of Science.

For proposals from Asia please contact Aninda Bose (aninda.bose@springer.com).

Kevin Daimi · Abeer Al Sadoon
Editors

Proceedings of the Second International Conference on Innovations in Computing Research (ICR'23)

Springer

Editors
Kevin Daimi
University of Detroit Mercy
Farmington Hills, MI, USA

Abeer Al Sadoon
Asia Pacific International College
Sydney, NSW, Australia

ISSN 2367-3370 ISSN 2367-3389 (electronic)
Lecture Notes in Networks and Systems
ISBN 978-3-031-35307-9 ISBN 978-3-031-35308-6 (eBook)
https://doi.org/10.1007/978-3-031-35308-6

This Springer imprint is published by the registered company Springer Nature Switzerland AG
The registered company address is: Gewerbestrasse 11, 6330 Cham, Switzerland

Preface

ICR 2023, the Second International Conference on Innovations in Computing Research, was held in Madrid, Spain, from September 4 to 6, 2023, at the Axor Hotel. ICR'23 was sponsored by the Spanish National Research Council (CSIC), Spain, Australian Computer Society (ACS), Australia, Polytechnic Institute of Porto, Portugal, University of Detroit Mercy, USA, Features Analytics, Belgium, and Flexens Ltd., Finland.

The 2023 International Conference on Innovations in Computing Research (ICR'23) is organized by the Institute for Innovations in Computer Science and Engineering Research (IICSER). The goal of this conference is to bring together researchers from academia, business, industry, and government to exchange significant and innovative contributions and research ideas and to act as a platform for international research collaboration. To this extent, ICR'23 sought submissions that furnish innovative ideas, techniques, methodologies, and applications.

The acceptance rate for ICR'23 is 27%. In addition, the Poster Chairs accepted three posters for graduate students. There were two presentation modes: remote (virtual) and in-person at Axor hotel. 19 papers were presented remotely, and 16 papers were presented in-person. ICR'23 deployed the hybrid synchronous presentation.

These proceedings contain the revised versions of the papers that took the comments of the reviewers into consideration. Only the Program Committee members were used as reviewers, and no secondary reviewers were allowed. The revisions were not re-reviewed. The authors assume full responsibility for the contents of their final papers. All papers were checked for plagiarism using the Turnitin App.

It gives us great pleasure to appreciate the great dedication of the Conference Chair, Advisory Committee, Organization Committee, and the Program Committee. This dedication greatly contributed to the success of ICR'23. Without the excellent papers that were accepted by the Program Committee, this conference would have not existed. Therefore, we are delighted to thank all the authors for their hard work to come up with excellent original papers and for their productive cooperation with us to incorporate the comments of the reviewers and editors that participated in improving their papers and submitting their camera-ready papers on time.

The proceedings are published by the Springer book series: Lecture Notes in Networks and Systems (LNNS). LNNS is currently indexed by SCOPUS, DBLP, INSPEC, Norwegian Register for Scientific Journals and Series, SCImago, WTI Frankfurt eG, and zbMATH.

It gives us great pleasure to thank Dr. Thomas Ditzinger, the editorial director in charge of the Springer book series: Lecture Notes in Networks and Systems (LNNS). We very much appreciate his valuable help and support. We would also like to thank

Ms. Varsha Prabhakaran, the coordinator of ICR'23 proceedings book project for her cooperation.

August 2023

Kevin Daimi
Abeer Al Sadoon

ICR 2023

The Second International Conference on Advances in Computing Research (ICR'23)
Madrid, Spain
September 4–6, 2023

Advisory Committee

Luis Hernandez Encinas	Spanish National Research Council (CSIC), Spain
Guilermo Francia III	University of West Florida, USA
Solange Ghernaouti	Swiss Cybersecurity Advisory & Research Group, Switzerland
Åsa Hedman	Flexens Ltd., Finland
Hiroaki Kikuchi	Meiji University, Japan
Slobodan Petrovic	Norwegian University of Science and Technology (NTNU), Norway
Stefan Pickl	University of the Federal Armed Forces Munich, Germany
Peter Schartner	Alpen-Adria-Universität Klagenfurt, Austria
Cristina Soviany	Features Analytics SA, Belgium

Organization Committee

Conference Chair

Luis Hernandez Encinas	Spanish National Research Council (CSIC), Spain

Program Chairs

Abeer Al sadoon	Charles Sturt University, Australia
Kevin Daimi	University of Detroit Mercy, USA

Posters Chairs

Flaminia Luccio	Ca' Foscari University of Venice, Italy
Esmiralda Moradian	Stockholm University, Sweden
Alisa Vorobeva	ITMO University, Russia

Sessions/Workshops Chairs

Pino Caballero-Gil	University of La Laguna, Spain
Luis Coelho	Polytechnic Institute of Porto, Portugal
Ioanna Dionysiou	University of Nicosia, Cyprus

Publicity Chairs

Anna Allen	IICSER, Australia
Carl Wilson	ZRD Technology, USA

Web Chair

Deshao Liu	Western Sydney University, Australia
Teresa Martinez	Kent Institute Australia, Australia

Program Committee

Data Science

Mahshid Lonbani	Kent Institute Australia, Australia
Farhad Ahamed	Western Sydney University, Australia
Nawzat Sadiq Ahmed	Duhok Polytechnic University, Iraq
Rawhi Alrae	UAE University, Al Ain, United Arab Emirates
Abdussalam Mohamad Ali	Melbourne Institute of Technology, Australia
Thair Al-Dala'in	Western Sydney University, Australia
Ghazi Al-Naymat	Ajman University, UAE
Suhair Amer	Southeast Missouri State University, USA
Ali Anaissi	Sydney University, Australia
Wolfgang Bein	University of Nevada, Las Vegas
Li-jing Arthur Chang	Jackson State University, USA
Saurav Keshari Aryal	Howard University, USA
Karim Baïna	Mohammed V University in Rabat, Morocco
Mahmoud Bekhit	University of Technology Sydney, Australia
Tru Cao	The University of Texas at Houston, USA
Ling Chen	National Yang Ming Chiao Tung University, Taiwan
António Dourado	University of Coimbra, Portugal
Iman M. A. Helal	Cairo University, Egypt
Waleed Ibrahim	Central Queensland University, Australia

Rodrigue Imad	University of Balamand, Lebanon
Fathe Jeribi	Jazan University, Saudi Arabia
Jonathan Kavalan	University of Florida, USA
Konstantinos Kolomvatsos	University of Thessaly, Greece
Dimosthenis Kyriazis	University of Piraeus, Greece
Jerry Chun-Wei Lin	Western Norway University of Applied Sciences, Norway
Thomas Morgenstern	HS Karlsruhe, Germany
Marian Sorin Nistor	Universität der Bundeswehr München, Germany
Mohammad Zavid Parvez	Australian Catholic University, Australia
Robert Polding	IE Business School, Spain
Khem Poudel	Middle Tennessee State University, USA
Sunny Raj	Oakland University, USA
Ahmed Salah	Zagazig University, Egypt
Karwan Jacksi	University of Zakho, Iraq

Computer and Network Security

Rouwaida Abdallah	CEA-LIST, France
Fawaz Alazemi	Kuwait University, Kuwait
Roberto Omar Andrade	Escuela Politécnica Nacional, Ecuador
Oli Buckley	University of East Anglia, UK
Khalil Challita	Notre Dame University-Louaize, Lebanon
Sammy Danso	The University of Edinburgh Medical School, UK
Feng Cheng	Hasso Plattner Institute, University of Potsdam, Germany
Ahmed Dawoud	Western Sydney University, Australia
George Dimitoglou	Hood College, USA
Ioanna Dionysiou	University of Nicosia, Cyprus
Levent Ertaul	California State University East Bay, USA
Luis Hernández Encinas	Spanish National Research Council (CSIC), Spain
Hicham H. Hallal	American University of Sharjah, United Arab Emirates
Stevens Fox	State of Washington Office of Cybersecurity, USA
Samuel Ndueso John	Nigerian Defence Academy, Nigeria
Chadi El Kari	University of the Pacific, USA
Ievgeniia Kuzminykh	King's College London, UK
Arash Habibi Lashkari	York University, Canada
Edison Loza-Aguirre	Escuela Politécnica Nacional, Ecuador
Maggie Mashaly	German University in Cairo, Egypt
Christophe Maudoux	Cnam Paris, France
J. Todd McDonald	University of South Alabama, USA

Computer Science and Computer Engineering Education

Ievgeniia Kuzminykh	King's College London, UK
Edison Loza-Aguirre	Escuela Politécnica Nacional, Ecuador
J. Todd McDonald	University of South Alabama, USA
Suzanne Mello-Stark	Rhode Island College, USA
Hoda M. O. Mokhtar	Egypt University of Informatics (EUI), Egypt
Nkaepe Olaniyi	Kaplan Open Learning, UK
Robert Polding	IE Business School, Spain
Razwan Mohmed Salah	The University of Duhok, Iraq
Karpoor Shashidhar	Sam Houston State University, USA
Nicolas Sklavos	University of Patras, Greece
Vasso Stylianou	University of Nicosia, Cyprus
Joane Jonathan	Kent Institute Australia, Australia
Mahshid Lonbani	Kent Institute Australia, Australia

Internet of Things

Hanady Hussien Issa	Arab Academy for Science, Technology and Maritime Transport, Egypt
Iness Ahriz	CEDRIC Lab Conservatoire National des Arts et Métiers, France
Ali Alwan Al-Juboori	Ramapo College of New Jersey, USA
Zakaria Benomar	Inria, France
Adrian Castillero Franco	IE Business School, UAE
Jide Edu	King's College London, UK
Hicham H. Hallal	American University of Sharjah, UAE
Marie Khair	Notre Dame University, Lebanon
Irene Kopaliani	Princeton University, USA
Lemia Louail	Université de Lorraine, France
Maggie Mashaly	German University in Cairo, Egypt
Mais Nijim	Texas A&M University - Kingsville, USA
Slobodan Petrovic	Norwegian University of Science and Technology (NTNU), Norway
Cathryn Peoples	Ulster University, UK
Sunny Raj	Oakland University, USA
Alessandro Ruggiero	University of Salerno, Italy
Amparo Fuster Sabater	Spanish National Research Council (CSIC), Spain
Sorin Soviany	National Institute for Research and Development in Informatics, Romania
Hailu Xu	California State University, USA
Suhad Yousif	Al-Nahrain University, Iraq
Sherali Zeadally	University of Kentucky, USA

Smart Cities/Smart Energy

Mohammed Akour	Yarmouk University, Jordan
Rouwaida Abdallah	CEA-LIST, France
Manuel I. Capel	Universidad de Granada, Spain
Adrian Castillero Franco	IE Business School, UAE
María del Mar Gómez	Universidad Rey Juan Carlos, Spain
Karina Kervin	IBM, USA
Sergio Ilarri	University of Zaragoza, Spain
Natarajan Meghanathan	Jackson State University, USA
Saraju Mohanty	University of North Texas, USA
Dmitry Namiot	Lomonosov Moscow State University, Russia
Mais Nijim	Texas A&M University - Kingsville, USA
Jun-Seok Oh	Western Michigan University, USA
Cathryn Peoples	Ulster University, UK
Alessandro Ruggiero	University of Salerno, Italy
Monica Siroux	INSA Strasbourg, France
Vivian Sultan	California State University, Los Angeles, USA
Hailu Xu	California State University, USA
Alberto Ochoa Zezzatti	Juarez City University, Mexico

Contents

Health Informatics and Biomedical Imaging

Computer Science and Engineering Education

Data Science

A Classification Algorithm Utilizing the Lempel-Ziv Complexity Score for Missing Data

Valerie Sessions[1](✉), Justin Grieves[1], and Stanley Perrine[2]

[1] Charleston Southern University, North Charleston, USA
{vsessions,jgrieves}@csuniv.edu
[2] Georgia Gwinnett College, Lawrenceville, USA
sperrine@ggc.edu

Abstract. Informative data analysis relies heavily on the quality of the underlying data. Unfortunately, often in our research, the data to be analyzed contains many missing values. While we have methods to mitigate the missing data – listwise deletion, multiple imputation, etc. - these methods are only appropriate for use when data are missing at random. When data are missing not at random, use of these methods leads to erroneous analyses. Determining whether a data set contains random or non-random missing data is an open challenge in our field. An algorithm to categorize missing data utilizing the Lempel-Ziv (LZ) complexity score is proposed by the authors and initial results from its use in both generated and publicly available data are analyzed. The authors' algorithm contains many positive features. It is useful with data sets of all compositions (string, numerical, graphics, mixed), yields easily interpreted results, and can be used autonomously to determine the type of missingness (random versus non-random). The authors review related literature, explain the algorithm, and interpret initial results of its use with data from canonical Bayesian networks, United States census data, and data sets from the University of California, Irvine machine learning repository. Further usages in the field of bioinformatics and pathways for future research are discussed.

Keywords: Data cleaning and preparation · data analysis · Missing Not at Random · Missing at Random · LZ Complexity Score · Informed Missingness

1 Introduction

Data cleaning and preparation for scientific research must contend with one common challenge: missing data. For example, as discussed in [1], data are routinely missing in electronic healthcare records. In certain data sets, the missingness itself can be quite informative. For example, if cholesterol measurements are frequently missing, we may infer a patient has not been adequately treated by their General Practitioner and therefore may indicate a future issue. Missing data is commonly categorized as Missing Completely at Random (MCAR), Missing at Random (MAR), and Missing Not at Random (MNAR)

K. Daimi and A. Al Sadoon (Eds.): ICR 2023, LNNS 721, pp. 3–12, 2023.
https://doi.org/10.1007/978-3-031-35308-6_1

[3]. The concept of Informative Missingness, which we have found used in bioinformatics, corresponds to the idea of Missing Not at Random, and in this paper, we will refer to these ideas as MNAR. When data sets are classified as having MAR and MCAR fields (i.e., randomized missingness) researchers have multiple methods at their disposal for either marginalizing or completing the missing fields. These include expectation maximization (EM), multiple imputation, list wise deletion, and other similar methods [4, 5]. These methods, however, are not appropriate for data that is MNAR and can lead to erroneous results when used to clean the data prior to input into machine learning algorithms. This was highlighted in healthcare data sets in [2], in which the authors discuss the issues of using a multiple imputation method on data that are MNAR. For a more thorough discussion of some of these issues, please refer to previous research work, regarding Bayesian Networks in particular [6]. Therefore, it should be clear from the above discussion that it is very important that we determine ***why*** the data is missing before utilizing data cleaning and preparation tools; one needs to make sure to use the appropriate method for the type of missingness exhibited in each data set, so that a data cleaning technique is not used in error. Furthermore, simply knowing that data is MNAR can yield dividends in terms of understanding and restricting the future data collection methods (revising a survey tool or recalibrating an instrument). Our goal here is to create a classification algorithm that can (1) determine whether there is an informative missingness to our data, (2) be applied to any type of data - text, numerical, graphical - and any data range, (3) be applied to any size data set, and (4) provide easily interpreted results. The paper is organized as follows: we present the current literature in data quality, explain the data sets used in this research, discuss the algorithm, present our results, and discuss our conclusions and future research avenues.

2 Related Work

A brief review of related literature in data quality is presented as well as practical review of the LZ Complexity score and review of Bayesian Networks used in the generation of test data sets.

2.1 Data Quality/Missing Data

Data and information quality is a growing field of research that seeks to classify types of data error, map data flows or Information Products (IP), create better business processes to minimize the risk of collecting poor quality data, and many other topics. For an overview of this large field the authors recommend [7]. For our purposes here, we will review the classifications of missing data and point to previous research and methods that seek to classify data as MAR or MNAR. Missing data, as classified by [1], can be MCAR, MAR, or MNAR. MCAR represents the case of a complete fluke – the missing mechanism is neither a result of the variable itself nor any other value in the distribution. MAR data can be missing because of its relationship to a particular variable in the model, but the missing mechanism has no relationship to other variables in the model. There is much research on how to account for both MCAR and MAR data. A good overview of these methods can be found in both [8] and [9]. As these methods are quite similar, we will in the remainder of this paper refer to data from either of these first two categories as MAR data. As noted previously, methods for handling MAR data are wholly inappropriate for data MNAR and have been shown to be unsuccessful when used on MNAR data [10]. There are some studies which seek to caragorize data as MNAR or MAR. For example, research conducted by [32] seeks to discover bias patterns in missing data using Association Rule Mining (ARM) algorithms and has done so with some success. This research seeks to find a bias or pattern for missingness, which would then enable the data set to be categorized as MNAR. In addition, biomedical informatics research by [11] incorporated missing data as an explicit classifier in BN modeling and found that in most cases the BN trained with the missing classifier performed better than those without. This is one method that may be able to be used for missing data that could be MNAR or MAR and still be used appropriately. Sebastiani and Remoni [36] make significant progress towards an estimation method that is appropriate under cases of both MAR and MNAR (which they refer to as Ignorable and Non Ignorable) data with the Bound and Collapse (BC) algorithm. Our algorithm, described in Section 3, expands upon this work but creating a classification algorithm that can be used on any type of data – numerical, text, images, blended – without significant changes to the data set itself.

2.2 Lempel-Ziv Complexity Score

The LZ Complexity Score is a measure named after its authors, Abraham Lempel and Jacob Ziv, first presented in their work [12]. It is used to measure the repetitiveness of a sequence of binary characters. The LZ score has been used to measure repetitiveness in various data sets including EEG data, neuroscience, and even musical lyrics [13–16] to determine the complexity of these strings. Data in each of these cases was first encoded as a binary string of 0's and 1's. Once encoded, the LZ Complexity score methodically read through the string to determine the number of substrings encountered from left to right. As an example, consider the string 1001111011000010. We can see that the unique substrings are 1 / 0 / 01 / 11 / 101 / 10 / 00 / 010 as we read the string from left to right in increasing number of characters. Thus, the LZ score for the binary string 1001111011000010 is 8. In contrast, a string with a repeating value, such as 010101010101, would have only the three unique substrings 0 / 1 / 01, and therefore a score of 3. While this is a small example, we see the power of the algorithm to distinguish complexity among strings. This scoring method, and modifications to this scoring technique, are the basis for many compression algorithms. We will leave the formal definition for the reader to discover in both their original work and [13].

2.3 Bayesian Networks

We utilize Bayesian Networks to generate the data sets for use in this research. BNs are used to model a domain of knowledge and are used in many machine-learning, bioinformatic, and scientific domains. A BN consists of a set of variables and directed edges between these variables. Together these form a directed acyclic graph (DAG). To each variable in the DAG there are attached possible states. If there exists a parent for this variable there is also a potential table. When new evidence was formed for a particular state in the DAG, the probabilities are then updated using Bayes Rule. If the reader desires a more detailed mathematical approach, we recommend [17–19]. To generate data used for verifying our algorithm, we use three canonical BNs further discussed in Sect. 3 of this paper.

3 Data Classification Algorithm (DCA) Rationale

The authors utilize the LZ complexity score to classify whether data are missing at random or missing not at random. If data is MNAR, presumably it will contain some pattern - either one field is primarily missing or two or more fields are missing in conjunction with one another, etc. If this is the case, there will be a substring that can be found often that mirrors this missingness mechanism, thus yielding a smaller LZ score. Conversely, if the data are missing randomly, then the score should be higher as this would be a more difficult string to encode and have no apparent substrings. The algorithm is defined below.

3.1 Data Classification Algorithm (DCA)

I. First, we take each individual "line" of data and encode it as a binary string. This is done simply by assigning a 1 to each entry which is non-empty and assigning a 0 to each entry that is missing For example, if we are encoding answers to a 20-question survey taken by 100 people, we would have 100 binary strings, each of length 20, in which a 1 would be assigned to each question having a response and a 0 assigned to each question that was left blank or was otherwise unusable.
II. We now place these binary strings end to end, attaching the beginning of a string to the end of the previous one in the set, to create one long binary string. If we did this process with the example given in 1, we would now have one binary string of length 2000.
III. We determine the LZ score for this long binary string using the work found in [31].
IV. We estimate an LZ score for a similar length binary string with the same percentage of missing data, but we ensure that this comparison string has data that is missing at random. (This is done by using the Python random number generator [35] to determine which data to delete. See the paragraph above Table 1 for a more detailed description of this process.)
V. We now compare the LZ score for our long binary string with the score for the randomly generated string of MAR data. If the LZ score for our long binary string is lower than the MAR data score by at least a factor of 10, we classify the original data that created the long binary string as MNAR. Otherwise, we classify it as MAR.

The full python program can be provided upon request.

3.2 DCA Testing Method

Our null and alternative hypothesis is as follows:

H_0: *The DCA cannot be used to distinguish the missingness mechanism of a given data set.*

Ha: The DCA can be used to distinguish the missingness mechanism of a given data set.

To test this hypothesis, we created data sets from the three canonical BNs in sets of 100, 1000, 10000, and 100000 records, resulting in 72 sets of generated data. Using the Hugin Expert software [20], we were able to generate data sets with various percentages of missing data that were missing at random (MAR). We then created the same size data sets with non-randomly generated missing data in correct percentages (5%, 10%, ... 50%). A non-random set with 8000 fields at 5% for example, would be created with 400 non-randomly generated missing fields. The non-random nature of this missingness is presented below.

The three BN data sets used to generate the data used to test are hypothesis are described here:

I. Chest Clinic - This is one of the most popular sample BNs. The network examines the possible causes of shortness of breath including tuberculosis, lung cancer, a visit to Asia, etc. A visit to Asia increases the risk of tuberculosis, while smoking increases the risk of lung cancer. A full explanation may be found in: [21]. This network has 8 fields. To generate the non-random data set, we extracted the appropriate number of fields in which "positive x-ray = no". This was the only field with missing data, therefore making it non-random. For randomly missing data, we used the Hugin random data generator and applied the appropriate amount of missing data (5%, 10%, etc.).

II. Fire - This network is used to predict the causes of forest fire - arson, picnic fire, smoking, etc. A full explanation may be found in [22]. This network has 6 fields. To generate the non-random data set, we extracted the appropriate number of fields in which "Electricity = working". This was the only field with missing data, therefore making it non-random. For randomly missing data, we used the Hugin random data generator and applied the appropriate amount of missing data (5%, 10%, etc.).

III. Year 2K - This is another canonical BN that describes various industries, such as electric grids or other utilities, that may have faced serious challenges if the year 2K software issues had gone unchecked. An explanation can be found here [23]. This network has 8 fields. To generate the non-random data set, we extracted the appropriate number of fields in which "Report = false". This was the only field with missing data, therefore making it non-random. For randomly missing data, we used the Hugin random data generator and applied the appropriate amount of missing data (5%, 10%, etc.).

We compare the LZ scores from these generated MAR and MNAR BN data sets to an estimated LZ score. This estimated LZ score was calculated by creating a data set of similar size – 100, 1000, 10,000, 100,000 rows, and similar fields 8 or 6. We then delete percentages of the data – 5, 10, 20, 30, 40, 50 using the Python random number generator [35] to determine which data to delete. We realize that random number generation can yield a variation in scores; therefore, to ensure the estimated LZ score and a score from an MNAR data set would be significantly divergent, we calculated the estimated score under each percentage of missing data 100 times and calculated the mean and the standard deviation of those scores. The results from this are shown in Table 1. We have confidence in this score estimation method because our standard deviation in each case, regardless of size and percent missing, is no greater than 8.5% of the score. This is significantly lower as the amount of data increases and well lower than our classification algorithm's cutoff of factor of 10 difference (or 100+%). We present these results in Table 1 in order to show that the natural deviations in the Python random number generator are not significant when compared to the resulting outcomes of the Data Classification Algorithm.

Table 1. Estimation Scores with Python Random Number Generator

Num records	Average score	Standard deviation	Percentage of score	95% prediction INT
100	15.326	1.300	0.085	(12.73, 17.92)
1000	98.304	2.237	0.023	(98.84, 102.76)
10000	768.940	5.528	0.007	(757.92, 779.96)
100000	1992.400	7.765	0.004	(1976.92, 2007.88)

Table 2. Data Classification Algorithm Results with Generated Data Sets

		Chest Clinic - 8 Fields		Year2K - 8 Fields		Fire - 6 Fields	
Percent Missing	Number of Rows	Algorithm Classification for MAR Data	Algorithm Classification for MNAR	Algorithm Classification for MAR Data	Algorithm Classification for MNAR	Algorithm Classification for MAR Data	Algorithm Classification for MNAR
5	100	Correct	**Incorrect**	Correct	**Incorrect**	Correct	**Incorrect**
	1000	Correct	Correct	Correct	**Incorrect**	Correct	Correct
	10000	Correct	Correct	Correct	Correct	Correct	Correct
	100000	Correct	Correct	Correct	Correct	Correct	Correct
10	100	Correct	**Incorrect**	Correct	Correct	Correct	**Incorrect**
	1000	Correct	Correct	Correct	Correct	Correct	Correct
	10000	Correct	Correct	Correct	Correct	Correct	Correct
	100000	Correct	Correct	Correct	Correct	Correct	Correct
20	100	Correct	**Incorrect**	Correct	**Incorrect**	Correct	Correct
	1000	Correct	Correct	Correct	Correct	Correct	Correct
	10000	Correct	Correct	Correct	Correct	Correct	Correct
	100000	Correct	Correct	Correct	Correct	Correct	Correct
30	100	Correct	Correct	Correct	**Incorrect**	Correct	Correct
	1000	Correct	Correct	Correct	Correct	Correct	Correct
	10000	Correct	Correct	Correct	Correct	Correct	Correct
	100000	Correct	Correct	Correct	Correct	Correct	Correct
40	100	Correct	Correct	Correct	**Incorrect**	Correct	Correct
	1000	Correct	Correct	Correct	Correct	Correct	Correct
	10000	Correct	Correct	Correct	Correct	Correct	Correct
	100000	Correct	Correct	Correct	Correct	Correct	Correct
50	100	Correct	Correct	Correct	**Incorrect**	Correct	Correct
	1000	Correct	Correct	Correct	Correct	Correct	Correct
	10000	Correct	Correct	Correct	Correct	Correct	Correct
	100000	Correct	Correct	Correct	Correct	Correct	Correct

As shown in Table 2 above, the algorithm correctly classified data as MAR in 100% of test cases and correctly for MNAR in 92.4% of the cases with our generated sets. The incorrectly classified data would be considered false negative – data that should be classified as MNAR but were classified as random. The instances where the DCA is incorrect are under very small amounts and percentages of missing data, therefore we would caution the user to use another mechanism if they are investigating a data set.of less than 8000 total fields with a small percentage missing. Because most practical data sets are larger than those smaller test cases, we believe average sized data sets will classify correctly.

From a practical standpoint, we believe a classification algorithm is useful if it correctly categorizes the data as MNAR or MAR in 85% of cases or more. This gives a researcher confidence that if they are using multiple imputation, listwise deletion, etc., they are using it correctly, especially if they have 1000 or more fields in their set.

We set $p =$ proportion of correctly categorized data. Ho: $p = 0.85$ versus Ha: $p > .85$. The proportion of correct classification is $133/144 = 0.924$. This gives a test statistic of $z = 2.474$ and a p-value of 0.00668 indicating strong evidence that this classification technique correctly classifies the type of missing data more than 85% of the time.

4 Results with Publicly Available Data Sets

After validating our approach using generated data sets, we then expanded to publicly available data sets from the University of California at Irvine (UCI) Machine Learning repository [24] as well as data from the US Census [25], to show the usage of this algorithm among "real-world" data. We do not know the missingness mechanism of these sets (missing at random or missing not at random), but the Data Classification Algorithm can guide us in determining this.

1. Adult Data Set – Predicts whether income is over 500K based on other classifiers [26].
2. Air Quality Data Set – Air quality measures from an Italian City.. [27].
3. Audit Data – An Indian audit firm's data from 2015–2016 collected to predict suspicious activity [28].
4. Credit Approval Data Set – Data collected from credit card applications [29].
5. Echocardiogram Data Set – Data collected to predict if a patient will survive at least a year after having a heart attack [30].
6. Small Area Income and Poverty Estimates Program (SAIPE) data – estimates government benefits and income information – from the US Census [25].

With the exception of the ECG data set, all data sets are large enough for confidence in the algorithm's classification of MNAR or MAR data. For ECG the overall number of records for ECG is small (fewer than 1600 total fields) and the percentage of missing is less than 5% percent. This would warrant another look at the data to determine it correctly was categorized MAR before using Multiple imputation, listwise deletion, etc.

The remaining datasets we have high confidence that they are correctly categorized based on size of data and an understanding of the collection methods. A review of the AIR data set shows that data were missing from the Nitrogen Oxides (NOx) and

Table 3. Classification Algorithm Results with Data Sets from UCI and US Census

	Records	Fields	Num Missing	Estimated LZ Score	DCA Score	Classification
ADULT	32562	15	4262	1676	1054	MAR
AIR	9358	15	16244	3782	180	MNAR
AUDIT	777	18	2334	659	227	MAR
CREDIT	690	15	67	39	29	MAR
ECG	132	12	74	44	30	MAR
CNTYSNAP	3205	30	231	171	25	MNAR

Nitrogen Dioxide (NO2) fields every day at 3:00AM, and for most fields for a few days. Presumably 3:00AM was a recalibration time for the nitrogen tester and there were a few days in which an entire instrument was down. This anecdotal review of the data would confirm that this data was missing because of instrument failure and MAR techniques should be avoided. Similarly, a review of the US Census data for county snap is missing entire rows from specific counties who did not report their numbers for the census. This also would be missing not at random and MAR techniques would be improperly used on this set.

5 Conclusions and Future Work

The DCA is a compelling method for determining the missingness mechanism of a data set. Knowing the presumed reason for missing data (either MAR or MNAR) allows the researcher to use only those data cleansing methods that are appropriate. The power of this algorithm to be used in a variety of data types through the simplicity of the 1 and 0 encoding scheme is not to be dismissed. By simplifying the data to 0s and 1s, we eliminate the need to massage the data in any further way and therefore lessen the possibility of introducing errors. Once the data is determined to be MAR or MNAR, it can be cleaned further using appropriate measures.

Future research has many possible avenues. From a practical standpoint, the Python program used for the LZ complexity score and MAR estimator are for testing and explanatory purposes only. They are not optimized and may have large run times with large amounts of data (>100,000). Simple optimization methods should speed this greatly and allow for scores within a much more reasonable time period. If very large data sets are used, one could alternately pull samples for testing to determine the missingness mechanism to save computational time. Parallelization schemes could also be employed.

A second direction for future research could be to incorporate data from a wider variety of fields, and to also use data sets that are known or suspected to be MNAR. After optimizing the Python program, running these tests on much larger data sets would further validate our results. The use of other complexity scores, such as Kolmogorov complexity, could also be an interesting avenue for future research.

Finally, it would be useful to show a practical application of this algorithm on a disputed set of data. For example, a study in the Journal of the American Medical

Assocation (JAMA) Psychiatry [33] regarding the effectiveness of a 1- day workshop for postpartum depression was recently criticized for its use of multiple imputation on missing data. A subsequent article [34] was written which questioned the use of this technique and therefore the results of the study. It would be an interesting case study to use our data classification algorithm with this data set to determine if multiple imputation was correctly utilized in the study. The authors have contacted the lead author for that research and have asked for the data set for this purpose. Similar case studies would be a useful avenue of future research.

References

1. Groenwold, R.H.H.: Informative missingness in electronic health record systems: the curse of knowing. Diagn. Progn. Res. **4**, 8 (2020). https://doi.org/10.1186/s41512-020-00077
2. Sterne, J.A., et al.: Multiple imputation for missing data in epidemiological and clinical research: potential and pitfalls. BMJ (2009)
3. Little, R., Rubin, D.: Statistical Analysis with Missing Data, 3rd edn. Wiley, Hoboken (2019)
4. Soley-Bori, M.: Dealing with missing data: key assumptions and methods for applied analysis (2013). https://www.bu.edu/sph/files/2014/05/Marina-tech-report.pdf
5. Swalin, A.: How to Handle Missing Data (2018). https://towardsdatascience.com/how-to-handle-missing-data-8646b18db0d4
6. Sessions, V., Perrine, S., Grieves, J.: A technique for incorporating data missing not at random (MNAR) into Bayesian networks. ICIQ 2016, Article 12, Publication date: June 22nd, 2016 (2016)
7. Yang Lee, L., Pipino, J.F., Wang, R.: Journey to Data Quality. The MIT Press, Cambridge (2006)
8. Horton, N., Klienman, K.P.: Much ado about nothing: a comparison of missing data methods and software to fit incomplete data regression models. Am. Stat. **61**, 79–90 (2007)
9. Patrick McKnight, K.M., McKnight, S.S., Figueredo, A.: Missing Data: A Gentle Introduction. Guilford Oress, New York (2007)
10. Almedar, M.: A Monte Carlo Study: The Impact of Missing Data in Cross-Classification Random Effects Models. Educational Policy Studies Dissertations. Paper 34 (2009)
11. Lin, J., Haug, P.: Exploiting missing clinical data in Bayesian network modeling for predicting medical problems. J. Biomed. Inform. **41**, 1–14 (2008)
12. Lempel, A., Ziv, J.: On the complexity of finite sequences. IEEE Trans. Inf. Theory **22**(1), 75–81 (1976)
13. Rosas, F., Mediano, P.: When and how to use Lempel-Ziv complexity Jun 26, 2019 (2019). https://information-dynamics.github.io/
14. Zhang, X.S., Roy, R.J., Jensen, E.W.: EEG complexity as a measure of depth of anesthesia for patients. IEEE Trans. Biomed. Eng. **48**(12), 1424–1433 (2001)
15. Gusev, V.D., Nemytikova, L.A., Chuzhanova, N.A.: On the complexity measures of genetic sequences. Bioinformatics **15**(12), 994–999 (1999)
16. Shmulevich, I., Povel, D.J.: Complexity measures of musical rhythms. In: Desain, P., Windsor, L. (eds.) Rhythm Perception and Production, pp. 239–244. Swets & Zeitlinger, Lisse (2000)
17. Robert Cowell, G., Dawid, S.L., Spiegalhalter, D.: Probabilistic Networks and Expert Systems. Springer, New York (1999). https://doi.org/10.1007/b97670
18. Jensen, F.: Bayesian Networks and Decision Graphs. Springer, New York (2001). https://doi.org/10.1007/978-0-387-68282-2
19. Neapolitan, R.: Learning Bayesian Networks. Pearson Education Inc, Upper Saddle River, NJ (2004)

20. Olesen, K., Lauritzen, S., Jensen, F.: aHUGIN: a system creating adaptive causal probabilistic networks. In: Proceedings of the Eighth Conference on Uncertainty in Artificial Intelligence, pp. 223–229 (1992)
21. Lauritzen, S., Spielgelhalter, D.J.: Local computation with probabilities in graphical structure and their applications to expert systems. J. Roy. Stat. Soc. B, **50**(2) (1988)
22. Sevinc, V., Kucuk, O., Goltas, M.: A Bayesian network model for prediction and analysis of possible forest fire causes. Forest Ecol. Manag. **457**, 17723 (2020). ISSN 0378-1127, https://doi.org/10.1016/j.foreco.2019.117723
23. Henrik Bengtsson Bayesian networks - a self-contained introduction with implementation remarks. https://citeseerx.ist.psu.edu/viewdoc/download?doi=10.1.1.100.6096&rep=rep1&type=pdf. Accessed 01 Dec 2022
24. Dua, D., Graff, C.: UCI Machine Learning Repository. Irvine, CA: University of California, School of Information and Computer Science (2019). http://archive.ics.uci.edu/ml
25. U.S. Census Bureau. SAIPE data sets (2020). https://www2.census.gov/programs-surveys/saipe/datasets/time-series/model-tables/
26. Kohavi, R.: Scaling up the accuracy of naive-bayes classifiers: a decision-tree hybrid. In: Proceedings of the Second International Conference on Knowledge Discovery and Data Mining (1996)
27. De Vito, S., Massera, E., Piga, M., Martinotto, L., Di Francia, G.: On field calibration of an electronic nose for benzene estimation in an urban pollution monitoring scenario. Sens. Actuators B: Chem. **129**(2), 750–757 (2008). ISSN 0925-4005
28. Hooda, N., Bawa, S., Rana, P.S.: Fraudulent firm classification: a case study of an external audit. Appl. Artif. Intell. **32**(1), 48–64 (2018)
29. Quinlan: Simplifying decision trees. .Int J. Man-Mach. Stud. **27**, 221–234 (1987)
30. Salzberg, S.: Exemplar-based learning: theory and implementation (Technical report TR-10–88). Harvard University, Center for Research in Computing Technology, Aiken Computation Laboratory (33 Oxford Street; Cambridge, MA 02138) (1988)
31. Kaspar, F., Schuster, H.G.: Easily-calculable measure for the complexity of spatiotemporal patterns. Phys. Rev. A **36**(2) (1987)
32. Tremblay, M., Dutta, K., Vandermeer, D.: Using data mining techniques to discover bias patterns in missing data. ACM J. Data Inf. Qual. **2**(1), Article 2 (2010)
33. Van Lieshout, R.J., Layton, H., Savoy, C.D., et al.: Effect of online 1-day cognitive behavioral therapy–based workshops plus usual care vs usual care alone for postpartum depression: a randomized clinical trial. JAMA Psychiatry (2021)
34. Toyomoto, R., Funada, S., Furukawa, T.A.: Some concerns about imputation methods for missing data. JAMA Psychiatry (2022)
35. The Python Standard Library. Python Software Foundation. https://docs.python.org/3/library/random.html
36. Ramoni, M., Sebastiani, P.: Learning conditional probabilities from incomplete data: an experimental comparison. In: Proceedings of the Seventh International Workshop on Artificial Intelligence and Statistics, pp. 260–265 (1999)

Overview of the Benefits Deep Learning Can Provide Against Fake News, Cyberbullying and Hate Speech

Thair Al-Dala'in and Justin Hui San Zhao(✉)

Western Sydney University, Sydney, Australia
t.aldalain@city.westernsydney.edu.au, justinzhao893@gmail.com

Abstract. Deep learning is a feasible technology and is the best replacement for traditional means to prevent fake news, cyberbullying and hate speech. Traditional methods to prevent fake news, cyberbullying, and hate speech include using real life personnel to go through messages and remove them. The research analyses other researchers' discoveries relative to deep learning. It is important to conduct this research so that we are all aware of how close we are to be able to protect our future generations of children and adults from having their mental and physical health affected. This research aims to analyse the current deep learning techniques used to prevent fake news, cyberbullying and hate speech. A comparison is included in this research to identify the state-of-the-art technique.

Keywords: Deep Learning · Machine Learning · DeepText · Word2Vec · FakeBERT

1 Introduction

Currently, the prevention of fake news, cyberbullying and hate speech has been addressed with Deep Learning techniques. Instagram and Facebook are both using DeepText to achieve lower rates of fake news, cyberbullying and hate speech [1] and [2]. Similar deep learning techniques can be used to create the same prevention mechanisms for Reddit, Discord, Twitter and other social media platforms [3]. Online gaming is an activity that many children are spending a lot of their time with daily, which is subject to a high quantity of constant hate speech and cyberbullying [4]. A major problem with previous methods handling fake news, cyberbullying and hate speech is the process of acting after the post has been posted and seen by the audience. This especially happens in online gaming, where the user's account is banned. However, this doesn't fix the problem that the audience has already absorbed the hate speech, and the damage is already received from cyberbullying. In some cases, companies don't even moderate the chat and don't ban players who are conducting cyberbullying and hate speech. This could be because the person has spent a lot of money in the game and on micro transactions, so it would be a loss if the person was banned from the game. This is more evident with games that are considered a live service, as there are many in-game purchases. Messages sent

K. Daimi and A. Al Sadoon (Eds.): ICR 2023, LNNS 721, pp. 13–27, 2023.
https://doi.org/10.1007/978-3-031-35308-6_2

between small groups of people that are cyberbullying aren't reported as they won't report each other. This causes issues as it could occur in a small high school Facebook group of students. Techniques created with deep learning lessen the need for a physical moderator to check every message and manually delete the message to provide a safe environment to users. Would you be satisfied if you knew the news you watched was fake? Would you be happy if your children were cyberbullied when they logged on to their favourite online game after completing their homework? Would you like it if your favourite musician or idol was subject to hate speech when you went to search for their name on Google? Detection of topics, extraction of entities, and analysis of sentiment are all part of what's provided when using deep neural networks, a part of deep learning, which has already proven to reduce the amount of fake news, cyberbullying and hate speech incidents on the internet [5]. A moderator is still required because the current deep learning techniques aren't good enough to completely remove the need of a moderator. However, these techniques make the moderator's jobs easier and creating a safer online environment for everyone. No other recent literature review compares all the techniques mentioned in the comparison together. Therefore, this study aims to evaluate recent literature on deep learning techniques for preventing fake news, cyberbullying and hate speech and identify their shortcomings. Shortcomings for DeepText, Word2Vec, ELMO, BERT and CNN have been identified. As of this moment, no research has identified shortcomings for FakeBERT. By identifying the shortcomings in this research, other researchers can improve the techniques by eliminating their shortcomings. The contribution of this research is to provide the comparison of the techniques analysed and shortcomings which allows future work on eliminating the shortcomings to be conducted by all researchers. The following research questions are addressed in the literature review: What is currently being done to prevent fake news, cyberbullying and hate speech?, How can deep learning be used to prevent fake news, cyberbullying and hate speech?, What are the benefits that deep learning can provide for the prevention of fake news, cyberbullying and hate speech?, What can be done to improve the prevention of fake news, cyberbullying and hate speech?. The document's structure includes a literature review, comparison, and summary and conclusions.

2 Literature Review

In the beginning, peer-reviewed papers are collected to create a literature review. Only peer-reviewed papers are collected because other papers that are not peer-reviewed may have incorrect information, which will interfere with the quality of this research and the comparison for the identification of the state-of-the-art technique. After the literature review is created, an evaluation to determine the best technique for improvement was conducted. The best technique will have shortcomings that can be addressed with the current technology. Once the best technique for improving is identified, the possible improvement for that technique can be identified.

2.1 Importance of Fake News, Cyberbullying and Hate Speech Prevention

Preventing fake news, cyberbullying, and hate speech is important for future generations. Fake news can spread faster than wildfire as people become more connected over the internet. Bullying is occurring online daily, and hate speech is occurring everyday online due to disputes. The mental wellbeing of future generations should be set at a high standard [6], and no one should feel excluded from using an online application.

2.2 Materials and Methods

Prevention of fake news, cyberbullying and hate speech is important. Thus, the literature review provides an analysis of sixty-two research articles between 2010 and 2023, such as [6–8]. These articles mainly focus on content related to preventing fake news, cyberbullying and hate speech. The articles are obtained from Google Scholar. The sixty-two research articles have been accepted based on the inclusion criteria of exposure of interest to the prevention of fake news, cyberbullying or hate speech, study design for conducting tests regarding specific techniques or population and conditions that are impacted by fake news, cyberbullying or hate speech. The literature review is split up into eleven subsections, including prevention of hate speech using DeepText, prevention of fake news using FakeBERT, prevention of cyberbullying, hate speech detection, deep learning types and techniques, Word2Vec, shortcomings of DeepText, shortcomings of Word2Vec, shortcomings of Embeddings from Language Models, shortcomings of Bidirectional Encoder Representations from Transformers and shortcomings of Convoluted Neural Networks. Deep learning types and techniques include Embeddings from Language Models, Bidirectional Encoder Representation from Transformers and Convolutional Neural Network (Table 1).

Table 1. Distinctions of the subsections within the literature review.

Subsection	Distinction
Prevention of Hate Speech Using DeepText	How DeepText is used in the context of hate speech prevention
Prevention of Fake News Using FakeBERT	How FakeBERT is used for fake news prevention
Prevention of Cyberbullying	How cyberbullying is prevented, and its impact to victims
Hate Speech Detection	How hate speech is detected and some techniques that have been used
Deep Learning Types and Techniques	Deep learning types and techniques covers the deep learning techniques that are used to prevent fake news, cyberbullying and hate speech and the introduces the types of deep learning techniques
Word2Vec	Covers some background history of Word2Vec
Shortcomings of DeepText	What are the shortcomings of DeepText
Shortcomings of Word2Vec	What are the shortcomings of Word2Vec
Shortcomings of ELMo	What are the shortcomings of ELMo
Shortcomings of BERT	What are the shortcomings of BERT
Shortcomings of CNN	What are the shortcomings of CNN

2.3 Prevention of Hate Speech Using DeepText

DeepText is currently being used by Instagram which is owned by Facebook to remove comments that violate Instagram's community guidelines. DeepText prevents hate speech in Facebook and Instagram by understanding what the comment is conveying. If the comment is conveyed as hate speech, it'll be removed automatically by the program. Currently, there is a filter combined with DeepText to scan for offensive comments, which will be removed. So, in short, DeepText is a product of deep learning which has benefited the prevention of hate speech in Facebook and Instagram by removing the need to have a human go through massive amounts of comments to manually remove the offensive comments [9]. This doesn't mean that all hate speech is removed from Facebook and Instagram, as some could get through, using a language that has not been filtered properly or obfuscated text. Obfuscated text means that the human brain can know what the person is saying. However, the program is unable to tell as the technology is not that capable as of this moment. Images are also being addressed currently in 2022 by a group of researchers [8].

2.4 Prevention of Fake News Using FakeBERT

FakeBERT is a deep learning approach based on Bidirectional Encoder Representation from Transformers applied to fake news, hence the name FakeBERT. Ambiguity is a major issue when trying to identify fake news, so BERT relies on filters and a variety of kernel sizes, which is feasible through combining various parallel blocks within a single layer deep convolutional neural network [5]. Instagram, Facebook and Twitter are all popular social applications that allow users to access and share information rapidly, news [9] and [10]. The data in these social media applications aren't all authentic, meaning that it's a good place to spread fake news [11] and [12]. It is important to address the prevention of fake news as it creates a significantly negative impact on the victim [11, 12] and [13], which can vary from being an idol to a politician. Fake news is often created to reap political or financial benefits by attempting to fool or mislead the audience and harming the reputation of an individual, product or organisation [13–16]. Therefore FakeBERT, a product of deep learning, is a benefit to the prevention of fake news.

2.5 Prevention of Cyberbullying

Cyberbullying victims have dire consequences that could result in anxiety, suicide or depression, depending on the severity. This serious problem requires intelligent systems to automatically prevent cyberbullying from occurring as much as possible [17]. Ever since web 2.0 existed, many adolescents spend most of their time online using social applications, thus exposing them to cyberbullying. Eighteen percent of children in Europe are related to cyberbullying, 20% aged 11 to 16 are related to cyberbullying [17], and teenagers make up 20 to 40% of victims [18]. This statistic highlights the importance of deep learning to put an end to cyberbullying. As it is impossible to have a moderator reading the posts twentyfour hours a day for every day, an intelligent, automated system must be created using deep learning techniques to detect and prevent these issues. These issues have been addressed, not with deep learning techniques, and require the user to read them. However, how many users spend time reading the pages of text? The YouTube Community Guidelines explain the systems YouTube uses to flag cyberbullying [17]. The Twitter Safety and Security page explain what to do with self-harm and suicidal thoughts on Twitter. Whilst both are great ideas and a step in the right direction of stopping cyberbullying, this requires the user's action. We can go beyond conventional methods to detect and prevent cyberbullying with deep learning. Previously conventional methods used to detect and prevent cyberbullying use machine learning models [17, 19] and [19]. Recently deep neural network-based models are being used for cyberbullying detection [20]. Researchers have completed tests which showed that the deep neural network-based model used was expanded to fit for a variety of social applications and the deep neural network-based model performed better than machine learning models. The researchers also stated that transfer learning had been used so that the deep neural network-based model worked on different data sets [20]. Based on this test, deep learning techniques are beneficial to the prevention of cyberbullying.

2.6 Hate Speech Detection

YouTube, Twitter and Facebook are social applications that grant users permission to post comments and opinions with anonymity. This results in some users posting hateful, threatening or aggressive comments, classified as hate speech because they feel it's safe to do so [21]. Hate speech basically means text that discriminates against a person's unique characteristics such as religion, race, sexual orientation, or gender [22] and [23]. So far, there are mechanisms in place to detect hate speech, and although not all hate speech is detected, it is an improvement. Government, law enforcement and large social application companies are working to remove accounts with hate speech on their services [24]. Currently, not all hate speech is being detected, thus requiring manual filtering by a moderator. This process is both tedious and long, which is how deep learning benefits the prevention of hate speech. Machine learning techniques currently used to prevent hate speech are not accurate enough, to remove the need for a moderator to do manual filtering. Deep learning is a part of machine learning, and it is very useful in natural language processing, which is used to classify text in comments [2]) and [26]. There are many techniques used to prevent hate speech. However, to keep it simple, there are machine learning techniques and deep learning techniques. Machine learning techniques include support vector machine, logistic regression and Naive Bayes classification algorithms, being used after manual text extraction [27] and [28]. Where deep learning provides a benefit to the prevention of hate speech, is it automatically extracts useful text by using multi-layer neural networks, basically attempting to mimic the human brain. Therefore, there are more researchers focusing on using deep learning to prevent hate speech [25].

2.7 Deep Learning Types and Techniques

Deep learning revolving around the topic of fake news, cyberbullying and hate speech is usually split up into two major types. The first type targets middle neural network processing, using character or simple word-based embedding technology. The second type attempts to improve the technology around word embedding by front-end processing. This is achieved using the bidirectional encoder representation from transformers and embeddings from language model methods. Embeddings from the language models' method use the context of the message to gather word vectors, which is vastly different to the bidirectional encoder representation which, as its name says, operates in both directions from the left and the right to conditionally join the context across all the layers [26, 29, 30] and [31].

1) Embeddings From Language Models

Embeddings from language models is a contextualised word representation that focuses on modelling the different contexts in which the word is used and the complex character of the word itself. ELMo uses context as a feature to customise the embeddings of words, Word2Vec uses a fixed embedding. A huge text corpus is used to train the word vectors that represent an input text's context. This allows ELMo to be implemented on a variety of task models. It also captures syntactic and semantic relationships, allowing ELMo to have higher accuracy than Word2Vec [21].

2) Bidirectional Encoder Representation from Transformers

Bidirectional Encoder Representation from Transformers is a machine learning technique for natural language processing based on transformers and trained by Google. The previous two methods, ELMo and Word2Vec, both require training from a model before use. Natural learning processing researchers are attempting to create a technique that doesn't require training from a model before use. It will use the objective of language modelling to train the neural network, which can eventually be assigned to a task with optimisation and supervision [32] and [33]. Bidirectional encoder representation from transformers is considered a massive accomplishment in the natural language processing area because it saves both computing resources and time for users who don't have the equipment or data to implement natural language processing to the desired task. Bidirectional encoder representation from transformers mainly consists of two major steps, training and optimisation. For training, a language model is being trained by an already existent unlabeled corpus. Google used both expensive machines and large-scale corpora to complete the training step for BERT. The training process took four days and utilised four cloud TPUs in pod configuration with Wikipedia and Books Corpus, which have two thousand five hundred million and eight hundred million words, respectively [21]. After training, BERT used the labelled data obtained from downstream tasks to optimise all the trained parameters. All the downstream tasks used contained various trained models but kept the same trained parameters. Task specific major architectural changes are not required for BERT to be operating at the state-of-theart standard, as it has an extra output layer for optimisation. This reason allowed BERT to break many records regarding its capability to handle tasks that are language based. BERT features parameter intensive settings, large and base [30] (Table 2).

Table 2. Difference in characteristics of bert base and bert large.

Large	Base
Layers × 24	Transformer Blocks × 12
Attention Heads × 16	Self-Attention Heads × 12
Parameters × 340 million	Parameters × 110 million

The learning rate of BERT large is clearly better than the learning rate of BERT base. However, it is not the clear winner as it also requires a stronger machine to handle the max batch size, which lowers the model accuracy when the machine is not powerful enough.

3) Convolutional Neural Network

Convolutional Neural Network: Convolutional neural network requires minimal processing because it uses a multi-layer perceptron variation. It is considered an architecture for the extraction of features, consisting of nonlinear activation functions with multiple Convolutional layers. This often makes CNN a significant building block for large networks. Useful results can only be obtained after training with classification layers. CNN originated as a tool used for the classification of images. Hence it can classify not only a sentence but also images [34]. CNN is proven to be the ideal model for quality and efficiency in the classification of text [35]. The model of CNN contains 4 segments, input, convolutional, pooling and full connection. The input contains concatenated word embeddings in a sentence format. Convolutional contains several filters. These filters are previously learned in the training process of the CNN so that it is customised for the task provided. Variable length feature maps are generated, and the filters convoluted the sentence matrix. The average or biggest number is recorded after the pooling is completed on every map. Hence, this creates the penultimate layer consisting of a feature vector which is derived from the concatenation of all the features in the uni-variate feature vectors. Finally, the SoftMax layer produces the classification of the text based on the penultimate layer's feature vector.

2.8 Word2Vec

A natural language processing technique is Word2Vec, existing since 2013. Automating the prevention process for fake news, cyberbullying and hate speech detection first requires the ability to represent text. A model called bag of words and a method named one hot coding are discrete representations that were used in the early days, being easy and simple to implement. The issue with those two discrete representations is that they do not assess the semantics of the text. This led to the development of Word2Vec, a commonly known technique. Word2Vec successfully proved to all researchers that it is possible to assess the semantics of the text being analysed using vectors [36]. Word2Vec can associate words together and remove the dimensional problem using a low dimensional space distributed representation. This allows Word2Vec to increase accuracy for semantic related vectors. But, Word2Vec does have a problem, struggling to represent the polysemy within various vectors. In simple English, this means that if a word has two different meanings used in different contexts, Word2Vec, is unable to represent the meaning. Unfortunately, this means that Word2Vec, is not able to provide a high accuracy result for tasks in natural language processing. Thus, ELMo is created to fix the context problem by training the word vectors with context [29].

2.9 Shortcomings of DeepText

DeepText is vulnerable to two adversarial sample attacks, both the white and black box attacks [37]. The white box attack also previously known as the fast gradient sign attack was first created by [38] and used to create adversarial image samples. These adversarial sample attacks create content that are both utility preserving and imperceptible perturbations. Utility preserving means that the adversarial sample still contains the semantics conveyed from the original message. If the semantics are changed, then humans may not be able to successfully understand the message [37]. Imperceptible perturbations mean that the adversarial sample needs to be unrecognisable by the human eye. Basically, if the original message is a spam message which advertises shampoo, then the adversarial sample will have to be a spam message which advertises the same shampoo and conveys the same meaning while bypassing the detection of DeepText [37]. Small perturbations can be detected by the human reading the message, so it's important that the perturbations are imperceptible to humans. If there are perturbations, the message will also be either misunderstood or completely make no sense to the reader, thus causing detection through the human eye [37]. Imperceptible perturbations are harder to achieve for text as the text does not tolerate perturbations due to it being discrete data. Audio and images are different though they are considered continuous data that can tolerate some perturbations [39]. These adversarial samples are created using DNNs, known as Deep Neural Networks, a deep learning technique. Both the white and black box attacks are used to gather exploitable knowledge for the generation of the adversarial samples. The perturbation is addressed by three strategies: removal, modification and insertion.

2.10 Shortcomings of Word2Vec

Word2Vec had a shortcoming of embedding each word with single word embedding. This problem was fixed by a researcher in 2014 though [40]. Embedding each word with single word embedding loses the polysemy between words, resulting in the inability to identify a phrase's true meaning correctly.

2.11 Shortcomings of ELMo

ELMo has a shortcoming in aspect sentiment analysis, but this has been overcome through the development of BERT [41]. Aspect sentiment analysis categorises data into aspects and identifies each one's sentiment.

2.12 Shortcomings of BERT

BERT has a shortcoming when practitioners are not being careful with fine tuning their data sets for use cases. If there is noise in the data set, BERT drops in performance [42]. Noise in the data set means that there are multiple languages, incorrect grammar, incorrect syntactic constructions, embedded metadata including hashtags and mentions and URLs, emojis, jargon, slang, abbreviations, colloquialism and typos in the text. It is important to process the data beforehand in natural language processing for applications to address this issue. Although the data has been processed beforehand, it is still not possible to eliminate noise completely from the data. This means that natural language processing models must address words that are out of vocabulary commonly.

2.13 Shortcomings of CNN

The shortcoming of Convoluted Neural Networks is its inability to extract contextual semantic information from texts that are long [43]. A method around this shortcoming is to use Bidirectional GRU to perform the extraction. However, this results in a lower quality of extraction as the Bidirectional GRU cannot extract the text's local features as well as Convoluted Neural Networks can. The channels in Bidirectional GRU are mainly used to capture the semantic information of the sentence's context, while the channels in CNN extract various local features from words in between sentences. There are three layers in each CNN channel, the first is embedding, the second is the attention mechanism, and the third is convolution. The embedding layer maps all input words to the vector representation. Attention mechanism layer extracts important information derived from words between sentences. Convolution layer extracts local features in between words. Bidirectional GRU channels each consist of four layers, word embedding, attention mechanism, forward GRU structures and backward GRU structures. Like the CNN channel, the word embedding layer of GRU does similar tasks as the CNN embedding layer. The attention mechanism layer extracts the sentence's important word information. The Bidirectional GRU model extracts each word's contextual semantic information from sentences. A comparison of all techniques discussed is included below.

3 Comparison

After discussing all the techniques, it is time to compare them against one another, to identify the best one. (Table 3).

Table 3. Techniques being used by which applications.

Application	Technique
Facebook and Instagram	DeepText
Instagram, Facebook and Twitter	FakeBERT
	Word2Vec
	ELMo
Google	BERT
	CNN

The table above shows the techniques that are currently being used in applications such as Facebook, Instagram and Twitter. DeepText is currently used in Facebook and Instagram. FakeBERT is used in Instagram, Facebook and Twitter. Bidirectional Encoder Representation from Transformers is used in Google. Word2Vec, Embeddings from Language Models and Convoluted Neural Networks are not used in applications currently as a standalone technique (Table 4).

Table 4. Characteristics of each technique.

Characteristics	Technique
Filters	DeepText
Uses BERT and CNN along with Filters and Parallel Blocks	FakeBERT
Uses Fixed Embedding, Vectors and Low Dimensional Space Distributed Representations	Word2Vec
Uses context and trained word vectors	ELMo
Uses the objective of language modelling and labeled data	BERT
Uses the variation of multi-layer perceptron, non-linear activation functions and filters	CNN

The table above shows each technique and their characteristics. DeepText operates on filters. FakeBERT is based on BERT and CNN with the combination of filters. Word2Vec, uses fixed embedding, vectors and low dimensional space distributed representations. ELMo uses context and trained word vectors. BERT focuses on language modelling and labeled data. CNN utilises multi-layer perceptron, non-linear activation functions and filters.

The Table 5 shows the test methods used for each technique and the accuracy of each technique. DeepText scored an accuracy of 0.85 and 0.83 F-measure in the ICDAR 2013 and 2011 benchmarks for robust text detection. FakeBERT scored an accuracy of 98.9% when tested using the Real-World Fake News Dataset. Word2Vec scored an accuracy of 93.48% when tested using IMDB movie review data set. Embeddings from Language Models scored an accuracy of 60.8% approximately when tested using two data sets namely by-article and bypublisher. BERT scored 68.4% F1-score when tested using two data sets namely by-article and by-publisher. Convoluted Neural Network was tested to have an accuracy of 99.86% with the TurkishSMS data set. The techniques currently being used in the real world all show a higher accuracy compared to those that aren't used in the real world. After comparing all the techniques, accuracy wise, it is apparent that CNN is the best method as it provides the highest accuracy.

The Table 6 below shows each technique and its corresponding shortcomings. DeepText is vulnerable to adversarial sample attacks. FakeBERT and Word2Vec, don't have any shortcomings as of this moment. ELMo struggles with aspect sentiment analysis. BERT has performance issues with noise. CNN cannot extract contextual semantic information within long texts and must use Bidirectional GRU to achieve that, which causes a lower quality result. Based on the accuracy and shortcoming comparison criteria, it's safe to conclude that FakeBERT is currently the state-of-the-art technique. Even though it comes in second for the highest accuracy it is only 0.96% lower than CNN which also has problems with extracting contextual semantic information from texts that are long. Using Bidirectional GRU to perform the extraction for CNN counteracts this problem but it also drops the quality of extraction as Bidirectional GRU cannot extract local features of text as well as CNN. Thus, FakeBERT is the state-of-the-art technique currently.

Table 5. Summary of all the techniques covered in this literature review.

Reference	Accuracy	Technique	Test Method
[37, 44–46]	0.85 and 0.83 F-measure	DeepText	ICDAR 2013 and 2011 benchmarks for robust text detection
[5, 7, 47, 48]	98.9%	FakeBERT	Real World Fake News data set
[49–53]	93.48%	Word2Vec	IMDB movie review data set
[26, 54–57]	60.8%	ELMo	2 data sets namely by-article and by-publisher
[30–32, 54] and [58]	68.4%	BERT	2 data sets namely by-article and by-publisher
[34, 46, 59, 60]	99.86%	CNN	TurkishSMS data set

Table 6. The table shows the shortcomings found in this literature review.

Shortcomings	Technique
Adversarial Sample Attacks	DeepText
	FakeBERT
	Word2Vec
Aspect Sentiment Analysis	ELMo
Nose and Performance	BERT
Inability to Extract Contextual Semantic Information from Long Texts	CNN

4 Conclusions

After the overview of techniques used to prevent fake news, cyberbullying and hate speech, it's safe to conclude that deep learning techniques are beneficial towards improving the prevention of fake news, cyberbullying and hate speech. FakeBERT and DeepText are deep learning techniques used to combat fake news, cyberbullying and hate speech on Facebook, Instagram and Twitter. Deep learning can be used to prevent fake news, cyberbullying and hate speech through natural language processing, using filters and analysing semantics between words. Deep learning can provide higher accuracy for preventing fake news, cyberbullying and hate speech, as shown in the comparison above. Deep learning techniques are significantly more accurate than the machine learning techniques. However, it is still possible to bypass these techniques. Therefore, an improvement to prevent fake news, cyberbullying, and hate speech would be to focus on removing some of the shortcomings identified in this research. Future work includes improving the prevention of fake news, cyberbullying and hate speech by removing existing Deep learning techniques shortcomings. This can be achieved through the proposal of a solution that eradicates a shortcoming or reduces the impact of a shortcoming. If a solution to the inability to extract contextual semantic information from texts that are long is proposed for CNN, this may result in CNN being the state of the art technique in the future.

References

1. Simpson, J.: How machine learning and social media are expanding access to mental health. Geo. L. Tech. Rev. **2**, 137 (2017)
2. Hammar, K., Jaradat, S., Dokoohaki, N., Matskin, M.: Deep text classification of Instagram data using word embeddings and weak supervision. In: Web Intelligence. IOS Press, vol. 18, no. 1, pp. 53–67 (2020)
3. Islam, M.R., Liu, S., Wang, X., Xu, G.: Deep learning for misinformation detection on online social networks: a survey and new perspectives. Soc. Netw. Anal. Min. **10**(1), 1–20 (2020). https://doi.org/10.1007/s13278-020-00696-x
4. Ibrahim, Y.: The social psychology of hate online: from cyberbullying to gaming. In: Technologies of Trauma, pp. 93–113. Emerald Publishing Limited (2022)

5. Kaliyar, R.K., Goswami, A., Narang, P.: "Fakebert: fake news detection in social media with a BERT-based deep learning approach. Multimedia Tools Appl. **80**(8), 11:765–11:788 (2021)
6. Guthold, R., et al.: The importance of mental health measurement to improve global adolescent health. J. Adolesc. Health **72**(1), S3–S6 (2023)
7. Agarwal, R., Gupta, S., Chatterjee, N.: Profiling fake news spreaders on twitter: a clickbait and linguistic feature based scheme. In: Rosso, P., Basile, V., Martínez, R., Métais, E., Meziane, F. (eds.) NLDB 2022. LNCS, vol. 13286, pp. 345–357. Springer, Cham (2022). https://doi.org/10.1007/978-3-031-08473-7_32
8. Kalkenings, M., Mandl, T.: University of Hildesheim at SemEval-2022 task 5: combining deep text and image models for multimedia misogyny detection. In: Proceedings of the 16th International Workshop on Semantic Evaluation (SemEval-2022), pp. 718–723. Association for Computational Linguistics, Seattle July 2022. https://aclanthology.org/2022.semeval-1.98
9. Del Vicario, M., et al.: The spreading of misinformation online. Proc. Natl. Acad. Sci. **113**(3), 554–559 (2016)
10. Kumar, S., Shah, N.: False information on web and social media: a survey. CoRR, abs/1804.08559 (2018). http://arxiv.org/abs/1804.08559
11. Gorrell, G., et al.: SemEval-2019 task 7: RumourEval, determining rumour veracity and support for rumours. In: Proceedings of the 13th International Workshop on Semantic Evaluation, pp. 845–854. Association for Computational Linguistics, Minneapolis June 2019. https://aclanthology.org/S19-2147
12. Vosoughi, S., Mohsenvand, M.N., Roy, D.: Rumor gauge: predicting the veracity of rumors on twitter. ACM Trans. Knowl. Discov. Data (TKDD) **11**(4), 1–36 (2017)
13. Zhou, X., Zafarani, R.: Fake news: a survey of research, detection methods, and opportunities. CoRR, abs/1812.00315 (2018). http://arxiv.org/abs/1812.00315
14. Ghosh, S., Shah, C.: Towards automatic fake news classification. Proc. Assoc. Inf. Sci. Technol. **55**(1), 805–807 (2018)
15. Ruchansky, N., Seo, S., Liu, Y.: CSI: a hybrid deep model for fake news detection. In: Proceedings of the 2017 ACM on Conference on Information and Knowledge Management, ser. CIKM '17, pp. 797–806. Association for Computing Machinery, New York (2017). https://doi.org/10.1145/3132847.3132877
16. Shu, K., Mahudeswaran, D., Wang, S., Lee, D., Liu, H.: FakenewsNet: a data repository with news content, social context, and spatiotemporal information for studying fake news on social media. Big Data **8**(3), 171–188 (2020)
17. Dadvar, M., Eckert, K.: Cyberbullying detection in social networks using deep learning based models. In: Song, M., Song, I.-Y., Kotsis, G., Tjoa, A.M., Khalil, I. (eds.) DaWaK 2020. LNCS, vol. 12393, pp. 245–255. Springer, Cham (2020). https://doi.org/10.1007/978-3-030-59065-9_20
18. Tokunaga, R.S.: Following you home from school: a critical review and synthesis of research on cyberbullying victimization. Comput. Hum. Behav. **26**(3), 277–287 (2010). https://www.sciencedirect.com/science/article/pii/S074756320900185X
19. Van Hee, C., et al.: Automatic detection of cyberbullying in social media text. PLoS ONE **13**(10), 1–22 (2018). https://doi.org/10.1371/journal.pone.0203794
20. Agrawal, S., Awekar, A.: Deep learning for detecting cyberbullying across multiple social media platforms. CoRR, abs/1801.06482 (2018). http://arxiv.org/abs/1801.06482
21. Zhou, Y., Yang, Y., Liu, H., Liu, X., Savage, N.: Deep learning based fusion approach for hate speech detection. IEEE Access **8**, 128:923–128:929 (2020)
22. De Gibert, O., Perez, N., García-Pablos, A., Cuadros, M.: Hate speech dataset from a white supremacy forum. arXiv preprint arXiv:1809.04444 (2018)
23. Davidson, T., Bhattacharya, D., Weber, I.: Racial bias in hate speech and abusive language detection datasets. arXiv preprint arXiv:1905.12516 (2019)

24. Cambria, E., Das, D., Bandyopadhyay, S., Feraco, A.: Affective computing and sentiment analysis. In: Cambria, E., Das, D., Bandyopadhyay, S., Feraco, A. (eds.) A Practical Guide to Sentiment Analysis. Socio-Affective Computing, vol. 5, pp. 1–10. Springer, Cham (2017). https://doi.org/10.1007/978-3-319-55394-8_1
25. Badjatiya, P., Gupta, S., Gupta, M., Varma, V.: Deep learning for hate speech detection in tweets. In: Proceedings of the 26th International Conference on World Wide Web Companion, pp. 759–760 (2017)
26. Bojkovsky, M., Pikuliak, M.: Stufiit at semeval-2019 task 5: multilingual hate speech detection on twitter with muse and elmo embeddings. In: Proceedings of the 13th International Workshop on Semantic Evaluation, pp. 464–468 (2019)
27. Waseem, Z., Hovy, D.: Hateful symbols or hateful people? Predictive features for hate speech detection on twitter. In: Proceedings of the NAACL Student Research Workshop, pp. 88–93 (2016)
28. Burnap, P., Williams, M.L.: Cyber hate speech on twitter: an application of machine classification and statistical modeling for policy and decision making. Policy Internet **7**(2), 223–242 (2015)
29. Sarzynska-Wawer, J., et al.: Detecting formal thought disorder by deep contextualized word representations. Psychiatry Res. **304**, 114135 (2021)
30. Devlin, J., Chang, M.-W., Lee, K., Toutanova, K.: BERT: pre-training of deep bidirectional transformers for language understanding. arXiv preprint arXiv:1810.04805 (2018)
31. Mozafari, M., Farahbakhsh, R., Crespi, N.: A BERT-based transfer learning approach for hate speech detection in online social media. In: Cherifi, H., Gaito, S., Mendes, J.F., Moro, E., Rocha, L.M. (eds.) COMPLEX NETWORKS 2019. SCI, vol. 881, pp. 928–940. Springer, Cham (2020). https://doi.org/10.1007/978-3-030-36687-2_77
32. Yin, X., Huang, Y., Zhou, B., Li, A., Lan, L., Jia, Y.: Deep entity linking via eliminating semantic ambiguity with BERT. IEEE Access **7**, 169:434–169:445 (2019)
33. Howard, J., Ruder, S.: Universal language model fine-tuning for text classification. arXiv preprint arXiv:1801.06146 (2018)
34. Zhang, Y., Wallace, B.: A sensitivity analysis of (and practitioners' guide to) convolutional neural networks for sentence classification. arXiv preprint arXiv:1510.03820 (2015)
35. Goldberg, Y.: Neural network methods for natural language processing. Synth. Lect. Hum. Lang. Technol. **10**(1), 1–309 (2017)
36. Mikolov, T., Chen, K., Corrado, G., Dean, J.: Efficient estimation of word representations in vector space. arXiv preprint arXiv:1301.3781 (2013)
37. Liang, B., Li, H., Su, M., Bian, P., Li, X., Shi, W.: Deep text classification can be fooled. arXiv preprint arXiv:1704.08006 (2017)
38. Goodfellow, I.J., Shlens, J., Szegedy, C.: Explaining and harnessing adversarial examples (2014). https://arxiv.org/abs/1412.6572
39. Goodfellow, I.J., Shlens, J., Szegedy, C.: Explaining and harnessing adversarial examples. arXiv preprint arXiv:1412.6572 (2014)
40. Salehi, B., Cook, P., Baldwin, T.: A word embedding approach to predicting the compositionality of multiword expressions. In: Proceedings of the 2015 Conference of the North American Chapter of the Association for Computational Linguistics: Human Language Technologies, pp. 977–983 (2015)
41. Yang, Y.-T., Feng, L., Dai, L.-C.: A BERT-based interactive attention network for aspect sentiment analysis. J. Comput. **32**(3), 30–42 (2021)
42. Srivastava, A., Makhija, P., Gupta, A.: Noisy text data: Achilles' heel of BERT. In: Proceedings of the Sixth Workshop on Noisy User-Generated Text (W-NUT 2020), pp. 16–21 (2020)
43. Cheng, Y., Yao, L., Xiang, G., Zhang, G., Tang, T., Zhong, L.: Text sentiment orientation analysis based on multi-channel CNN and bidirectional GRU with attention mechanism. IEEE Access **8**, 134:964–134: 975 (2020)

44. Zhong, Z., Jin, L., Huang, S.: Deeptext: a new approach for text proposal generation and text detection in natural images. In: 2017 IEEE International Conference on Acoustics, Speech and Signal Processing (ICASSP), pp. 1208–1212 (2017)
45. Zhong, Z., Jin, L., Huang, S.: Deeptext: a new approach for text proposal generation and text detection in natural images. In: 2017 IEEE International Conference on Acoustics, Speech and Signal Processing (ICASSP), pp. 1208–1212. IEEE (2017)
46. Karasoy, O., Ballı, S.: Spam SMS detection for Turkish language with deep text analysis and deep learning methods. Arab. J. Sci. Eng. **47**(8), 9361–9377 (2022)
47. Khan, R.H., Shihavuddin, A., Syeed, M.M., Haque, R.U., Uddin, M.F.: Improved fake news detection method based on deep learning and comparative analysis with other machine learning approaches. In: 2022 International Conference on Engineering and Emerging Technologies (ICEET), pp. 1–6. IEEE (2022)
48. Devika, S., Pooja, M., Arpitha, M., Ravi, V.: BERT transformer-based fake news detection in Twitter social media. In: Jacob, I.J., Kolandapalayam Shanmugam, S., Izonin, I. (eds.) Data Intelligence and Cognitive Informatics. Algorithms for Intelligent Systems, pp. 95–102. Springer, Singapore (2022). https://doi.org/10.1007/978-981-19-6004-8_8
49. Jang, B., Kim, M., Harerimana, G., Kang, S.-U., Kim, J.W.: Bi-LSTM model to increase accuracy in text classification: combining word2vec CNN and attention mechanism. Appl. Sci. **10**(17), 5841 (2020)
50. Di Gennaro, G., Buonanno, A., Palmieri, F.A.: Considerations about learning word2vec. J. Supercomput. **77**(11), 12:320–12:335 (2021)
51. Lilleberg, J., Y., Zhu, Y., Zhang, Y.: Support vector machines and word2vec for text classification with semantic features. In: 2015 IEEE 14th International Conference on Cognitive Informatics and Cognitive Computing (ICCI* CC), pp. 136–140. IEEE (2015)
52. Church, K.W.: Word2vec. Nat. Lang. Eng. **23**(1), 155–162 (2017)
53. Rong, X.: Word2vec parameter learning explained. arXiv preprint arXiv:1411.2738 (2014)
54. Huang, G.K.W., Lee, J.C.: Hyperpartisan news and articles detection using BERT and ELMO. In: 2019 International Conference on Computer and Drone Applications (IConDA) , pp. 29–32. IEEE (2019)
55. Li, B., Zhou, H., He, J., Wang, M., Yang, Y., Li, L.: On the sentence embeddings from pre-trained language models. arXiv preprint arXiv:2011.05864 (2020)
56. Peng, Y., Yan, S., Lu, Z.: Transfer learning in biomedical natural language processing: an evaluation of BERT and ELMO on ten benchmarking datasets. arXiv preprint arXiv:1906.05474 (2019)
57. Ethayarajh, K.: How contextual are contextualized word representations? Comparing the geometry of BERT, ELMO, and gpt-2 embeddings. arXiv preprint arXiv:1909.00512 (2019)
58. Jwa, H., Oh, D., Park, K., Kang, J.M., Lim, H.: exbake: Automatic fake news detection model based on bidirectional encoder representations from transformers (BERT). Appl. Sci. **9**(19), 4062 (2019)
59. Huang, Q., Inkpen, D., Zhang, J., Van Bruwaene, D.: Cyberbullying intervention based on convolutional neural networks. In: Proceedings of the First Workshop on Trolling, Aggression and Cyberbullying (TRAC-2018), pp. 42–51 (2018)
60. Zhang, Z., Robinson, D., Tepper, J.: Detecting hate speech on twitter using a convolution-GRU based deep neural network. In: Gangemi, A., et al. (eds.) ESWC 2018. LNCS, vol. 10843, pp. 745–760. Springer, Cham (2018). https://doi.org/10.1007/978-3-319-93417-4_48
61. Ajao, O., Bhowmik, D., Zargari, S.: Fake news identification on twitter with hybrid CNN and RNN models. In: Proceedings of the 9th International Conference on Social Media and Society, pp. 226–230 (2018)

Surface Area Estimation Using 3D Point Clouds and Delaunay Triangulation

Helia Farhood[1,3(✉)], Samuel Muller[1,2], and Amin Beheshti[3]

[1] School of Mathematical and Physical Sciences, Macquarie University, Sydney, Australia
{helia.farhood,samuel.muller}@mq.edu.au

[2] School of Mathematics and Statistics, University of Sydney, Sydney, Australia

[3] School of Computing, Macquarie University, Sydney, Australia
amin.beheshti@mq.edu.au

Abstract. Estimating the surface area of a stockpile is a crucial challenge in several fields, including in construction projects. While modern remote sensing platforms are increasingly popular, their utility in indoor stockpiles is limited, and their use in outdoor settings can be cost-prohibitive. This study presents a straightforward and cost-effective approach for estimating the surface area of both indoor and outdoor stockpiles using 3D point cloud data and the Delaunay triangulation technique. A mobile phone camera is used to capture a video of the stockpile, from which a 3D point cloud is generated, followed by the production of a mesh to reconstruct its surface via Delaunay triangulation. The proposed method's output is the stockpile's surface area, which is estimated by summing the surfaces of individual triangles. Experimental results from a laboratory setting on small-scale stockpiles indicate that this method is an effective approach to measuring stockpile surface areas and has the potential for widespread use in various stockpiles in different settings.

Keywords: 3D Point Cloud · Image and Video Processing · Surface Area Estimation · Delaunay Trian-gulation · Smart 3D Model Reconstruction

1 Introduction

A stockpile is a place to keep objects in an open or closed area, which is then removed, processed, or utilised [1]. Stockpiles store different materials, including construction materials such as sand, cement, and stone. Monitoring stockpiles and keeping as accurate a record as possible of raw material stockpiles is crucial to enhancing the success and efficiency of building site activities [2]. The capability to accurately measure stockpiled materials can have a profound impact on various aspects of a project [2, 3]. One important quantitative parameter for stockpile measurement is the surface area because the discrepancies in stockpile measurement are primarily attributable to the diverse three-dimensional (3D) surface modelling [2]. The monitoring of the surface area of a stockpile has numerous advantages. For instance, in the case of stockpiling topsoil, expanding the surface area of the stockpile can aid in preserving the viability of certain seeds and rhizomes [4].

K. Daimi and A. Al Sadoon (Eds.): ICR 2023, LNNS 721, pp. 28–39, 2023.
https://doi.org/10.1007/978-3-031-35308-6_3

Although modern aerial and ground remote sensing platforms are gaining widespread popularity, they are not suitable for measuring stockpiles stored indoors and can be excessively costly for outdoor stockpiles. Additionally, while laser scanning can gather 3D coordinates of the stockpile surface for quantification, it can be challenging to measure stockpiles that have irregular shapes, sizes, heights, and ground conditions and are overlapped with one another [5]. Furthermore, measurement accuracy of stockpiles can be compromised, for example, when the actual shape of the rock does not align with the assumed spherical shape [6].

To address these challenges, this study presents a method for estimating the surface area of stockpiles using 3D point cloud data and the Delaunay triangulation method. We show this effective method to be a simple and cost-effective solution for both indoor and outdoor stockpiles. As a result of advancements in sensor technology and computer science, the utilisation of 3D point cloud data has been adopted to improve the precision of measurement and to provide a more comprehensive understanding of the spatial morphology of stockpiles [5]. Significant scholarly efforts have been dedicated to exploring the utilisation of 3D point clouds for monitoring and modelling in various applications [6, 7]. Our work leverages the power of data science and processes information from video data to develop a novel approach for efficient surface area estimation of stockpiles using mobile phone camera footage.

Therefore, in this work, we start the process in a lab environment by capturing a video of the stockpile with a mobile phone, which is then used to produce a 3D point cloud. The Delaunay triangulation method is then applied to the point cloud to create a mesh, and the surface area of the stockpile is estimated by summing the individual triangle surfaces. Triangulation is a technique that is utilised to partition discrete and disordered sets of points in 3D space into a mesh grid [8]. This is typically accomplished by projecting the point cloud onto a two-dimensional plane, resulting in a discrete point set within the plane area [8]. Subsequently, an irregular triangulated network of the point set is established. Among the various methods for generating triangle meshes, the Delaunay triangulation method [9] is considered to be the most effective, as it eliminates the presence of poorly-conditioned triangles [8]. The Delaunay triangulation process involves connecting three-dimensional points into triangles according to specific criteria, resulting in a high level of stability [8]. In this research, the Delaunay triangulation method is employed to create a mesh of the stockpile. The surface area of the stockpile is then calculated by summing the surface areas of the individual triangles that make up the mesh. This method of estimating surface area is an effective solution for measuring stockpiles, and it has the potential to be applied in various industries.

To further elaborate on the problem statement, we intend to address the challenges experienced by engineers and site managers in precisely measuring the surface area of stockpiles, particularly those with irregular shapes and sizes, using a mobile phone or another similar device. Our objective of this work is to propose a simple and cost-effective approach for estimating the surface area of stockpiles using 3D point cloud data and the Delaunay triangulation method that applies to both indoor and outdoor stockpile environments. By doing so, we make a step towards increasing the accuracy of measurements and improving stockpile monitoring.

To the best of our knowledge, while the utilisation of 3D point cloud data and the Delaunay triangulation method is established, no previous research has specifically focused on utilising the combination of the particular steps outlined in this article for the precise measurement of the stockpile surface area in both indoor and outdoor settings. We contribute to the existing literature by introducing a cost-effective and straightforward approach that combines the use of a mobile phone or similar device for the capturing of the video, processing that data into a point cloud using Agisoft [10], and then using Delaunay triangulation for creating the mesh and measuring the surface area. We believe that our proposed method has the potential to significantly improve the efficiency of stockpile measurement, which could ultimately lead to cost savings and better project outcomes.

The subsequent sections of this article are organized as follows: In Sect. 2, relevant literature and the unique contributions of this study are examined. The proposed framework is discussed in Sect. 3. Section 4 presents the results of the experimental evaluation. Lastly, in Sect. 5, the study's conclusions are summarized, and potential avenues for future research are proposed.

2 Related Work

Literature on stockpile measuring can be broadly categorised into the following three main categories.

2.1 Traditional Methods

This category includes traditional methods of stockpile measuring, such as manual measurements using tape measures and total station surveying equipment. A total station theodolite is an electronic and optical device utilised in surveying [11]. It combines an electronic theodolite with an electronic distance meter to measure slope distances from the instrument to a specific point [11, 12]. Stockpile surveys using a total station involve the manual measurement of a few strategically placed points using the device and determining volumes based on the created polyhedral surface [3]. The surveyor must ascend the stockpile to position a target prism pole over the measurement sites, which include the stockpile's perimeter [3].

2.2 Digital Imaging Techniques

This category encompasses approaches for measuring stockpiles that involve taking photographs or videos of the stockpile and utilising software to obtain measurements from the images. In this way, digital image processing techniques can be used to gather information about an image, such as the volume of an item derived from the three-dimensional reconstruction of real stockpiles [1]. Image matching technique is an example of this category and operates based on the principle of parallax, requiring multiple overlapping images to generate 3D information [3]. Putra et al. [1] utilised the Structure from Motion (SfM) approach as a 3D reconstruction technique to estimate the volume of a sand material stockpile using Euclidean Distance. Another approach to determining the 3D model involves using extracted geometry and genetic algorithms to corresponding points and restrictions [13].

2.3 Remote Sensing Techniques

This group covers methodologies that involve the use of satellite imagery, Unmanned Aerial Vehicles (UAVs) based remote sensing, airborne laser scanning and Light Detection and Ranging (LIDAR), and using these technologies to measure stockpiles remotely. Several studies have utilised remote sensing technology, such as satellite imaging, for construction waste management [14]. In some studies [11, 15], the use of photogrammetry from unmanned aerial vehicles has been documented for capturing point cloud data and measuring stockpiles. In research works [16, 17], 3D laser scanning technology was utilised to obtain point cloud data for landslide analysis and to calculate earthwork volume. Ashtiani et al. [18] offered a method for calculating the volume of stored materials using Google Earth Pro as an example of employing satellite imagery for stockpile volume estimation.

2.4 Restrictions of Current Methods

Each of the methods listed above has certain restrictions. Traditional approaches pose risks to survey crews as they should work directly on or near the stockpiles, exposing them to potential hazards such as moving heavy machinery, noise, falls, and construction dust [3]. In addition, total station techniques are laborious and require the expertise of highly competent and careful surveyors [19]. Some digital imaging methods may face challenges in image overlap. For example, to achieve accurate 3D models, SFM necessitates con- siderable overlap between captured images [20]. Remote sensing and LIDAR techniques are known to be cost-prohibitive, which makes them unattainable to users with limited funds [3].

3 Methodology

To address the aforementioned issues, we present an effective approach for estimating the surface area of a stockpile using a 3D point cloud and Delaunay triangulation, which is more efficient and reduces the likelihood of human error compared to traditional methods. Our method, which can be accomplished using a standard video recording camera, is cost-effective and makes it a practical solution for the management of construction materials and measuring the stockpiles in construction projects. Unlike some UAVs, this method can also be used in indoor environments. Then, the proposed method is applicable to both indoor and outdoor stockpiles and is characterized by being fast, non-invasive, straightforward, and low-cost. In order to assess the effectiveness of using video processing, a 3D point cloud, and a Delaunay triangulation mesh to measure the surface area of stockpiles in the construction field, our research work involved creating various small-scale stockpiles of randomly arranged stones in a laboratory setting. Our proposed method was then applied to these small stockpiles, demonstrating its capability to be extrapolated to large-scale data. Subsequently, we provide a detailed description of each step involved in the process.

Figure 1 shows the key steps in estimating the surface area of stockpiles.

3.1 Setting up the Lab Environment

Arrange the small stones to form a stockpile randomly, as shown in Fig. 2(a), and use a standard video recording camera so that it can capture the entire stockpile.

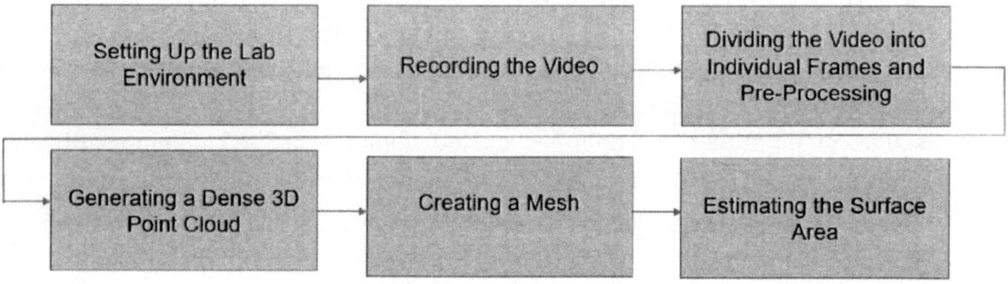

Fig. 1. Primary steps in our suggested method for estimating the surface area of a stockpile.

3.2 Recording the Video

The first step in measuring the surface area of a stockpile in our proposed method is to record a video of the stockpile from multiple angles using a standard video recording device, such as a mobile phone. It is important and challenging to be mindful of the way the video is captured, such as having a distinct starting and ending point, avoiding recording the same scene multiple times, and taking the video as smoothly and steadily as possible.

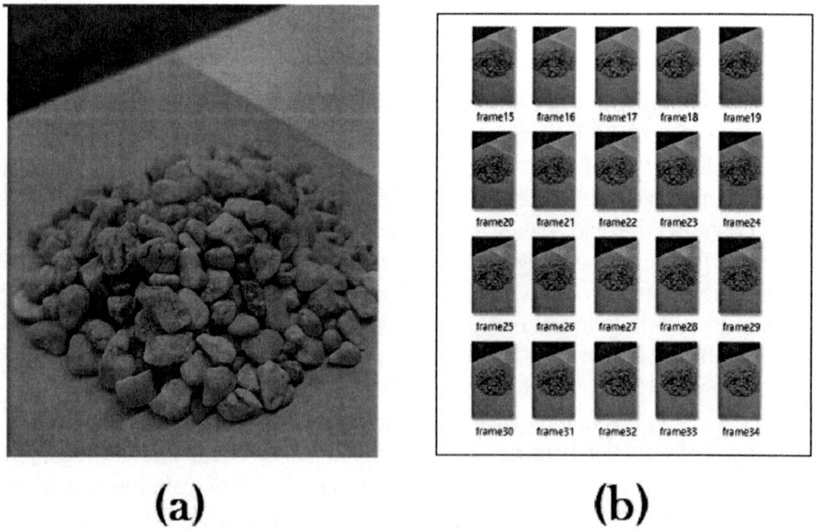

Fig. 2. Capturing a video from a small pile of stone in the lab setting. (a) A randomly generated pile. (b) Separated frames of the video.

3.3 Dividing the Video into Individual Frames and Pre-processing

After the video has been captured, the frames should be extracted and transformed into individual images as shown in Fig. 2(b). To obtain individual frames from the video, we employed the VideoCapture function from the Open-Source Computer Vision (OpenCV) library [21] to read the video and subsequently utilised the imwrite [22] function from the same library to separate the frames as individual images. In some cases, the images captured by the mobile phone camera may contain significant noise, which can affect the accuracy of the point cloud generation and subsequent surface area estimation. Therefore, a pre-processing step that involves denoising the images can be employed. The Non-local Means algorithm from OpenCV library [23] is a popular denoising technique that might be used in such cases. This algorithm is particularly suitable for denoising images corrupted by Gaussian noise.

3.4 Generating a Dense 3D Point Cloud

The dense 3D point cloud was produced using Agisoft Metashape Standard version 1.8.4. The input for this stage is the images obtained from the previous stage, and the output is a dense 3D point cloud. Creating a dense 3D point cloud involves three key steps in Agisoft [10], including uploading photos, aligning images, and producing a dense point cloud, which involves creating a depth map and then a point cloud. The 3D input and the dense output of using Agisoft are depicted in Fig. 3 for EXP1.

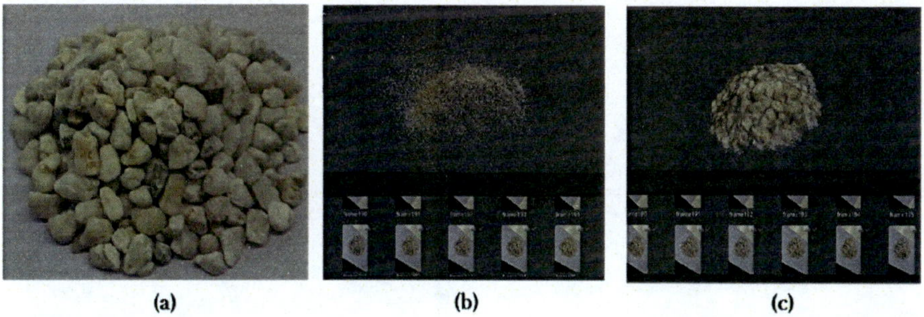

Fig. 3. Creating a 3D point cloud with Agisoft. (a) One of the frames of the input of the software. (b) A scatter 3D point cloud. (c) A dense 3D point cloud.

3.5 Creating a Mesh

In order to determine the surface area of a stockpile, it is not sufficient to simply estimate it from the point cloud data. Rather, a mesh should be generated from the point cloud, and the surface area must be computed from this mesh. Our proposed method employs the use of a triangulation algorithm, specifically the Delaunay triangulation method [9], which has been found to be the most efficient and accurate among various methods for generating triangle meshes [8]. Triangulation is a technique that is utilized to partition discrete and disordered sets of points in three-dimensional space into a mesh grid [8]. The Delaunay triangulation algorithm is a common technique for generating a triangulation [24], which creates a mesh grid by connecting 3D points into triangles based on specific rules and has high stability [8]. We have implemented this method in our proposed solution through Python code, following relevant work, to generate the mesh [24, 25] and [26]. A sample of the mesh generated using the Delaunay triangulation method for the stones stockpile in a lab setting is shown in Fig. 4. In Python, the Delaunay triangulation has been implemented using the SciPy library, which is a free and open-source library and contains a module named scipy.spatial, which provides a Delaunay triangulation function to compute the Delaunay triangulation of a set of points in 2D or 3D [26].

Voxel-based downsampling can be utilized as a pre-processing step for point cloud processing in order to reduce the number of points in the point cloud [27]. This is achieved by applying a standard voxel grid to the input point cloud to generate a consistently downsampled point cloud [27]. Then, in this work, the downsampling process was implemented prior to creating the mesh using the Delaunary method.

3.6 Estimating the Surface Area

The surface area of the stockpile will be determined by summing up the surface area of each triangular face, which is calculated by considering the area of the respective triangular face. The Open3D library, which is an open-source library that facilitates the development of software that processes 3D data, includes a function for computing the surface area of a mesh [28].

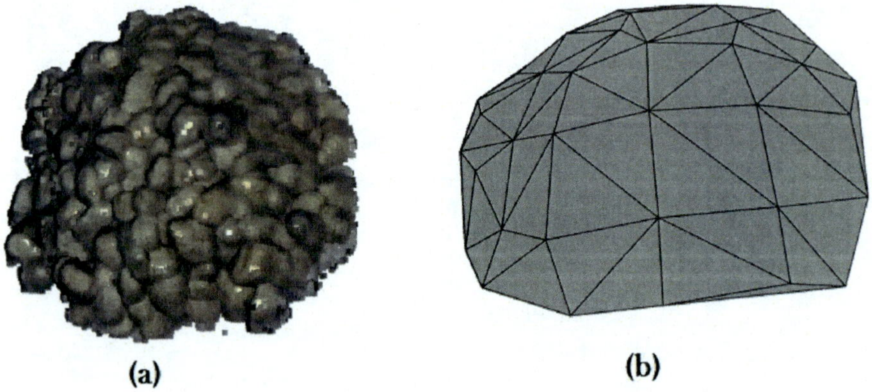

Fig. 4. Creating mesh based on the Delaunay triangulation method. (a) The created 3D point cloud by Agisoft. (b) The generated mesh by the Delaunay triangulation method.

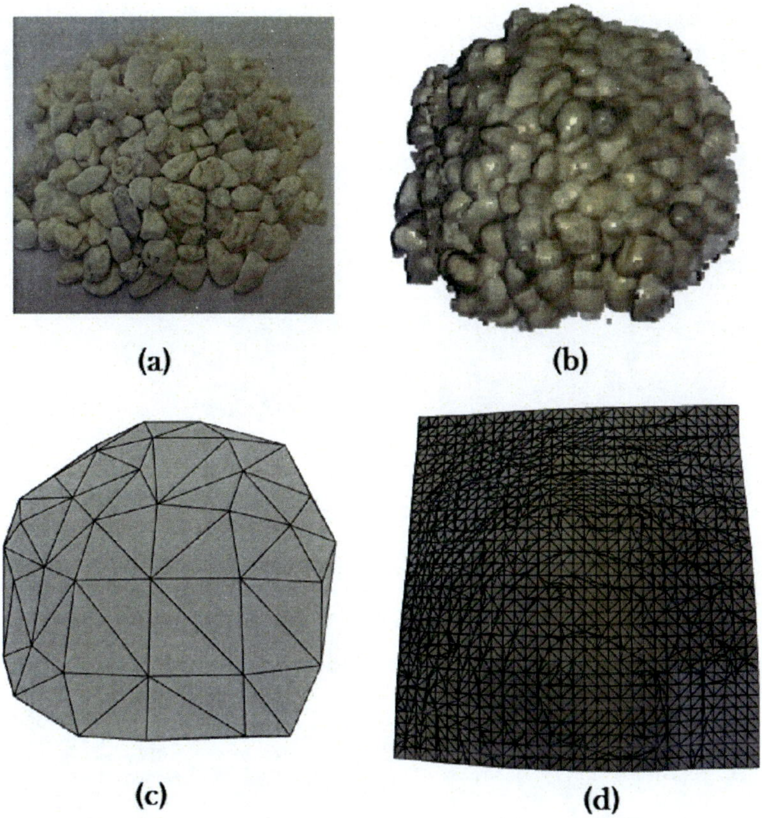

Fig. 5. EXP1: Estimating the surface area. (a) The original image. (b) The created 3D point cloud. (c) The mesh generated by the Delaunay triangulation method. (d) The generated mesh is based on the Poisson Surface Reconstruction method.

4 Experimental Results

The experiments aimed at evaluating the surface area estimation of a stone stockpile in small-scale and lab settings using 3D point clouds and the Delaunay triangulation method were conducted with satisfactory results. The point cloud data was collected from the stockpile and processed through Delaunay triangulation to generate a mesh representation of the surface. The surface area was calculated from this mesh representation. The results obtained from Delaunay triangulation were compared with those obtained from Poisson surface reconstruction [29], another widely used method for creating the 3D mesh. The process of creating a mesh model of a 3D point cloud using the Poisson surface reconstruction method was accomplished by utilizing the Open3D library in Python [30]. The results of two experiments conducted using both the De-launay triangulation method and the Poisson surface reconstruction algorithm are presented in Fig. 5 and Fig. 6. We included Poisson surface reconstruction in our comparison because it is one of the commonly used methods for generating a smooth surface mesh from point cloud data, for example, see [31].

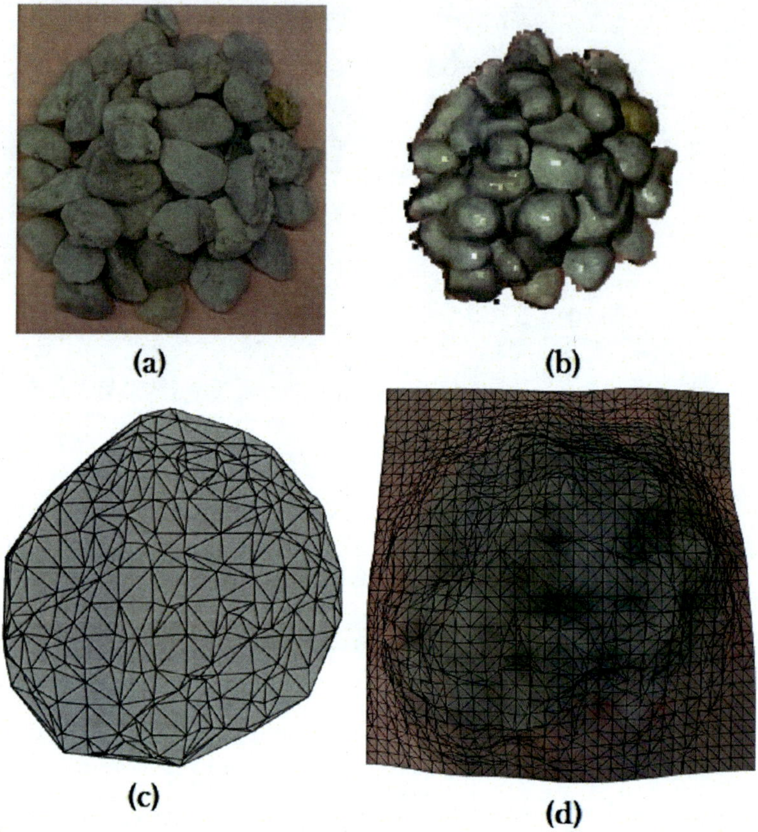

Fig. 6. EXP2: Estimating the surface area. (a) The original image. (b) The created 3D point cloud. (c) The mesh generated by the Delaunay triangulation method. (d) The created mesh is based on the Poisson Surface Reconstruction method.

The experiments used the same voxel size for downsampling in both methods, and the results were compared to the approximately measured real size of the stockpiles by hand. In the pre-processing stage of the 3D point cloud, the determination of the voxel size is contingent upon the desired spatial resolution and the intended use of the stockpile measurement. Currently, the selection of voxel size is performed visually; however, in future work, a more robust method of determination can be employed. Table 1 displays the outcome of two experiments using different methods and compares them to the result obtained through manual approximation. The comparison indicated that the Delaunay triangulation method was more accurate than the Poisson surface reconstruction algorithm, highlighting its value for accurate surface area estimation in small-scale and lab settings, with the potential to be applied to large-scale data. For example, in the first experiment, the relative error of using the Delaunay triangulation compared to manual approximation was 5.6%, whereas it was 69.4% for Poisson surface reconstruction. The Delaunay triangulation method provides a robust and efficient way to estimate the surface area of complex, irregularly shaped objects like stockpiles of stones.

Table 1. Comparison of results obtained from the Delaunay triangulation method and Poisson surface reconstruction algorithm.

Method	Surface Area of EXP1 Surface Area of EXP2	
Delaunay triangulation	391.7 cm^2	34.7 cm^2
Poisson Surface Reconstruction	628.3 cm^2	49.9 cm^2
Manual Approximation	370.9 cm^2	38.2 cm^2

5 Conclusion and Future Work

This study introduced a practical method for estimating the surface area of indoor and outdoor stockpiles using 3D point cloud data and the Delaunay triangulation method in a laboratory setting on small-scale stockpiles. The method involves capturing a video with a mobile phone and using Delaunay triangulation to sum the surface of individual triangles in a mesh created from the video. This method is characterized by its simplicity, affordability, and versatility, promising to be advantageous compared to other methods, such as aerial and ground remote sensing platforms, which are either unsuitable for indoor stockpiles or prohibitively expensive for outdoor stockpiles. The results of two laboratory experiments indicate that this proposed method holds the potential to measure the surface area of stockpiles in a rapid, straightforward, and cost-efficient manner. This study highlighted the importance of measuring stockpiles and demonstrated the potential of using the technology of computer vision to enhance the efficiency and success of construction projects and other industries that rely on stockpiles.

We expect future work to demonstrate that the proposed method has the potential for widespread use across various industries. However, further research and experiments are needed to evaluate the accuracy and performance of the method in large-scale real-world settings and to identify other potential areas of application. We plan to conduct additional experiments to test the method's performance on a larger scale and in diverse environments. These experiments will involve field testing of the method's accuracy and testing the performance under different conditions, including various surface types and lighting conditions.

References

1. Putra, C.A., Syaifullah, J.S.W., et al.: Approximate volume of sand materials stockpile based on structure from motion (SFM). In: 2020 6th Information Technology International Seminar (ITIS), pp. 135–139. IEEE (2020)
2. Sălăgean, T., Şuba, E.E., Pop, I.D., Matei, F., Deak, J.: Determining stockpile volumes using photogrammetric methods. Scientific papers. Series e. land reclamation, earth observation & surveying. Environ. Eng. **8**, 114–119 (2019)
3. Mora, O.E., et al.: Accuracy of stockpile estimates using low-cost SUAS photogrammetry. Int. J. Remote Sens. **41**(12), 4512–4529 (2020)
4. Mackenzie, D.D., Naeth, M.A.: Native seed, soil and atmosphere respond to boreal forest topsoil (LFH) storage. PLoS ONE **14**(9), e0220367 (2019)
5. Yang, X., Huang, Y., Zhang, Q.: Automatic stockpile extraction and measurement using 3D point cloud and multi-scale directional curvature. Remote Sens. **12**(6), 960 (2020)
6. Shishido,H., Wanzhi, Z., Jang, H., Kawamura, Y., Kameda, Y., Kitahara, I.: Clustering method of 3D point cloud of muck-pile based on connectivity of adjacent surface. In: 2019 IEEE 8th Global Conference on Consumer Electronics (GCCE), pp. 770–774. IEEE (2019)
7. Farhood, H., Perry, S., Cheng, E., Kim, J.: Enhanced 3D point cloud from a light field image. Remote Sens. **12**(7), 1125 (2020)
8. Yongbing, X., Liu, K., Ni, J., Li, Q.: 3D reconstruction method based on second-order semiglobal stereo matching and fast point positioning delaunay triangulation. PLoS ONE **17**(1), e0260466 (2022)
9. Delaunay, B., Spherevide, S.: A la memoire de georges voronoi. Bulletin de l'Académie des Sciences de l'URSS, Classe des Sciences Mathématiques et Naturelles **6**, 793–800 (1934)
10. Agisoft. https://www.agisoft.com/. Jan 2023
11. Arango, C., Morales, C.A.: Comparison between multicopter UAV and total station for estimating stockpile volumes. Int. Arch. Photogram. Remote Sens. Spat. Inf. Sci. **40**(1), 131 (2015)
12. Kavanagh, B.F., Bird, S.J., et al.: Surveying: principles and applications (1984)
13. Annich, A., El Abderrahmani, A., Satori, K.: Fast and easy 3D reconstruction with the help of geometric constraints and genetic algorithms. 3D Res. **8**, 1–21 (2017)
14. Jiang, Y., et al.: Automatic volume calculation and mapping of construction and demolition debris using drones, deep learning, and GIS. Drones **6**(10), 279 (2022)
15. Tamin, M.A., Darwin, N., Majid, Z., Ariff, M.F.M., Idris, K.M., et al.: Volume estimation of stockpile using unmanned aerial vehicle. In: 2019 9th IEEE International Conference on Control System, Computing and Engineering (ICCSCE), pp. 49–54. IEEE (2019)
16. Lu, T.-F., Zhao, S., Xu, S., Koch, B., Hurdsman, A.: A 3D of system for3 dimensional stockpile surface scanning using laser. In: 2011 6th IEEE Conference on Industrial Electronics and Applications, pp. 1–5. IEEE (2011)
17. Jia-Chong, D., Teng, H.-C.: 3D laser scanning and GPS technology for landslide earthwork volume estimation. Autom. Constr. **16**(5), 657–663 (2007)
18. Ashtiani, M.Z., Muench, S.T., Gent, D., Uhlmeyer, J.S.: Application of satellite imagery in estimating stockpiled reclaimed asphalt pavement (rap) inventory: a Washington state case study. Constr. Build. Mater. **217**, 292–300 (2019)
19. Carrera-Hernandez, J.J., Levresse, G., Lacan, P.: Is UAV-SFM surveying ready to replace traditional surveying techniques? Int. J. Remote Sens. **41**(12), 4820–4837 (2020)
20. Shalaby, A., Elmogy, M., El-Fetouh, A.A.: Algorithms and applications of structure from motion (SFM): a survey. Algorithms **6**(06) (2017)
21. Opencv-VideoCapture. https://docs.opencv.org/3.4/d8/dfe/classcv11VideoCapture.html. Accessed Feb 2023

22. Opencv library imwrite. https://docs.opencv.org/3.4/d4/da8/groupimgcodecs.html#gabbc7ef1aa2edfaa87772f1202d67e0ce. Accessed Feb 2023
23. Opencv-Denoising. https://docs.opencv.org/3.4/d1/d79/groupphotodenoise.html. Accessed Jan 2023
24. Liu, Y., Zheng, Y.: Accurate volume calculation driven by Delaunay triangulation for coal measurement. Sci. Program. 1–10 (2021)
25. Jose-Llorens. Stockpile volume with Open3D. https://jose-llorens-ripolles.medium.com/stockpile-volume-with-open3d-fa9d32099b6f/. Accessed Feb 2023
26. Delaunay. https://docs.scipy.org/doc/scipy/reference/generated/scipy.spatial.Delaunay.html. Accessed Jan 2023
27. Yusheng, X., Tong, X., Stilla, U.: Voxel-based representation of 3D point clouds: methods, applications, and its potential use in the construction industry. Autom. Constr. **126**, 103675 (2021)
28. Open3d surface area. http://www.open3d.org/docs/release/pythonapi/open3d.geometry.TriangleMesh.html. Accessed Feb 2023
29. Kazhdan, M., Bolitho, M., Hoppe, H.: Poisson surface reconstruction. In: Proceedings of the Fourth Eurographics Symposium on Geometry Processing, vol. 7 (2006)
30. Open3D Poisson surface reconstruction. http://www.open3d.org/docs/latest/tutorial/Advanced/surfacereconstruction.html#Poisson-surface-reconstruction. Accessed Feb 2023
31. Xu, X., Jiang, M.: 3D meteorological radar data visualization with point cloud completion and Poissonsurface reconstruction. In: Yu, S. et al. (eds.) PRCV 2022. LNCS, vol. 13536, pp. 137–150. Springer, Cham (2022). https://doi.org/10.1007/978-3-031-18913-5_11

Descriptive Analysis of Gambling Data for Data Mining of Behavioral Patterns

Piyush Puranik(✉), Kazem Taghva, and Kasra Ghaharian

University of Nevada, Las Vegas, USA
{piyush.puranik,kazem.taghva,kasra.ghaharian}@unlv.edu

Abstract. The use of data analytics methods for behavioral analysis of gamblers has been of interest in the gambling field. Most of the research on this topic has been conducted using self-reported survey data due to the limited availability of quantitative data such as behavioral tracking data. To fill in this gap, we describe a dataset comprising financial payments records for modeling behavioral patterns of gamblers using quantifiable variables. This data has been obtained from a digital payments provider, which acts as an intermediary between customers' banks and gambling merchants. In this paper, we provide a descriptive analysis of this data comprising its distribution with respect to transaction volume and amounts, outlier analysis, auto-correlation analysis, and stationarity analysis. From this analysis, we conclude that this data is right skewed with the largest number of transactions taking place after 2019. We also conclude that the data is non-stationary and does not exhibit any significant auto-regressive characteristics. Stationarity and seasonality for this data will need to be addressed for applying statistical time-series forecasting models. It is worth noting that this data is limited to customers in the USA and only includes details on money committed to gambling and not detailed betting behavior. It also does not take account other methods of payments available to customers and the possibility of customers having multiple accounts with the same payments provider. Additionally, since merchant IDs and customer IDs have been obfuscated, further analysis on merchants and specific customers could be impacted.

Keywords: responsible gambling · descriptive analysis · financial transactions · data mining · time-series analysis

1 Introduction

A considerable body of work has leveraged data science methods to support gambling-related harm prevention and minimization efforts; commonly termed *responsible gambling*. Several promising studies have been published that use self-reported survey data and betting-related behavioral tracking data to model the behavior of gamblers and preemptively identify at-risk groups or individuals [5]. The use of payment-related behavioral tracking data has been far less common. From the perspective of data analytics, financial data has historically

K. Daimi and A. Al Sadoon (Eds.): ICR 2023, LNNS 721, pp. 40–51, 2023.
https://doi.org/10.1007/978-3-031-35308-6_4

been used by financial institutions for fraud detection [1] and risk assessment [4] of customers. In the scope of responsible gambling, these methods can potentially be tweaked to obtain insights on problematic gambling behavior and risky financial behavior.

A study by Muggleton et al. demonstrated that analyzing customers' retail banking transactions can provide valuable insight regarding the impacts of gambling, while at the same time highlighting its advantages over self-report data [10]. Data analysis is often used in the field of responsible gambling, however the lack of publicly available raw financial data impedes granular analysis in this area. Haeusler et al. published a study in 2016 which uses payment-related behavioral tracking data, similar to what we present here, to model an artificial neural network for predicting future self-exclusion from gambling (presumably due to gambling addiction) [6].

The data we analyse here primarily comprises financial transactions conducted using a "digital wallet", which acts as an intermediary between banks, other financial institutions, and gambling merchants. Features of this data include clearly labeled withdrawals and deposits, successful and failed transactions with reasons for failure clearly stated, every transaction conducted by a customer using their digital wallet from the year 2015 to 2021, and unique merchant ID for each merchant with whom the transaction was conducted. In the following sections we provide a detailed descriptive analysis of this data for data mining of behavioral patterns.

2 Data Features

This data described here was provided by a single payments technology provider (PTP) whose identity shall remain anonymous and will be referred to as PTP henceforth. It comprises two types of transactions: financial and non-financial. Non-financial transactions comprise user account related transactions such as address update, phone number updates, and other personally identifiable information linked to the customer's account. These non-financial transactions have not been described in this paper. We solely focus on the financial transactions present in the data for this descriptive analysis.

PTP is an organization that acts as an intermediary between merchants and a customer's financial organization such as bank, credit union, etc. This relationship is illustrated in Fig. 1.

Originally, this data was provided to us in the form of comma separated values (CSV) files with partially cleaned personally identifiable information. In addition, the provided data contained several null entries and invalid transactions. We first uploaded this data into a Spark Cluster in order to perform a cleaning and preliminary analysis. Following is an overview of the data after clean-up and storage in a relational database.

- The time frame for this dataset ranges from **January 01, 2015 to December 31, 2021**.

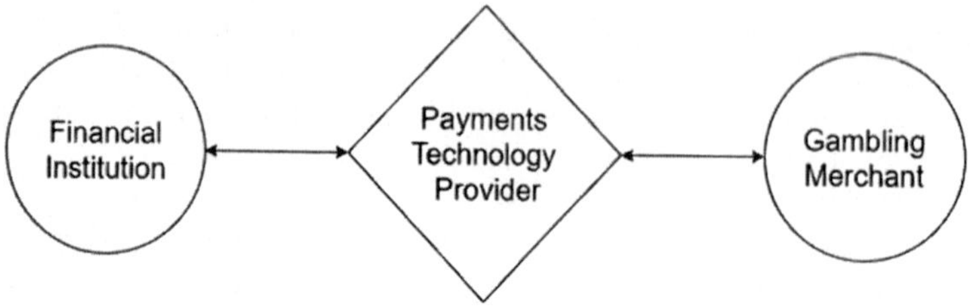

Fig. 1. Relationship between financial institutions, PTP and gambling merchants.

- There are a total of **53,445,398 financial transactions** in this data.
- **251,043 unique customers** are involved in these transactions. Actual customer IDs have been obfuscated to protect their identity.
- **206 unique merchants** are involved in these transactions. Actual merchant codes have been obfuscated to protect their identity.
- There are **51,542,349 approved** transactions, **1,886,572 declined** transactions, **15,648 failed** transactions, and 829 transactions with system errors.
- Of all transactions, there are **24,182,509 deposits** to the PTP digital wallet, **28,954,493 withdrawals** from the digital wallet (i.e., deposits to a gambling merchant), and **308,396 balance checks** (indicates that customer checked their digital wallet balance). Deposits to the digital wallet from credit cards and credit accounts are recorded separately from deposits from debit cards and bank accounts.

All features included as part of this data are described in Table 1. `MerchantTransactionID` and `EncodedTransactionID` can potentially be null in some cases so they are not valid unique identifiers for each transaction.

Table 1. Features included in the data

Feature	Description
ReqTimeUTC	Timestamp of transaction
MerchantID	Obfuscated unique merchant ID
ServiceMethod	Indicates, deposit/withdrawal/balance check
AccountID	Obfuscated unique customer account ID
MerchantTransactionID	Unique transaction ID assigned by merchant
EncodedTransactionID	Unique transaction ID assigned by PTP
TransactionType	Indicates credit or debit for loyalty card
TransactionAmount	Amount of transaction
Status	Approved/Declined/Failed/Unknown
ErrorMessage	Error shown for Declined/Failed/Unknown Status
FriendlyMessage	Human readable version of ErrorMessage

3 Descriptive Analysis

From the features present in this data, it is evident that certain aggregate features in this data can be treated as time series. There are 3 key features that we analyze for this data:

1. **Amounts of approved transactions.** Money spent for each transaction can give us valuable insight into the cash flow through PTP.
2. **Value of transactions conducted monthly.** This is the sum of the amount of all transactions for each month. Only approved transactions are considered for this test. Failed and declined transactions have been disregarded since they do not contribute to any cash flow.
3. **Number of transactions conducted monthly.** This determines the frequency of transactions conducted using PTP. In this case the value of transactions are not considered. However, declined and failed transactions have been considered in this situation because they contribute to the overall volume of transactions conducted each month.

3.1 Distribution

The largest chunk of transactions in this dataset are between 2019 and 2021. This is evident from the representation in Fig. 2. This figure illustrates the number of transactions recorded by month and year for the entire dataset.

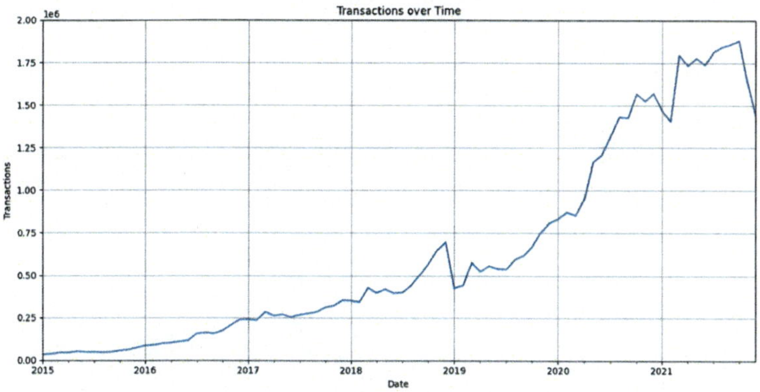

Fig. 2. Number of transactions over time (non-cumulative).

Similarly, the largest value of transactions are also within the same period. Figure 3 illustrates the amount of transactions taking place each month between 2015 and 2021. The similarity between these graphs also shows a direct correlation between the volume of transactions and the amount of transactions.

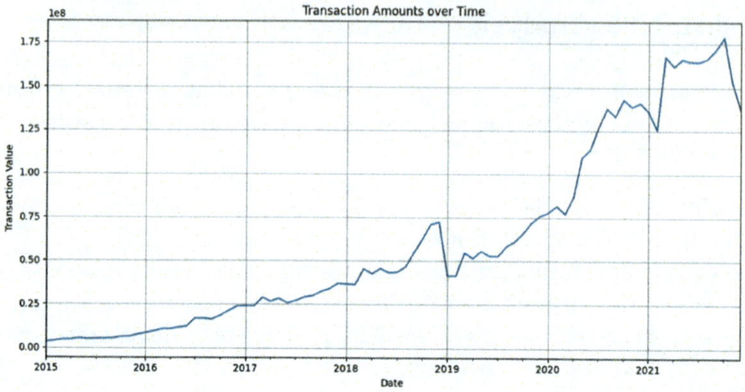

Fig. 3. Value of transactions each month over time (non-cumulative)

There are a total of 51,235,927 transactions that fit our criteria of being approved and over \$0. The minimum, maximum, and percentile figures for transaction amounts is given in Table 2. Observing the 95th percentile of this data indicates that only 5% of the transactions in this dataset are above \$360.

Table 2. Minimum, maximum, and percentiles for transaction amounts (in USD)

Index	Amount
Minimum	0.01
5%	10.00
10%	10.00
25%	20.00
50%	50.00
75%	100.00
90%	200.00
95%	360.00
Maximum	100000.00

From these figures, we can infer that the transaction amounts in this dataset are left skewed. To better understand the most significant chunk of this data, we will first have to remove outliers and explain them separately. Based on the above percentile figures, we can use the Interquartile Range Rule to remove these outliers to get the data described in Table 3. This data now has a mean of **56.02** and a standard deviation of **49.30**.

A histogram of this data is given in Fig. 4. On observing this histogram, we can conclude that the largest number of transactions in this data set are between \$20 and \$30.

Table 3. Minimum, maximum, and percentiles for transaction amounts (in USD) after outlier removal.

Index	Amount
Minimum	0.01
10%	10.00
25%	20.00
50%	40.00
75%	94.00
90%	108.95
Maximum	220.00

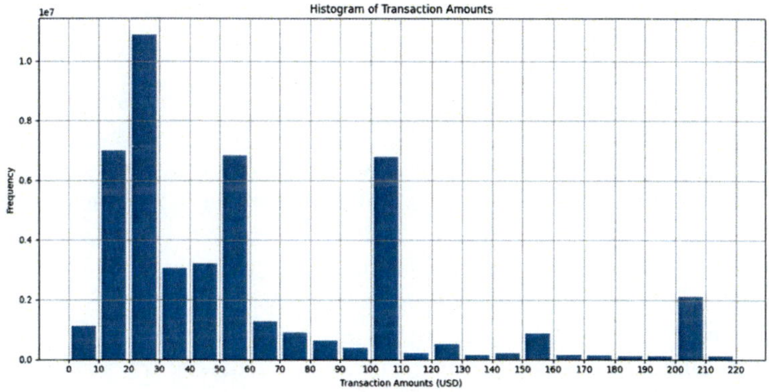

Fig. 4. Histogram of amounts after outlier removal.

We can represent all transactions between \$220 and \$1000 as a histogram illustrated in Fig. 5. This histogram shows that among transactions above \$220, transactions of values between \$300 and \$400 are the most prevalent. Transactions between \$500 and \$600 also show a very high frequency after which the frequency drops rather drastically.

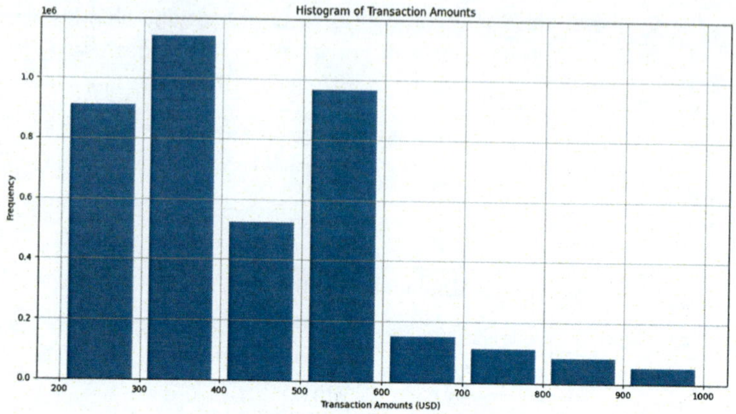

Fig. 5. Histogram of amounts between $220 and $1000.

Of all transactions, **1.17%** of the transactions are above $1000. These are represented by a pie chart given in Fig. 6 along with the raw transaction values.

3.2 Autocorrelation Plots

Both autocorrelation function (ACF) and partial autocorrelation (PACF) functions can help determine seasonality and the process of a time-series. This is useful when designing models for forecasting or analysing this time-series effectively.

The ACF plot and PACF plot for number of transactions over time is given in Fig. 7.

The ACF graph shows a gradual declining trend while the PACF shows significance only for the first lag. This indicates that this time-series is an autoregressive process with a lag of 1 i.e. AR(1) process. From the PACF plot, we can also observe that there is no seasonality present in this data.

Similar plots for monthly values of transactions over time are given in Fig. 8. Since the data for both these aggregate features are similar, the ACF and PACF plots are also very similar.

Index	Amount
Minimum	0.01
10%	10.00
25%	20.00
50%	40.00
75%	94.00
90%	108.95
Maximum	220.00

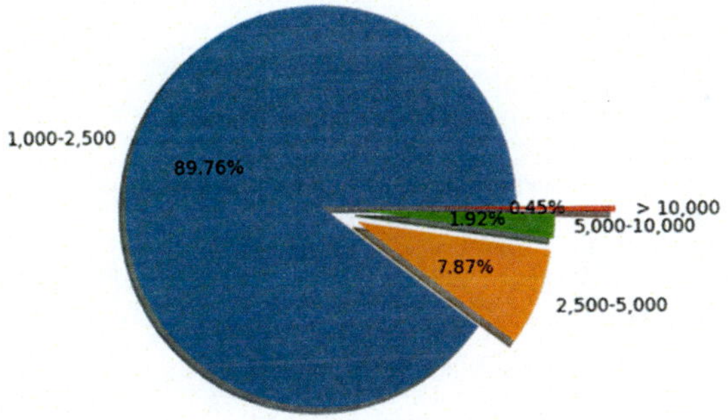

Fig. 6. Transactions above $1000.

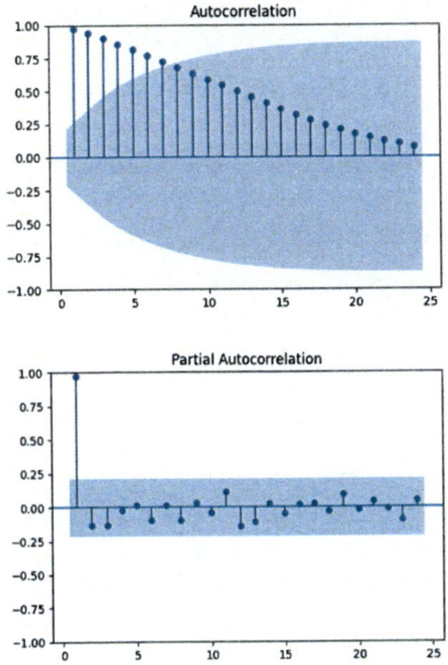

Fig. 7. ACF and PACF plot for number of transactions over time

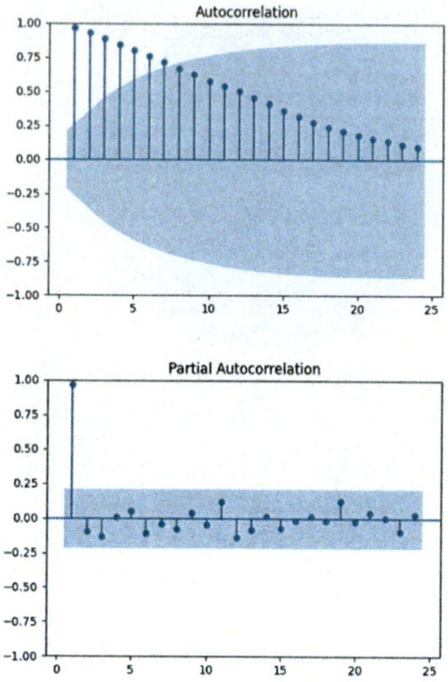

Fig. 8. ACF and PACF plot for values of transactions over time

3.3 Stationarity

A stationary time series is defined as data which does not have any seasonality or trend component in it. In other words, the properties of the time series are independent of the time at which it is observed [7]. Stationarity of this data can be determined for aggregate features described at the beginning of Sect. 3. To determine the stationarity of these features we performed a unit root test using the Augmented Dickey-Fuller (ADF) test [11] and the Kwiatkowski-Phillips-Schmidt-Shin (KPSS) test [8].

The ADF test determines whether a time-series has a unit root or not with the null hypothesis being that a unit root is present in the time-series function. The threshold for rejecting the null hypothesis for this test is a p-value less than 0.05. This means that if a p-value less than 0.05 is obtained, then the series can be said to have no unit roots and is potentially stationary. However, even in the presence of a unit root, a series can still be stationary around a deterministic trend or around a mean. For such a series, we apply the KPSS test for which the null hypothesis assumes that the time-series is stationary around a deterministic trend.

1) Number of transactions Plot for the number of transactions conducted each month is already demonstrated in Fig. 2. ADF and KPSS tests are performed on this time-series and the results of both tests are given in Table 4.

Table 4. ADF and KPSS results for transactions over time.

(a) ADF Test

Index	Value
Test Statistic	−0.299447
p-value	0.925583
Lags Used	1.000000
No. of Observations	82.000000
Critical Value (1%)	−3.512738
Critical Value (5%)	−2.897490
Critical Value (10%)	−2.585949

(b) KPSS Test

Index	Value
Test Statistic	0.313977
p-value	0.010000
Lags Used	5.000000
Critical Value (10%)	0.119000
Critical Value (5%)	0.146000
Critical Value (2.5%)	0.176000
Critical Value (1%)	0.216000

The ADF test for transactions over time has a p-value of 0.926 which is greater than the critical value for accepting the null hypothesis. This means that we can say with high confidence that this time-series does in fact have a unit root. The low p-value of the KPSS test suggests that this time-series is not stationary around a constant mean or a deterministic trend. Therefore, we can conclude that our data is non-stationary.

2) Monthly Value of transactions Due to the similarity between the transactions over time and transaction values over time graphs, the results of the ADF and KPSS test are also similar with the conclusion also being the same. The results for these tests performed on value of transactions over time is given in Table 5.

Table 5. ADF and KPSS results for transaction values over time.

(a) ADF Test

Index	Value
Test Statistic	−0.342481
p-value	0.919269
Lags Used	1.000000
No. of Observations	82.000000
Critical Value (1%)	−3.512738
Critical Value (5%)	−2.897490
Critical Value (10%)	−2.585949

(b) KPSS Test

Index	Value
Test Statistic	1.331583
p-value	0.010000
Lags Used	5.000000
Critical Value (10%)	0.347000
Critical Value (5%)	0.463000
Critical Value (2.5%)	0.574000
Critical Value (1%)	0.739000

From the perspective of forecasting, these aggregate features will need to first be made stationary using differencing and transformations before they can be used in any time-series forecasting models. Any seasonality components will also have to be accounted for.

4 Research Scope

In our systemic review of the use of machine learning in the field of responsible gambling [5] we showed that there is interest in the gambling research community for using machine learning and data science tools for responsible gambling. In addition to this, the chronological nature of this data present an opportunity to apply forecasting methods and markov models to predict gambling behavior for financial transactions. Several time-series analysis and forecasting methods are applicable for data of this nature with more popular methods illustrated by Chris Chatfield [2] [3]. Lim et al. have also demonstrated the use of hybrid deep learning models for time-series forecasting [9].

Certain aggregate characteristics of this data such as frequency of gambling, win-loss characteristics which can be derived from withdrawals and deposits made by customers within a specific time-frame, declined transactions and their reasons, and other such features can be used to create markov models and variations of AR models for time-series analysis. Along with dynamic time warping, this data can potentially be used to predict future behavioral patterns of gamblers [12].

5 Limitations

There are several limitations inherent to this data that future researchers should be made aware of and we acknowledge some of these here. Firstly, this data represents gamblers' digital wallet payment transaction records only, this imposes limits in terms of what may be inferred from any analyses. For example, while one can determine the amount of money a certain customer has committed to a gambling merchant during a specified time period, there is no information related to the betting-related activity that same customer engaged in with the gambling merchant (e.g., number of wagers made, what types of bets were made, etc.). Secondly, gambling merchants provide a multitude of payment options to their customers, and this digital wallet may be just one of the options available. Therefore, if aggregated data is calculated per customer - for example, the win-loss of a customer - one cannot assume that this value represents a complete picture of a customer's gambling payments activity. Similarly, in many jurisdictions individuals have the option to gamble via a variety of outlets (i.e., at both virtual and physical locations), so the transactions of a customer contained herein may represent only a portion of one's gambling payments activities. Thirdly, a significant strength of this financial transactions data is that it contains payments records from multiple gambling merchants including, for example, casino-focused brands, sports-betting brands, and state lotteries. This allows for comparative analysis between gamblers who have different preferences. However, unique identifiers for each customer are only applicable per gambling merchant. In other words, it is plausible that a single person could hold multiple "unique" accounts across several merchants. Finally, PTP operates and provides its services to gambling merchants located in the United States, therefore the generalizeability of any analyses based on this data are constrained to this locale.

In addition to the above limitations, the obfuscation of merchant and customer identifications could potentially affect any further analysis of individual merchants and customers. This measure was necessary to maintain confidentiality of all parties involved in this dataset.

6 Availability

The data described in this paper is a subset of a larger dataset. Access to this subset can be provided by contacting the authors.

References

1. Al-Hashedi, K.G., Magalingam, P.: Financial fraud detection applying data mining techniques: a comprehensive review from 2009 to 2019. Comput. Sci. Rev. **40**, 100402 (2021)
2. Chatfield, C.: Time-Series Forecasting. Chapman and Hall/CRC (2000)
3. Chatfifield, C., Xing, H.: The analysis of time series: an introduction with r (2019)
4. Chen, N., Ribeiro, B., Chen, A.: Financial credit risk assessment: a recent review. Artif. Intell. Rev. **45**, 1–23 (2016)
5. Ghaharian, K., et al.: Applications of data science for responsible gambling: a scoping review. International Gambling Studies **0**(0), 1–24 (2022). https://doi.org/10.1080/14459795.2022.2135753
6. Haeusler, J.: Follow the money: using payment behaviour as predictor for future self-exclusion. Int. Gambl. Stud. **16**(2), 246–262 (2016)
7. Hyndman, R.J., Athanasopoulos, G.: Forecasting: principles and practice. OTexts (2018)
8. Kwiatkowski, D., Phillips, P.C., Schmidt, P., Shin, Y.: Testing the null hypothesis of stationarity against the alternative of a unit root: how sure are we that economic time series have a unit root? J. Econometr. **54**(1–3), 159–178 (1992)
9. Lim, B., Zohren, S.: Time-series forecasting with deep learning: a survey. Phil. Trans. R. Soc. A **379**(2194), 20200209 (2021)
10. Muggleton, N., Parpart, P., Newall, P., Leake, D., Gathergood, J., Stewart, N.: The association between gambling and financial, social and health outcomes in big financial data. Nat. Hum. Behav. **5**(3), 319–326 (2021)
11. Mushtaq, R.: Augmented dickey fuller test (2011)
12. Oates, T., Firoiu, L., Cohen, P.R.: Clustering time series with hidden markov models and dynamic time warping. In: Proceedings of the IJCAI-99 workshop on neural, symbolic and reinforcement learning methods for sequence learning. vol. 17, p. 21. Citeseer (1999)

A Taxonomy for Car Accidents Predication Model Using Neural Networks

Ghazi Al-Naymat[1](✉), Qurat ul Ain Nizamani[2], Shaymaa Ismail Ali[3], Anchal Shrestha[4], and Hanspreet Kaur[2]

[1] Artificial Intelligence Research Center (AIRC), College of Engineering and Information Technology, Ajman University, Ajman, UAE
ghazi.n@gmail.com
[2] Kent Institute Australia, Melbourne, Australia
{Qurat.Nizamani,Hanspreet.Kaur2}@kent.edu.au
[3] Cihan University, KRG, Erbil, Iraq
shayma.ali@duhokcihan.edu.krd
[4] Catholic University, Fitzroy, Australia
Anchal.Shrestha@kent.edu.au

Abstract. Traffic accident is a serious problem worldwide, causing human losses every year. Significant contributors to road accidents are road conditions, climate, unusual driving behaviors, drowsiness, and distraction while driving. In order to mitigate this problem, drivers can be facilitated with a prediction model that can assist them in avoiding accidents. There have been many developments in vehicle crash prediction, but they can be improved in terms of performance and accuracy. This paper suggests an accident prediction model based on Long short-term Neural Networks (LSTM) and Deep Convolution Neural Network (DCNN) Models. The proposed taxonomy allows the creation of a prediction model based on the components such as data, view, and prediction technique. Raw data captured from the gyroscope, speedometer, and smartphone camera is processed for speed estimation. Road facility detection is done through a smartphone-based intelligent Driving Device Recorder (DDR) system consisting of LSTM and CNN. DCNN model is used to analyse different kinds of road components such as traffic lights, crosswalks, stop lines, and pedestrians. Hence, this research critically analyses the works available on vehicle crash prediction using deep learning systems. Furthermore, an enhanced solution that can accurately predict the possible vehicle crash by analyzing the crash dataset using a deep neural network is proposed.

Keywords: Driving data recorder · Smartphone · Deep Learning · Speedometer · Scene understanding · LSTM · Deep Convolution Neural Network (CNN) · Compress Convolution Neural Network

1 Introduction

Road Traffic accident is a major problem all around the world. According to the statistics by World Health Organization, crashes kill about 1.2 million people, and 137000 people are injured every day. Accidents also cause economic losses, marked at 43 billion

K. Daimi and A. Al Sadoon (Eds.): ICR 2023, LNNS 721, pp. 52–63, 2023.
https://doi.org/10.1007/978-3-031-35308-6_5

dollars, due to traffic accidents. With the advancements in technology, computer-guided vision techniques and deep learning neural networks can be used to develop prediction models that help avoid accidents. AI deep learning neural network technology for crash prediction trains the machine and accurately predicts the crash. The limitation of this technology is that it can only predict the data from a certain place and the same algorithm cannot be applied to a different location as data varies from place to place. For instance, some of the algorithms can only be applied to snowy areas but cannot be generalized. Also, it cannot process different types of data. This research aims to propose a taxonomy that can provide a robust and precise prediction for vehicle crashes. This taxonomy comprises three components, i.e., data, view, and prediction technique. Based on this taxonomy, the framework will be able to address the limitations of existing systems and handle different types of data from different places and time zones.

Classifying the components is essential to analyse the proposed solution and its feasibility. The proposed technique provides a sophisticated solution, but it has limitations. The methodology could be applied to other roadway networks if only appropriate attribute variables are available. Further, it does not consider the weather data which directly affects the crash prediction. There was a limited literature review on weather data, so it could not be part of the current methodology. The prediction technique has two parts: one is the speed estimation model, which is estimated with the help of Gyroscope, and an Accelerometer with the implementation of the LTSM. The other part is Object detection model using a compressed convolution neural network. With the help of a camera from the smartphone and CNN algorithm, the traffic lights status, distance to the critical area, sidewalk, traffic light detection, etc., can be done. There are other conventional approaches for driving speed estimation. However, the proposed approach has a robust and precise prediction in crowded and complicated areas such as urban and busy roadways. Considering the requirement and the limitations of smartphones' processing resources, a road facility detection network can be developed using a lightweight architecture.

Around 30 papers were considered and further filtered to 12 used for extracting our components. The selection of the papers is based on the technique (i.e., deep learning) used and the accuracy provided by the model. The criteria used for verifying the system components can be accuracy, performance, capability, and completeness, but for majority of the works, the focus is on accuracy. The paper is divided as follows; Sect. 2 is about literature review, Sect. 3 presents system components, and Sect. 4 provides validation and evaluation of the system. Finally, Sect. 5 provides a discussion and a conclusion in Sect. 6.

2 Literature Review

The work presented in [1] predicts vehicle crashes by using the deep learning neural network. More specifically, the integration of high-order feature interaction and low-order feature interaction is used to do the predictions. This solution is promising but could be enhanced by using information such as weather-related data and driver-related information. We believe that the resulting system can be used in real-time to provide driver safety. In [2], the authors collected traffic data sets and passed them through various algorithms step by step. The algorithms used for this purpose are multi-setup genetic algorithms, decision trees, and Non-Dominated Sorting Genetic Algorithm (NSGA-II). The results are used to identify comprehensibility metrics. Overall, the accuracy metric is increased by 4.5%. However, it only uses accident instances, making it unsuitable for all scenarios. It should add feature section and extraction methods such as Linear Discriminant Analysis (LDA) and Principal Component Analysis (PCA) to improve the applicability. [3] takes the sample data from 100 car crashes, provides real-time monitoring of the driving behaviors, and alerts the driver accordingly. This work has used L1/L2 non-negativity autoencoder and is promising. However, it has filtering redundancy and large inference costs, which could be eliminated by using different functions like constrained network cost and issue clustering. The suggested solution uses deep CNN to detect traffic lights, stop lines, crosswalks, and other critical areas using a smartphone. The idea is promising, however, the use of more robust devices instead of smartphones for image processing and object detection would have given better results. Furthermore, a video recording and processing system can also be implemented to improve efficiency. Similar to [3, 4] predicts the vehicle crash using Multi-stream CNN and multi-scale information fusion. It extracts multi-scale features by filtering the image with different kernel sizes and deploying different fusion strategies to predict the vehicle crash. The presented work is good as it can extract all the features from the original image for the prediction but it does not emphasize much about the video-based solution. The work can be improved by providing video-based driving behavior recognition to make the correct prediction.

In contrast to [3] and [4, 5] have used a slightly different way to predict vehicle crashes. The traffic data set is run through a web-based tool Machine Learning Assisted Image Annotation (MAIA). With the help of the ANNS model, the system is trained with the sample data, resulting in accurate computation. This methodology provides the accurate result, and authors have planned to develop flexibility and scalability by integrating self-model prediction ability, which is very innovative, but the events should be incorporated to get dynamic results. [6] have used traffic dataset and used it to train the system by utilizing Deep Brief Network Based algorithm to predict the risk of vehicle crash in snow and ice environment basically on the freeways. The algorithm used by the author is very promising and competitive compared to other methodologies. The algorithm processes the accurate result for the snowy area; however, results cannot be generalized. There are lots of blind areas that cannot be implemented in the broken road and complex traffic situations. If the technique can be applied for all scenarios, it will be a promising solution for crash predictions. The work presented in [7] used a sample dataset from traffic crashes and broke it down into different pieces. The data is then run through the K-Means algorithm and Random Forest model to get an accurate result.

Using clustering algorithm and support vector model, the accuracy is measured and the prediction gives the output of 78%. The result of the three different models elaborate that the variable selection clustering algorithm have an extra support for vehicle crash prediction. The proposed methodology is great but lacks the data like driver information and weather data which is a disadvantage of the proposed system. Without weather and driver information, the predictions would not be accurate enough. The data from various sources can be used to ensure it can be implemented everywhere. Finally, the better solution would be [4], that used LSTM neural network model to calculate vehicle speed and data sequence of accelerometer, gyroscope and then DCNN model to detect traffic lights, stop lines, crosswalks and other critical areas using smartphone. Arvin et al. [12] offered the best accuracy with high precision in determining the crash and nearly crash vehicle prediction by using the 1DCNN-LSTM technique over the multi-stream data by extracting the different features. The previous state-of-the-art publications has proposed several deep learning-based methods. However, they have not concentrated on a unified approach to predict the occurrence or avoidance of road accidents. This can be problematic as drivers cannot apply different techniques and suggestions given by different sources in real-time. The proposed solution will allow drivers to get a prediction based on this comprehensive solution that has considered many different patterns and techniques and provided predictions accordingly.

3 System Components

The taxonomy of data, view, and prediction method has been developed based on the deep learning-based system for vehicle crash prediction. The system uses two different types of neural networks: 1. LSTM network-based model to estimate vehicle speed from accelerometer and gyroscope, 2. Deep CNN-based model to detect traffic lights, crosswalks and stop lines. Based on the literature review, the factors that are considered for the proposed model are Data, Prediction, and View. These components presented in Fig. 1 and are explained below.

Data: The data types considered for our work are raw data, raw image data, trained dataset and other datasets. The data is first reviewed, analysed and then transferred to the next process. Raw data can be further categorized as crash data, police office data and traffic data. The raw data are collected for a specific period from different places like local police stations. The data formats that are allowed are numerical data, video, or images and can be 2D image, jpg, png, HD camera image, RGB, greyscale, and low light images. Similarly, the trained dataset includes the same kind of data as the raw image data. In the other datasets, their data includes video and image from the vehicle's blind spot. Hence, data used in this paper is traffic crash data, which consists of the data from the past crash and real-time crash data. The data consist of images and video from the surrounding, describing the traffic in that area in that specific time. The purpose of using crash data is to give a close idea about the surroundings at the time of the accident.

The crash data will provide image and video before the crash so that the algorithm can predict the crash by scene understanding.

Prediction Technique: The prediction technique is the methodology used to predict accidents. There are a lot of prediction techniques available, but two prediction techniques out of those are used in this model. They are Long short-term memory (LSTM) neural networks and DCNN. These two methods work together to predict a crash. The technique is the primary important factor in this paper as it is responsible for predicting the vehicle crash accurately and precisely. LSTM neural network-based model estimates vehicle speed and acceleration from accelerometer and gyroscope. DCNN based model detects traffic lights, crosswalks and stop lines.

View: View is another component that displays the prediction output. The prediction can be displayed in various ways, such as smart phone or vehicle screen. Various other tools can be used to get the output other than mention above. Hardware and virtual interaction tools can be used for the better viewing experience. The main purpose of the view is to display the result to the end user so that they could implement in the real-time and predict the crash before it happens. The result can be seen in different output device such as smartphone, car screens, etc. Table 1 presents the selected works and related classification:

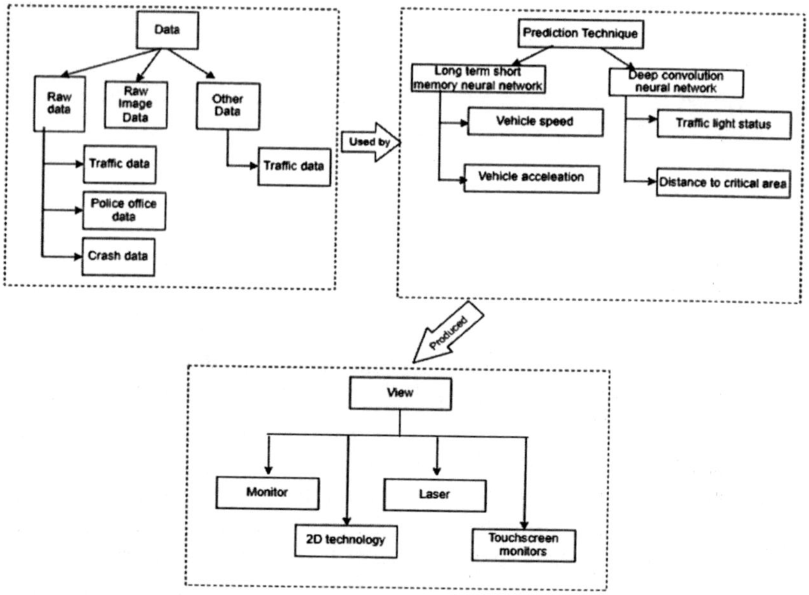

Fig. 1. Components of the proposed vehicle crash prediction model

Table 1. Classification of Crash prediction in different roadway

Reference	Area	Data		Prediction		Learning
		Raw data	Processed data	Technique	Algorithm	
M. S. et al., (2022)	Car Crash Detection	Dash cam data	Image, video	CNN	Machine Learning & Deep Learning	Parameter evaluation
Arvin et al., (2020)	Prediction of the occurrence of the crash	Multiple data stream	Real time data	1DCNN-LSTM	Extraction of the features from input data by kernel	Feature extraction and prediction
Gu et al., (2019)	Traffic Scene Understanding	Raw data, Image, Video	Traffic signs, crosswalk, stop lines	CNN and LSTM	Scenario based recording function	Cost effective since smartphones is used
Zhao et al., (2019)	Driving safety prediction	Raw data	Traffic data, Normalized data	Factorization Machine Combined Neural Network (FMCNN)	Normalization	Low-order and high-order feature interaction
Hashmienejad et al., (2017)	Rural and urban roads in Tehran	Crash data	Traffic data	(NSGA-II) Classification and decision tree	Genetic Algorithm	Decision tree for precision, recall and accuracy will correctly identify traffic incident
Hu et al., (2018)	Driving behaviour recognition	Raw image	Trained image data	Multi Stream CNN and Multi-scale information Fusion	Fusion Algorithm	Pattern detection
Meddeb et al., (2017)	Object and obstacle detection	Images, videos	Motion data, video, images	Augmented Reality Head-Up Display (AR-HUD) and CNN	Deep learning road obstacle detection and scene understanding	Reduce errors from background detection
Wang et al., (2017)	Freeway exit ramps	Raw data	Sensor data	Model Prediction Method Collision based conflict metric	Conflict risk index	Crash prediction in real time

(*continued*)

Table 1. (*continued*)

Reference	Area	Data		Prediction		Learning
		Raw data	Processed data	Technique	Algorithm	
'Zhao et al., (2018)	Icey and snowy area	Raw data	Trained dataset	Deep learning Deep belief network	Rough sets technique	Use multi sensors to detect the obstacle
Yu et al., (2018)	Driver drowsiness in roadway	Face image data	Sensor and camera data	Condition adaptive representation leaning framework, 3D-deep CNN	Feature fusion, Scene Understanding	Drowsiness detection
Sun et al., (2016)	Urban Expressways	Sample dataset	Trained dataset	Support vector machine model, Random Forest model	K-means clustering algorithm	Better crash prediction outcome by using support vector model and k-means algorithm and random forest
Ma et al., (2016)	Single and multivehicle crashes	Sample data	577 crashes and 5794 non-crashed datasets	Bayesian Program Learning model	Random Forest model	Better prediction outcome using BPL model

4 Validation and Evaluation

Validation and evaluation for all the components is presented in Table 2. The focus is given on the accuracy of the prediction results as it is important for the vehicle crash prediction to work correctly and accurately. People's life depends on the prediction; there would be a life-and-death situation in case of inefficient prediction. An important parameter that we have considered in the prediction model is accuracy. Among all of the works considered, none of the works has evaluated the weather and driver behaviour data which directly affects the prediction. Most of the researchers focused either on algorithm or technique. A fully robust system hasn't been proposed yet. Most of the papers have used the traffic and crash data, and some have used data and processed data before the crash. However, road parameters data like length to the stop lines, traffic signs has not been used most of the times. Most of the published papers have considered the same form of the data for crash prediction, just like raw, image, video, traffic and crash data.

According to Zhao et al. [1], the prediction of driving safety can be measured by implementing Factorization Machine Combined Neural Network (FMCNN) over the raw, traffic and normalized data but accuracy is just better than others. In most of the publications, other road data such as traffic signs, crosswalks, stop lines and pedestrians have not been considered in real time for crash prediction. Hashmienejad et al. [2] showed that predication of the vehicle crash could be improved by 4.5% in terms of accuracy metrics proposed by themselves using the Generic Algorithm like C4.5, ID3, CART, KNN, ANN, Naıve Bayes, and SVM over the crash data, traffic data. Sun et al. [7] proposed the crash prediction outcome over the sample and trained dataset to measure the accuracy using K-means clustering algorithm, giving 78% accuracy. Gu et al. [3] presented the traffic scene understanding by implementing LSTM and CNN to provide high-accuracy detection up to 2 FPS by considering traffic signs, crosswalk, stop lines and raw data. The results demonstrate that traffic scene understanding can be implemented for vehicle crash prediction for high accuracy. Data received from the camera (traffic light and distance to critical area), gyroscope, and accelerometer (speed and acceleration of the vehicle) will be used to predict the crash. As there are many sources of data including raw data, crash data, video, image, and traffic data that can be used to determine the predication of the crash of the vehicle, but still prediction needs some real time data, which plays an essential role in identifying the crash such as weather data, driver related data, road condition data such as stop sings, crossovers, traffic lights etc.

Table 2. Validation and Evaluation of crash prediction in different roadway

Date and author	Data		Prediction Technique		Component validated and evaluated	Results
	Field of study	Data type	Criteria of study	Validation Technique		
M. S. et al., (2022)	Identifying accident on time	Dash cam data	Accuracy, Precision, Recall, FI, Sensitivity and Specificity	Deep learning utilizing unique Visual Geometry	Crash Prediction accuracy with precision	Provides high accuracy for point of impact, to check if the car is damaged or not, and severity
Arvin et al., (2020)	Driving behaviour	Multi-dimensional data stream	Accuracy, Precision, Recall, Harmonic average to precision and recall	Extracting the features from the raw data by applying kernel(filter)	Crash Prediction accuracy	Provides high accuracy up to 95.45%
Gu et al., (2019)	Traffic Scene Understanding	Raw data, Image, Video, Traffic signs, crosswalk, stop lines	Accuracy and Precision	Scenario based recording function	Vehicle Crash accuracy	Provides high accuracy detection: 2FPS

(*continued*)

Table 2. (*continued*)

Date and author	Data		Prediction Technique		Component validated and evaluated	Results
	Field of study	Data type	Criteria of study	Validation Technique		
Zhao et al., (2019)	Driving safety prediction	Raw data Traffic data, Normalized data	Accuracy	Factorization Machine Combined Neural Network (FMCNN)	Accuracy rate	Provides better accuracy than other state of art
Hashmienejad et al., (2017)	Rural and urban roads in Tehran	Crash data Traffic data	Traffic incident	Generic Algorithm	correctly identify traffic incident	Result of the proposed method with C4.5, ID3, CART, KNN, ANN, Naive Bayes, and SVM algorithms revealed that the proposed method yielded promising results and improved the value of Accuracy metric by 4.5%
Hu et al., (2018)	Driving behavior recognition	Raw image Trained image data	Vehicle behavirous	Fusion Algorithm	Pattern detection	Excels in vehicle behaviours prediction using image
Meddeb et al., (2017)	Object and obstacle detection	Images, videos Motion data, video, images	Accuracy	Deep learning road obstacle detection and scene understanding	background detection	Real-time superior and better than any other technique
Wang et al., (2017)	freeway exit ramps	Raw data Sensors data	Conflict prediction	Conflict risk index	Crash prediction in real time	Better than any other methodology
Zhao et al., (2017)	Icey and snowy area	Raw data Trained dataset	Obstacles	Rough sets technique	detect the obstacle	Beneficial for snowy and Icey environment
Yu et al., (2018)	Driver drowsiness in roadway	Face image data Sensor and camera data	Drowsiness prediction	Feature fusion Scene Understanding	Drowsiness detection	Better performance and outperforms other methods and improve accuracy

(*continued*)

Table 2. (*continued*)

Date and author	Data		Prediction Technique		Component validated and evaluated	Results
	Field of study	Data type	Criteria of study	Validation Technique		
Sun et al., (2016)	Urban Expressways	Sample dataset Trained dataset	Accuracy	K-means clustering algorithm	crash prediction outcome	The accuracy of the crash prediction model can be as high as 78.0%. The results of the transferability of the 3 different model explains that the variable selection clustering algorithms both have an advantage for crash prediction
Ma et al., (2016)	Single and multivehicle crashes	Sample data 577 crashes and 5794 non-crashed dataset	Better and accurate	Random Forest model	Better prediction outcome	Run it though through K-Means algorithm and later on Random Forest model to gain the accurate result

SVM: Support Vector Machine
FMCNN: Factorization Machine Combined Neural Network

5 Discussion

Most of the papers have focused on object detection, as it is crucial for crash prediction. Scene understanding scans the surroundings and object detection detects the objects around. It all depends on the image quality and visibility. Lack of visibility of the object will result in inaccurate results. For this kind of phenomenon, Yu et al. [8] have used drowsiness detection, feature fusion, and scene understanding to detect the object where visibility doesn't affect the result.

Similarly, [9] used deep learning road obstacle detection and scene understanding with the help of sensors and video where the video is captured in decent quality and night vision included. All the paper has chosen neural network technique for crash prediction. Most of the papers have used the neural network as their base technique for crash detection, although every paper has a different source of data. Hu et al. [4] examine the driving behavior recognition by Multi-Stream CNN to learn the patterns and its relationship with vehicle behavior. Gu et al. [3] demonstrate the ability to understand the traffic scene by using deep CNN and LSTM network models to reflect high accuracy.

M.S. et al. [11] implemented the Deep leaning technique to identify the accident on time by using a dash cam to provide high accuracy for the point of impact and to check how severely the car had been damaged.

Similarly, Arvin et al. [12] applied the 1DCNN-LSTM to predict the crash with high accuracy, nearly 95.45%, with high precision, where new features were extracted by applying the kernel in multi-dimensional data. In our proposed model of vehicle crash prediction, Deep CNN and LSTM are the key techniques to determine vehicle crash prediction. LSTM will process the data related to the vehicle's speed and acceleration captured by the gyroscope and accelerometer. Deep CNN will use the traffic light status and distance to the critical area. In the selected publications, different display devices were used. The primary purpose of the display device is to display the prediction of the crash to the end users, which will happen if the real-time data is accessed from gyroscope, accelerometer, and camera. The prediction output can be projected to the car screen, smart screen, or smartphone.

6 Conclusion

This paper discusses the best deep-learning neural network algorithm to predict vehicle crashes in real-time. 12 state of art papers were selected, discussed, analysed in detail, and compared to determine the best possible solution for the vehicle crash. LSTM and CNN are more accurate than the rest of the state-of-the-art papers regarding crash prediction. The three components presented in this paper are data, prediction technique, and view, which describe what kind of data is required, what type of prediction technique is used, and where it is visualized for the end user. The proposed system is efficient and outperforms other methodologies discussed in the literature review. However, some limitations are found during the verification, validation, and evaluation process. The object detection system plays a vital role in crash prediction; therefore, it could be upgraded for better performance. In the future, the system could use an intelligent Driving Device Recorder with a more robust device for driving data recording. The proposed system should be able to use all sort of data from different places and use it for crash prediction. It currently accepts all the data from the busy highway to the urban area. The proposed methodology has an object detection system, such as detecting traffic lights and sidewalks. To make the object detection system more reliable dynamic object detection (by accepting videos) can be used in the future for better performance.

Acknowledgment. We would like to thank Maharjan Dinesh for his participation in collecting some information.

References

1. Zhao, H., Mao, T., Duan, J., Wang, Y., Zhu, H.: FMCNN: a factorization machine combined neural network for driving safety prediction in vehicular communication. IEEE Access **7**, 11698–11706 (2019)
2. Hashmienejad, S.H.-A., Hossein, S.M.: Traffic accident severity prediction using a novel multi-objective genetic algorithm. Int. J. Crashworthiness, 425–440 (2017)

3. Gu, Y., Wang, Q., Kamijo, S.: Intelligent driving data recorder in smartphone using deep neural network-based speedometer and scene understanding. IEEE Sens. J. **19**(1), 287–295 (2019)
4. Hu, Y., Lu, M., Lu, X.: Driving behaviour recognition from still images by using multi-stream fusion CNN. Mach. Vis. Appl. **30**(5), 851–865 (2018). https://doi.org/10.1007/s00138-018-0994-z
5. Wang, T., Wang, C., Qian, Z.: Development of a new conflict-based safety metric for freeway exit ramps. Adv. Mech. Eng. **9**(9), 1–10 (2017)
6. Zhao, W., Xu, L., Bai, J., Ji, M., Runge, T.: Sensor-based risk perception ability network design for drivers in snow and ice environmental freeway: a deep learning and rough sets approach. Soft. Comput. **22**(5), 1457–1466 (2017). https://doi.org/10.1007/s00500-017-2850-x
7. Sun, J., Sun, J.: Real-time crash prediction on urban expressways: identification of key variables and a hybrid support vector machine model. IET Intell. Transport. Syst. **10**(5), 331–337 (2016)
8. Yu, J., Park, S., Lee, S., Jeon, M.: Driver drowsiness detection using condition-adaptive representation learning framework. IEEE Trans. Intell. Transport. Syst. 1–13 (2018)
9. Abdi, L., Meddeb, A.: Driver information system: a combination of augmented reality, deep learning and vehicular ad-hoc networks. Multimedia Tools Appl. **77**(12), 14673–14703 (2017). https://doi.org/10.1007/s11042-017-5054-6
10. Ma, X., Chen, S., Chen, F.: Correlated random-effects bivariate poisson lognormal model to study single-vehicle and multivehicle crashes. J. Transport. Eng. **142**(11) (2016)
11. Supriya, M.S., Shankar, S.P., BJ, H.J., Narayana, L.L., Gumalla, N.: Car crash detection system using machine learning and deep learning algorithm. In: 2022 IEEE International Conference on Data Science and Information System (ICDSIS), pp. 1–6 (2022). https://doi.org/10.1109/ICDSIS55133.2022.9915889
12. Arvin, R., Khattak, A.J., Qi, H.: Safety critical event prediction through unified analysis of driver and vehicle volatilities: application of deep learning methods. Accident Anal. Prevent. **151**, 105949 (2021). ISSN 0001-4575, https://doi.org/10.1016/j.aap.2020.105949

DCPV: A Taxonomy for Deep Learning Model in Computer Aided System for Human Age Detection

Nischal Maskey[1], Salma Hameedi[2], Ahmed Dawoud[3(✉)], Karwan Jacksi[4], Omar Hisham Rasheed Al-Sadoon[5], and A B Emran Salahuddin[6]

[1] Study Group Australia, Darlinghurst, Australia
[2] University of Technology, Baghdad, Iraq
Salma.h.abdullah@uotechnology.edu.iq
[3] University of South Australia, Adelaide, Australia
ahmed.dawoud@unisa.edu.au
[4] Department of Computer Science, University of Zakho, KRG, Zakho, Iraq
karwan.jacksi@uoz.edu.krd
[5] Al Iraqia University, Baghdad, Iraq
[6] Crown Institute of Higher Education (CIHE), Sydney, Australia
emran.salahuddin@kent.edu.au

Abstract. Deep Learning prediction techniques are widely studied and researched for their implementation in Human Age Prediction (HAP) to prevent, treat and extend life expectancy. So far most of the algorithms are based on facial images, MRI scans, and DNA methylation which is used for training and testing in the domain but rarely practiced. The lack of real-world-age HAP application is caused by several factors: no significant validation and devaluation of the system in the real-world scenario, low performance, and technical complications.

This paper presents the Data, Classification technique, Prediction, and View (DCPV) taxonomy which specifies the major components of the system required for the implementation of a deep learning model to predict human age. These components are to be considered and used as validation and evaluation criteria for the introduction of the deep learning HAP model. A taxonomy of the HAP system is a step towards the development of a common baseline that will help the end users and researchers to have a clear view of the constituents of deep learning prediction approaches, providing better scope for future development of similar systems in the health domain. We assess the DCPV taxonomy by considering the performance, accuracy, robustness, and model comparisons. We demonstrate the value of the DCPV taxonomy by exploring state-of-the-art research within the domain of the HAP system.

Keywords: Deep Learning · Classification · Taxonomy · Human Age Prediction · Pattern Recognition · Feature Extraction · Neural Network

K. Daimi and A. Al Sadoon (Eds.): ICR 2023, LNNS 721, pp. 64–79, 2023.
https://doi.org/10.1007/978-3-031-35308-6_6

1 Introduction

Deep learning age prediction technique is one of the major fields of research in the medical domain for the prevention, treatment, and extension of life expectancy. Also, these techniques and algorithms are used for classification, prediction, feature and pattern recognition, and training purposes. Deep learning prediction algorithms have improved the accuracy and performance in the estimation of human age from complex multi-dimensional data [1]. Human aging is a constant growth in the aging process that is influenced by the living environment, genetic factors, and diseases. This aging process can be predicted using various mechanisms and applied for the betterment of crucial areas. Also, human age prediction plays a vital role in the medical domain where the acute estimation of age could prevent the patient from dying and save many lives. The prediction of human age is based on various criteria including face image, brain MRI, DNA methylation, chest plate radiographs dental image etc. [2]. Various techniques and algorithms based on deep learning were proposed for the highly accurate prediction of human age including algorithms like Convolutional Neural Network (CNN) is one of the methods for faster prediction of human age [3, 4].

The main contribution of this research is highlighted below

- propose a taxonomy for detail analysis, evaluation, verification, and validation of the deep learning prediction model
- obtain better knowledge regarding crucial components of deep learning estimation techniques.
- to understand the algorithm process, reduce errors, achieving better performance in deep learning prediction systems.

The rest of this paper is organized as follows. Section 2 provides a discussion of previous state-of-art approaches and a current literature review. We discuss our proposed DCPV taxonomy and its major components in Sect. 3. Section 4 elaborates on the verification process of the DCPV taxonomy. Finally, the conclusion of the work is given in Sect. 5.

2 Literature Review

Previous prediction models and taxonomies have a typical focus on minimal aspects of the prediction: e.g., data type, tools used, specific techniques, and model. Moreover, most of the publications failed to achieve its goal or faced a maximum error rate. However, we explore a wide range of proposed prediction taxonomies in the following section and focus on the emphasized prediction methodology. Several journal papers have performed research and development in human age prediction based on various aspects. Although, most of them have described only one or two aspects of the prediction technique and failed to focus on all the major factors required for significant output. Mostly the papers reviewed prediction techniques or algorithms with few drawbacks, but only limited papers explored the in-depth process explaining the inputs, outputs, datasets, pattern recognition, and feature extraction which is the most essential factor of prediction and classification through deep learning. Xu et al. presented a regression model-based gradient boosting (GBR) feature [5]. The author proposed the prediction of human age with the DNA methylation data sample datasets as the input and further made clusters to obtain the estimated age as output. The creation of age predictors in relation to DNA methylation of human blood tissues with a more accurate estimation for the beneficiary in the field of disease prevention, treatment, forensics, and life extension has overcome the low-performance regression models. Li et al. used the GBR model where he has made an in-depth study on the validation criteria where the results showed that the correlation between age and DNA methylation was 0.97 for the gradient boosting regressor [6]. The correlation coefficient between predicted age and real age was 0.85, and the MAD was 2.1 years (training) and 5.3 years (independent) showing the robustness of the GBR model on non-blood tissue. The error was 5.2 years in the multiple linear regression model on the other hand the average error is 3.76 years in GBR Model which is more specific. Here, the author has taken the human blood dataset as the input and estimated the age in relation to CpG sites. Therefore, Li et al. claim that the GBR Model has comparatively better prediction accuracy for blood samples than the other linear methods leading to a close relationship between DNA methylation and aging and higher performance [6]. However, the author did not consider the impact of gender on age prediction as the age–related methylation may be different in gender. Similarly, Becker et al. also proposed a regression approach naming Gaussian process regression (GPR) predictors [7]. This regression algorithm obtained better performance - sampled (with replacement) 95% of the training cases but retained only one instance of each individual case, which enhanced the prediction performance. Also, the computation of mean absolute deviation (MAE) using the multivariate models resulted in MAEs of 6.3 years showing the strongest correlation between chronological age and estimated age. Zhu et al. proposed a multi-label sorting algorithm that analyses facial images which shows an achievement of high accuracy where the mean absolute error was only recorded 4.35 where on the other hand AGES method showed 6.77, SVM method showed 7.25 mean absolute error [8]. This proposed sorting model has simplified the tedious steps and reduced the time for training model. Xing et al. has proposed a deep multi-task age estimation model from a single image [9]. The author presents a significant change in performance compared to the previous paper with mean absolute error of 2.96 on the MORPH II dataset. The solution has outperformed most of the previous solutions on two of the largest benchmark datasets. However, there needs to be focus on the age-specific age estimation problem, the author tends to find a principled way to learn age-dependent optimization objectives for the deep age estimation model. While Qawaqneh et al. introduced a backpropagation algorithm where depth features based on image super pixels and their relations are used for age classification from face images [10]. The scored accuracy was 63.78% for the Adience [10] database. Moreover, this approach lessens the possibility of overfitting error during training and testing while utilizing additional features to represent age and gender information. Zaghbani et al. proposed an autoencoder Adaboost algorithm based on deep learning providing high efficiency model capable of extracting high level features and learning facial expressions [1]. The Mean Absolute Error (MAE) presents the best result with less than 2.88 and 3.92 for the FG-NET dataset and 3.26 for the MORPH one. Also, the cumulative scores of proposed age estimation at error levels from 0–20 years on the FG-NET dataset is impressive with 0.8 scores. Chen et al. presented a Ranking - Convolutional Neural Network (CNN) – based framework with error between two adjacent iterations less than 0.001 [4].

Duan et al. used. Feature enhancement via excavating the correlations among age-related attributes and estimation over different group schemes [11]. The author claimed achieving an accuracy of 0.6978 of age prediction on Adience. Liao et al. also proposed divide and rule estimator based on a convolution neural network which showed a significant accuracy with 3.77 mean absolute error [12]. This proposed model is more likely to get less estimation errors in comparison to multiclass classification approaches. Aderinola et al. used Part-Adaptive Residual Graph Convolutional Neural Network (PairGCN) for age classification, they claimed to achieve 99% accuracy on Multimedia University Gait Age and Gender dataset (MMU GAG) [13]. However, the authors used handcrafted features.

Tan et al. proposed Age Group-n encoding (AGEn) method which is presented as a novel age grouping method [2]. Moreover, this research paper has proposed an age group-n encoding strategy to group ages and again achieved an exact age output after decoding the classification results. Similarly, the proposed solution has the best performance with less computational error for the estimation of human age. Also, the proposed method achieves an average mean absolute error (MAE) of 2.86 the and best performance as the MAE is reduced by 0.17. Sajedi et al. proposed Brain Age Estimation (BAE) based on Magnetic Resonance Imaging (MRI) images [14]. The author has used C-SVDDNet and Complex Network which has provided a remarkable accuracy, where the input of classification (raw data) has 75.34% accuracy and features extracted from C-SVDDNet shows 22.78%. This model takes a single MRI image in the one-dimensional format as input and provides feature vector classified age information with satisfactory performance. This solution has increased the possibility of calculating the brain age by brain MRI images with remarkably accurate outcomes which could be reliable for BAE and neurological disease detection. Fang et al. presented multi–stage learning technique itheiris paper for the prediction of gender and age [15]. The model accepts raw images as input and provides estimated age after regression. The author derives an acceptable range of accuracy along with avoidance of interferences and noises of complex background data. Also, this method predicts the precise gender and age based on facial images leading to better performance in human age estimation. Tan et al. explained the effectiveness of deep learning prediction techniques in achieving performance and accuracy through efficient training and testing methods [2]. The authors introduced an age group-n-encoding strategy to group ages and again achieved an exact age output after decoding the classification results. The author has systematically arranged the classification and prediction process in four stages: pre-processing of raw images, age grouping, age group classification, age decoding. The author has proposed a deep learning solution for age estimation based on a single network where classification is implemented in a CNN with multiple outputs and recovery of the exact age for each face image is achieved by decoding the classification results.

3 DCPV Components

Figure 1 depicts the major components of our proposed taxonomy; Data, Classification, Prediction, View, and the relationships between these components. The taxonomy of Data, Classification technique, Prediction, and View (DCPV) has been developed on the basis of the current and past deep learning-based prediction algorithms and methodologies based on Human Age Prediction (HAP). The taxonomy was generated including all the relevant factors in association with this research for the creation, evaluation as well as validation of the system.

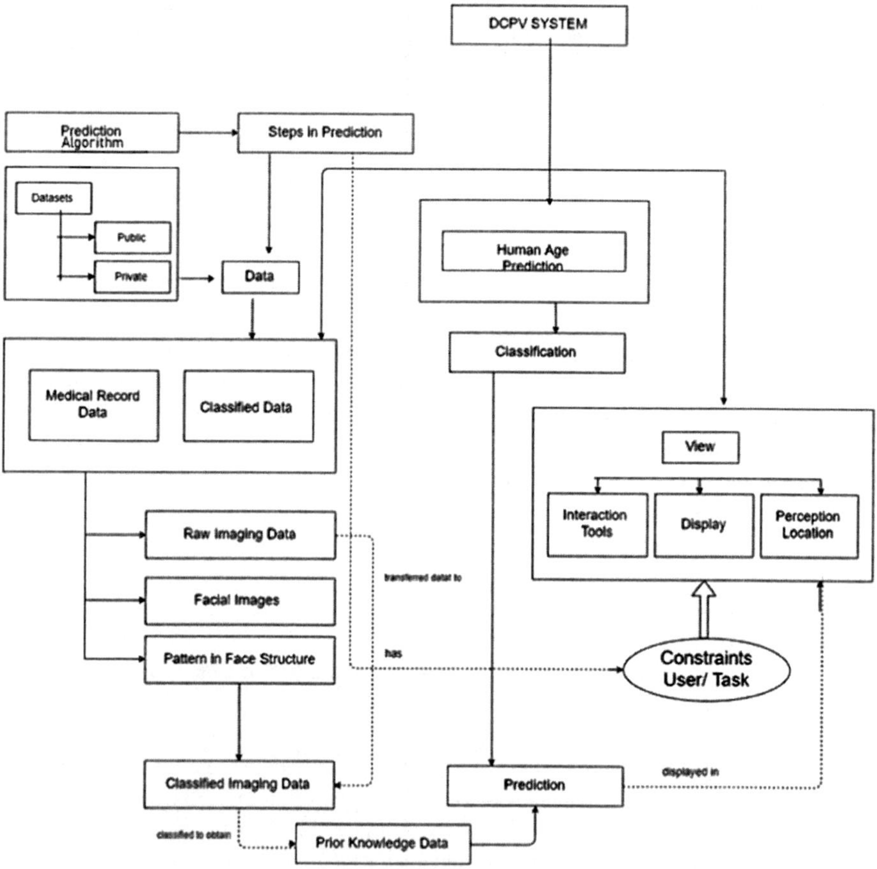

Fig. 1. Components of our proposed Taxonomy; Data, Classification, Prediction, View and the relationships between them.

Data The first factor of our DCPV taxonomy is data. The data includes information of human facial images or datasets with the properties of dimensionality, data modality, and whether the data are implemented for testing and training for the classification step. Such factors are used in the classification of various prediction systems. Secondly, the classification process is where the raw data is further classified with use of different techniques or algorithms and grouped based on rank or applied scenario. It enhances performance accuracy via deep learning approaches. Thirdly, there is a prediction step where the classified data is further manipulated to achieve a final prediction with the use of definite formula or algorithm in the deep learning process. Lastly, the classification of the model is based in the view which is the final component of the prediction model, which provides the end user with final real-time predicted output. The components and the classes are explained in detail in Table 1. The above-reviewed journal papers outlined facial images as an input for the system. Also, few journal papers have worked on medical records and DNA samples as input. Among all the reviewed papers majority of the journal papers classified the prior data which is then used for the prediction of human age. Facial image for the prediction of human age is majorly used for the prediction. MRI Images and DNA Methylation is also majorly used to convert into classified data. Also, this research focuses on blood datasets and electronic medical records as raw input for the estimation of human age. Figure 2 shows different data attributes considered for the taxonomy.

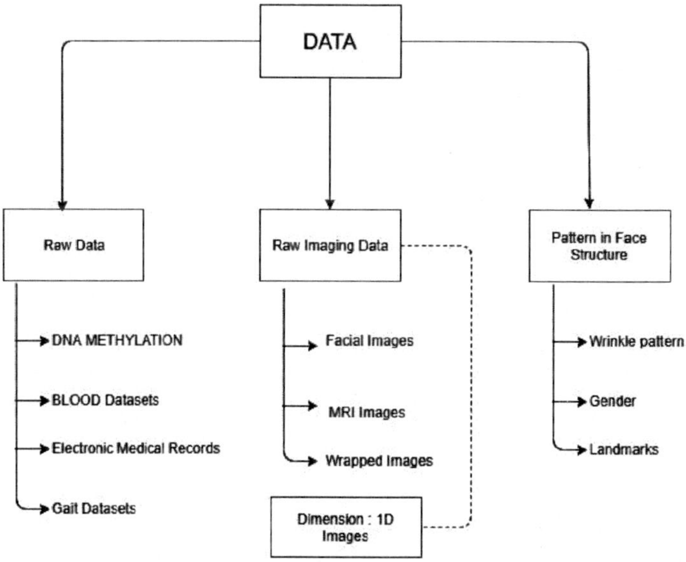

Fig. 2. Data Attributes and their examples.

Several classification algorithms and approaches were encountered in the reviewed journals where the deep convolutional neural network (DCCN) method was widely used for the accurate classification of the data [16–19]. The authors employed a convolutional neural network (CNN) as a classifier to classify raw data and estimate the human age. Also, a Support Vector Machine (SVM) combined with various other functional and statistical tools for the classification [21, 22]. However, the SVM lacks processing speed for training data. Similarly, the reviewed publication discussed on other classification approaches like Gait – based human age classification, Binary Classifier and detection of relation approach, Age group-n encoding (AGEn), Auto Encoder etc. these contributions described the classification technique and algorithm to achieve significant output with optimal performance.

Prediction Technique The prediction technique is the major method the paper has discussed. The evaluated journals have various approaches and models to predict the age from classified data. The following figure shows the various models applied in human age prediction among which regression modeling for the estimation process was applied. The Regression model is used to predict and estimate the age of humans after using the classified data as input into the model. Gradient Boosting Regressor (GBR) to estimate the aging process through the input of classified DNA samples into the prediction model, which was successful in portraying a remarkable accuracy rate in age prediction. Also, Fine Tuning, Multi-label Sorting, Support Vector Regression Algorithms, Encoding and Decoding algorithms, and Back Propagation algorithms are some of the proposed prediction techniques implemented in the research. Figure 3 shows prediction technique components with various models and algorithms for the taxonomy.

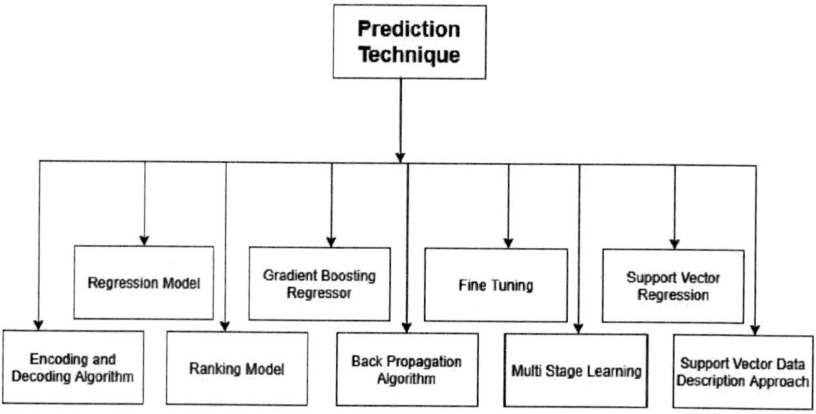

Fig. 3. Prediction techniques components with various models and algorithms

View The perception of a view is the area of focus, where the prediction technique is viewed for the offered system. Various types of perception locations such as training, testing environment and digital display is discussed. The specific technology of display is portrayed to present data to the users. The prediction algorithm takes place on the computer screen itself, so the display unit discussed are monitor, digital screen, and other usual devices. The perception location is subdivided into the different forms of perception i.e., image database, sample datasets or training and testing datasets. Moreover, the tools are classified into hardware and software tools, where the software could be the system software, application software or programming tools. Similarly, the statistical tools and computer components are listed under the hardware section. The main components and class view of the view component along with various subclasses is presented in Fig. 4.

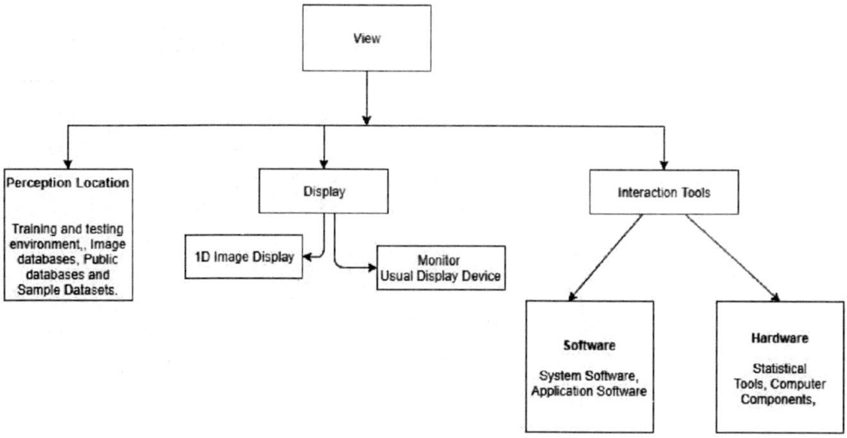

Fig. 4. Major components of class view with its sub classes.

4 Discussion

Table 1 summarizes and compares the current state of art solutions. We considered two important factors for systems selection, firstly the effectiveness, our major concern was on the accuracy and execution time which determines the effectiveness of the system. All the components were not under the standard procedure of system verification as most of the reviewed papers do not consider training and testing lag during the prediction process. However, the prediction process could not be fully automated since the components and data were dependent on the context. Secondly the completeness, the state-of-the-art papers were deeply analyzed, and their components were compared with our proposed taxonomy to compare the completeness of out DCPV taxonomy.

We prepared a review that considers the different relevant factors associated with this research. The initial search out-turned 211 results, of these only 31 satisfied the stated inclusion criteria. The included publications were considered based on their scope and domain which was prediction of human age. Moreover, the publications were selected on terms of technology and algorithms applied which was deep learning. Also, the paper had to include the algorithm for prediction and the techniques implemented for the output. However, 71 publications were neglected due to irrelevant domain, other 43 because they studied the age prediction of animals rather than human age, 18 were rejected as they did not meet the standard of journal which is Q1 and Q2, the remaining 48 were not included because the technique applied to predict the output was not based on deep learning. We shortlisted the journal publications matching the scope and goal which are newly published in Q! an Q2 list with our model. Most of the publications contain raw data, sample data, classified imaging data. Moreover, the terms and expression that help the goal of the framework lead to high beneficial complete framework in specific domain. The figure below demonstrates the components stated in terms of percentage from reviewed publications.

The reviewed papers have used facial images, medical records, and DNA Methylation in the form of input data. Few papers are also based on MRI images. The reviewed paper

Table 1. DCPV table of Human Age Prediction System

Ref	Predection		Data		Classification/Feature Detected	Predection Technique	View			Evaluated and Validated Components	Study Criteria	Evaluation / Validation Method And / OR DATASETS	Results
	Type	Area	Raw	DT			PL	DP	IT				
[5]	AE	GBR on DNA Datasets	DNA Methylation of human blood tissues	SD	Extraction of methylation level	Regression Model-Gradient Boosting Regressor (GBR)	SD	DS	PLT, OS, ST	Prediction method	Performance	MATLAB R2014b v8	Performance in independent datasets the MAD = 6.11 years for GBR; 9.57 years for Bayesian ridge; 7.58 years
[1]	AE	Face extraction using AdaBoost framework	Human facial images	1D pixel images	Autoencoder	Face features to age regression	IDB	DD	OS, ST	Estimation method	Robustness, Effectiveness, Performance	MORPH & Face and Gesture Recognition Research Network (FGNET) Datasets	MAE (Mean Absolute Error) presents the best result with less than 2.88 and 3.92 for the FG-NET dataset and 3.26 for the MORPH one
[14]	AP	Aging Scenario of brain and human age	Human brain MRI images	One MRI Image – 1D	SVDD (Support Vector Data Description) approach clusters the features and sets feature maps	Brain Age Estimation (BAE) based on Magnetic Resonance Imaging (MRI) images	N/S	DD	PLT, ST, OS	Magnetic Resonance Imaging (MRI) in Age Estimation	Accuracy, Error Rate	MRI Images Public Datasets	Classification (raw data) has 75.34% accuracy and features extracted from C-SVDDNet shows 22.78%

(continued)

Table 1. *(continued)*

Ref	Predection		Data		Classification/Feature Detected	Predection Technique	View			Evaluated and Validated Components	Study Criteria	Evaluation / Validation Method And / OR DATASETS	Results
	Type	Area	Raw	DT			PL	DP	IT				
[9]	AP	GBR on DNA Datasets	Human blood tissues datasets	SD	MAD (Mean Absolute Deviation), MSE (Mean Square Error), RMSE (Root Mean Square Error)	Gradient Boosting Regressor (GBR)	SD	DS	AS, ST,	Gradient Boosting Algorithm (GBR) for Age Prediction	Accuracy, Robustness, Performance	MATLAB R2014b	Correlation between age and DNA methylation was 0.97 for the gradient boosting regressor. The average error is 3.76 years in GBR Model which is more specific
[4]	AR	Pretraining with facial images and fine tuning with age labelled faces	Facial Images	Raw Face images from IDB	Ranking - Convolutional Neural Network (CNN) – based Framework	Binary rankings and feature maps via cascade classifiers to extract features	IDB	DD	PLT, ST, OS, HWT	Ranking Framework for estimation of Age	Accuracy, Error Bound	SoftMax	Error between two adjacent iterations is less than 0.001
[7]	AE	Predicting epigenetic changes in DNA	Intervertebral disc (IVD) samples Epiglottis (EPI) samples	SD	Fit a model for mapping between the features and the target variable which is chronological age	Gaussian process regression (GPR) predictors	SD	N/S	PLT, ST	Gaussian process regression (GPR) Age predictors	Performance, Accuracy	MATLAB	Sampled 95% of he training cases but retained only one instance enhancing the performance. Mean Absolute Error (MAE) using the multivariate models resulted in MAEs of 6.3 years

(continued)

Table 1. *(continued)*

Ref	Predection		Data		Classification/Feature Detected	Predection Technique	View			Evaluated and Validated Components	Study Criteria	Evaluation / Validation Method And / OR DATASETS	Results
	Type	Area	Raw	DT			PL	DP	IT				
[2]	AE	Human age prediction from single face image	Facial Images	Fixed Dimension Face Image	Age group-n encoding strategy to group ages and obtain an exact age after decoding the classification results	Age group-n encoding (AGEn) method	IDB	DD	HWT, ST, AS	Age Group Encoding and Decoding method	Accuracy, Performance	FG-NET, Morph Datasets	Average Mean Absolute Error (MAE) = 2.86 Decreased the decoding speed by 10 times
[8]	AE	Age Estimation Algorithm of facial image based on multi–label sorting	Age Label	Facial Age Datasets	Construct binary classifier and detect relation between age and samples	Multi-label Sorting	IDB	DS	ST, OS	Multi- Label Sorting based age prediction	Accuracy	FG-NET Morph Datasets	MAE (Mean Absolute Error) results of FG-NET dataset of Multi-label is 4.35
[12]	AE	Estimate the human age with the use of divide – and – rule strategy	Extraction of face age descriptor	Image as datasets from public databases	Convolutional Neural Network (CNN)	Extraction methodology based on superior image representation capability of depth convolutional neural network	SD	DD	ST, OS, AS, PLT	Prediction Method	Accuracy	Age Network (AgeNet)	The Mean absolute Error (MAE) is derived the lowest of 3.77 with highest accuracy
[15]	AE	encoder-decoder based segmentation	Real world images	1D Face Image	Extraction of classes in segmentation with enhancement in image representation	Multi – Stage Learning	SD	DS	HWT, PLT, OS, ST	Encoding and Decoding Network	Accuracy, Performance	VGG19-Net based net- work	They achieve 4.42% and 7.73% increments in terms of g.caaa than that of MA respectively due to powerful capability in visual feature extraction

(continued)

Table 1. (*continued*)

Ref	Predection		Data		Classification/Feature Detected	Predection Technique	View			Evaluated and Validated Components	Study Criteria	Evaluation / Validation Method And / OR DATASETS	Results
	Type	Area	Raw	DT			PL	DP	IT				
[16]	AE	Label distribution approach to exploit real and adjacent ages	Extraction of facial image features and sequential features to achieve age patterns	Facial Image	Convolutional Neural Network (CNN)	Recurrent Age Estimation (RAE) which uses Long short-term Memory (LSTM) architecture	IDB	N/S	ST, OS, PLT	Prediction method based on appearance features as well as ageing pattern	Performance, Accuracy	MORPH and FG-NET Datasets	The Mean Absolute error on MORPH and FG_NET Datasets are recorded 1.32 and 2.19 respectively which is a remarkable performance
[17]	AE	Training of age estimation model for classification	Label of age groups represented by a range	Face Image	Deep Convolutional Neural Network (DCNN)	Transfer Learning	SD	DS	OS, ST, PLT	Prediction method based on deep learning algorithm	Performance	Age estimation dataset-Images of Groups of People	System performance is measured through the confusion matrix which shows, age ranges0–2 and 66+ are easier to predict with better performance

(*continued*)

Table 1. *(continued)*

Ref	Predection		Data		Classification/Feature Detected	Predection Technique	View			Evaluated and Validated Components	Study Criteria	Evaluation / Validation Method And / OR DATASETS	Results
	Type	Area	Raw	DT			PL	DP	IT				
[18]	AE	Age estimation by learning the association of the face attributes and components	Face Attributes and Regions	Facial Image- 1D	Multi Task Learning	Attribute-Region Association Network (ARAN)	IDB	DS	N/S	Attribute-Region Association Network (ARAN) Prediction Method	Performance	MORPH Album II and FG-NET Datasets	The Mean Absolute Errors (MAE) are decreased to 2.51 years compared to the state-of-the-arts on the MORPH Album II dataset
[19]	AE	Deep Expectation of Real and Apparent age from single image	Single image without facial landmarks	Single Face Image	Convolutional Neural Network (CNN)	Formulation of age regression for robust face alignment	SD	DD	PLT, ST, OS, HWT	Prediction method with the use of facial landmarks	Performance, Robustness	IMDB-WIKI dataset, the largest public dataset of face images	Best performance on pre-training. 0.282 error (MAE 3.252) compared to 0.456 error (MAE 5.369) Above 40% occlusion the MAE performance rapidly deteriorates
[20]	AE	Representation of face under deep convolutional neural network framework	Facial images in public database	Batch Image Data	Study of discriminative feature descriptor per image directly from raw pixels from image datasets	Group-aware Deep Feature Learning (GA-DFL) Technique	IDB	N/S	PLT, ST, OS, HWT	Prediction Method based on Feature Learning Technique	Performance	MATLAB & VGG-16 Face Net	The proposed model showed the lowest MAE – 3.93 which has upgraded the overall performance

is lacking preceding knowledge data and real-world implementation of the solution on the patients and real people. The solutions are just limited to datasets and computer-aided systems performing statistical calculations for huge image datasets or sample databases. The prediction approach determines the accuracy and performance of the system; therefore, it has a crucial role. However, the practical implementation of the system on real patients is essential. Most of the authors mostly used raw facial image data from public databases.

The prediction techniques component of the proposed system gives emphasis on the deep learning approach that can be achieved through classified data to gain the predicted output through deep learning methodologies. The classification model classifies the features extracted from raw imaging data then the classified data is decoded through prediction techniques or algorithms to gain accurate output. Numerous layers of classification and prediction modeling along with statistical formulation are carried out for down sampling to achieve maximum values in each process. Primarily, the prediction technique in our presented system uses a classification approach that classifies the raw imaging data and encodes the actual classified data which is then decoded and categorized by the prediction algorithm to estimate the actual age of humans which will help us in the prevention, treatment and extend life expectancy. The Regression model and GBR are used to predict and estimate the age of humans after using the classified data as input into the model. Similarly, Ranking Model is another widely proposed prediction algorithm used with increased performance.

The view component of the system is a mixture of the display, interaction tools, and perception locations involved the d in the prediction process which estimates the human age accurately. The majority of the research papers fail to provide the interaction tools; however, they use the perception and display technology. All three components were discussed in very few papers. The prediction algorithm takes place on the computer screen itself, so the display unit discussed are monitor, digital screen, and other usual devices. The perception location is subdivided into the different forms of perception i.e. image database, sample datasets, or training and testing datasets. Moreover, the tools are classified into hardware and software tools, where the software could be system software, application software, or programming tools. Similarly, the statistical tools and computer components are listed under the hardware section. Therefore, special consideration should be taken when displaying the output to the end user. In our prediction model, we have found very little information on interaction tools. As interaction tool plays a vital role in prediction and lack of this component may negatively affect the system's performance and fail to perform age prediction. Therefore, we have to construct these factors with significant consideration and further examine them for the efficient prediction of human age.

5 Conclusion

There is an increasing deployment of deep learning algorithms for human age prediction. However, there is a lack of real-world practical applications that could be used for practical, and commercial purposes. DCPV predictions include various components of a deep learning model for human age prediction. It emphasizes the worth of deep learning practices rather than existing machine learning methods based on performance, accuracy, and efficiency in the prediction approach for the estimation of human age. The study introduces a review of the prediction approach based on deep learning to estimate the human age. Also, it emphasizes the worth of deep learning practices rather than existing machine learning methods based on performance, accuracy, and efficiency in the prediction approach for the estimation of human age.

References

1. Zaghbani, S., Boujneh, N., Bouhlel, M.S.: Age estimation using deep learning. Comput. Electric. Eng. (2018)
2. Tan, Z., Wan, J., Lei, Z., Zhi, R., Guo, G., Li, S.Z.: Efficient group-n encoding and decoding for facial age estimation. IEEE Trans. Pattern Anal. Mach. Intell. (2017)
3. Rathor, S., Ali, D., Gupta, S., Singh, R., Jaiswal, H.: Age prediction model using convolutional neural network. In: 2022 IEEE 11th International Conference on Communication Systems and Network Technologies (CSNT) (2022)
4. Chen, S., Zhang, C., Dong, M.: Deep age estimation: from classification to ranking. IEEE Trans. Multimedia (2017)
5. Xu, Y., Li, X., Yang, Y., Li, C., Shao, X.: Human age prediction based on DNA methylation of non-blood tissues. Comput. Methods Programs Biomed. (2019)
6. Li, X., Li, W., Xu, Y.: Human age prediction based on DNA methylation using a gradient boosting regressor. Genes (2018)
7. Becker, J., Mahlke, N.S., Reckert, A., Eickhoff, S.B., Ritz-Timme, S.: Age estimation based on different molecular clocks in several tissues and a multivariate approach: an explorative study. Int. J. Legal Med. (2020)
8. Zhu, Z., Chen, H., Hu, Y., Li, J.: Age estimation algorithm of facial images based on multi-label sorting. EURASIP J. Image Video Process. **2018**(1), 1 (2018). https://doi.org/10.1186/s13640-018-0353-z
9. Xing, J., Li, K., Hu, W., Yuan, C., Ling, H.: Diagnosing deep learning models for high accuracy age estimation from a single image. Pattern Recogn. (2017)
10. Qawaqneh, Z., Mallouh, A.A., Barkana, B.D.: Deep neural network framework and transformed MFCCs for speaker's age and gender classification. Knowl.-Based Syst. (2017)
11. Duan, M., Li, K., Ouyang, A., Win, K.N., Li, K., Tian, Q.: EGroupNet: a feature-enhanced network for age estimation with novel age group schemes. ACM Trans. Multimedia Comput. Commun. Appl. (TOMM) (2020)
12. Liao, H., Yan, Y., Dai, W., Fan, P.: Age estimation of face images based on CNN and divide-and-rule strategy. Math. Probl. Eng. (2018)
13. Aderinola, T.B., Connie, T., Ong, T.S., Teoh, A.B., Goh, M.K.: Gait-based age group classification with adaptive graph neural network. arXiv preprint arXiv:2210.00294 (2022)
14. Sajedi, H., Pardakhti, N.: Age prediction based on brain MRI image: a survey. J. Med. Syst. (2019)
15. Fang, J., Yuan, Y., Lu, X., Feng, Y.: Muti-stage learning for gender and age prediction. Neurocomputing (2019)
16. Zhang, H., Geng, X., Zhang, Y., Cheng, F.: Recurrent age estimation. Pattern Recogn. Lett. (2019)
17. Dong, Y., Liu, Y., Lian, S.: Automatic age estimation based on deep learning algorithm. Neurocomputing (2016)
18. Chen, Y., He, S., Tan, Z., Han, C., Han, G., Qin, J.: Age estimation via attribute-region association. Neurocomputing (2019)

19. Rothe, R., Timofte, R., Van Gool, L.: Deep expectation of real and apparent age from a single image without facial landmarks. Int. J. Comput. Vision (2018)
20. Liu, H., Lu, J., Feng, J., Zhou, J.: Group-aware deep feature learning for facial age estimation. Pattern Recogn. (2017)
21. Tian, Q., Chen, S.: Joint gender classification and age estimation by nearly orthogonalizing their semantic spaces. Image Vision Comput. (2018)
22. Ouafi, A., Zitouni, A., Ruichek, Y., Taleb-Ahmed, A.: Two-stages based facial demographic attributes combination for age estimation. J. Vis. Commun. Image Represent. (2019)

Augmenting Character Designers' Creativity Using Generative Adversarial Networks

Mohammad Lataifeh(✉), Xavier Carrasco, Ashraf Elnagar, and Naveed Ahmed

Department of Computer Science, University of Sharjah, Sharjah, United Arab Emirates
{mlataifeh,ashraf,nahmed}@sharjah.ac.ae

Abstract. Recent advances in Generative Adversarial Networks (GANs) continue to attract the attention of researchers in different fields due to the wide range of applications devised to take advantage of their key features. Most recent GANs are focused on realism; however, generating hyper-realistic output is not a priority for some domains, as in the case of this work. The generated outcomes are used here as cognitive components to augment character designers' creativity while conceptualizing new characters for different multimedia projects. To select the best-suited GANs for such a creative context, we first present a comparison between different GAN architectures and their performance when trained from scratch on a new visual character's dataset using a single Graphics Processing Unit (GPU). We also explore alternative techniques, such as transfer learning and data augmentation, to overcome computational resource limitations, a challenge faced by many researchers in the domain. Additionally, mixed methods are used to evaluate the cognitive value of the generated visuals on character designers' agency conceptualizing new characters. The results discussed proved highly effective for this context, as demonstrated by early adaptations to the characters' design process. As an extension for this work, the presented approach will be further evaluated as a novel co-design process between humans and machines to investigate where and how the generated concepts are interacting with and influencing the design process outcome.

Keywords: Generative Adversarial Networks · Creative Design Process · Character Generations · Cognitive Scaffolding · Human Machine Co-creation

1 Introduction

The introduction of the first GAN [1] caught the attention of many researchers due to the novel algorithmic approach it introduced. The model includes two networks competing adversely to generate new images indistinguishable from the original dataset. However, there has been no consensus on clear measures to evaluate the quality of GANs output [2], researchers often rely on Fréchet Inception Distance (FID) score [3] as an objective metric used to assess the quality of the generated images compared to ground truth. The FID score calculates the distance between two multivariate Gaussian distributions, one representing the original data, and the other for the generated output. Hence, the

K. Daimi and A. Al Sadoon (Eds.): ICR 2023, LNNS 721, pp. 80–92, 2023.
https://doi.org/10.1007/978-3-031-35308-6_7

lower the FID score, the higher the similarities between the original and output samples. Nonetheless, the development of new and more complex architectures required new datasets as existing ones maintained low image resolutions between (32 × 32) [4] and (256 × 256) [5, 6]. Such a need motivated the creation of CelebA-HQ [7] and the Flickr-Faces-HQ (FFHQ) [8]. Consequently, more complex architectures to deal with high-resolution images also implied the demand for higher computational resources dedicated to performing the training process. Networks such as StyleGAN2-ada require 8 GPUs working in parallel for days to get the results shared in the work [9]. Despite being plausible to obtain good results with a single GPU, the consumed time and output results are far from state-of-the-art, such limitation was addressed by using a technique called transfer learning [10] and [11], which has proven to be effective when working with limited computational resources, reducing the training time and the number of features to learn. Transfer learning is effectively used if sufficient details are made available about the previous network. Such information is shared as snap-shots or ".pkl" files or pickles that contain weights and features of networks often trained for a considerable time over large numbers of parallel GPUs, such as the case of StyleGAN2, which offers the possibility to use their pre-trained snaps for the FFHQ dataset by as a transitional starting point for the training process on a different dataset. Transfer learning will be used in this work to compare the performance and results of pre-trained pickle and newly trained models from scratch. The remainder of the paper is organized as follows: research objectives and contributions are listed in Sect. 2. Related work is presented in Sect. 3. Section 4 describes the datasets and models used. Followed by the details of the experiments and results in Sect. 5, and we conclude in Sect. 6.

2 Research Objectives

Reaching lower FID scores has been one of the primary goals when developing a new GAN since it implies closer similarities, details, and fidelity of the output compared to the original dataset. However, the nature of GANs enabled further adaptation due to their ability to create something new based on a random procedure, extending their applications to different fields where novelty and creativity are sought. Indeed, innovating a new design concept for a character is much more than being novel. It must also fit a specific narrative or context. Therefore, despite the gallant strides of success in a wide range of implementations, creating a realistic result of lifelike visual scenes and characters does not work for this creative domain. Most recent advances in other generative models such as Stable Diffusion models [12] and Semantic Image Synthesis with Spatially Adaptive Normalization [13] are deployed with open platforms such as Midjourny [2] which is raising concerns on the responsible and ethical use of these models, as thousands of designers contested the use of their creations on ArtStation [14] as training materials [15, 16] for Midjourney diffusion models. In reality, the astonishing outputs of these models are nothing but computed syntheses of human creative work. Hence, while we acknowledge the value of computational intelligence, we see this work as a proof of concept to set things in perspective on how these models can serve such a creative domain by providing cognitive aid for a human-led process. In light of the continuous creative demand for various multimedia projects, even the most talented designers may reach a high level of exhaustion in their creative production and exhibit some limitations in their work, falling within analogical or stylistic similarities of the previously presented concepts. Designers, therefore, employ different strategies to step into fresh grounds that can inform their creative process while creating novel outputs. As such, the generated visuals in this work are proposed as a non-verbal depiction of a design brief, which is a starting point for designers to synthesize, formulate, evaluate, reflect, and create novel concepts far from being a rehash of old concepts. Furthermore, designers' perception stimulated by a visual proposition has been proven sharper compared to mental images composed from remembered representations of features, objects, structures, and semantics [17, 18]. Most of the common datasets mentioned earlier contained 30k and more images, which means a larger variety and features for the network to learn. But to provide a relevant dataset for this work, we constructed a new visual dataset to evaluate the performance of the models working with a smaller collection of images using a single GPU, this hardware limitation is not present in other works so the results obtained cannot be comparable. Our contributions can be summarized as follows: Exploring the performance of different GAN architectures when trained on a context-focused dataset for characters. Reviewing correlations between the FID scores and human-observed perceptual quality of the generated images. Evaluating the performance of the models when trained on limited GPU resources compared to leveraged transfer learning. Paving the way toward a novel co-design process between humans and machines.

3 Related Work

Since its inception, the Vanilla GAN proposed in 2014 by Goodfellow [1] caught the interest of many researchers for the new algorithmic directions offered. Most of the initial improvements were related to the techniques and type of networks used in training, notably integrating the Convolutional Neural Networks [19] referred to as Deep Convolutional GAN (DCGAN); despite its distinguished output, DCGANs had three main limitations: impossibility to deal with high-resolution images, mode collapse [20] and somewhat reliance on conditioned output instead of a completely random image. Addressing the main issue of mode collapse, works like Wasserstein GAN (WGAN) [21], WGAN with Gradient Penalty (WGAN-GP) [22] or SparseGAN [23] proposed changes in the loss function and the training process, providing an effective way to avoid mode collapse, despite increasing the training time; further details on GANs and their different versions can be seen in [24, 25]. Fundamentally, the use of common datasets allowed researchers to benchmark the performance of new GANs. Early attempts were occupied with improving FID scores for the models trained on the previously noted low-resolution datasets [4–6]. The first successful attempt working with an image resolution of 512×512 was BIGGAN and BIGGAN-deep [26] trained on ImageNET and JFT-300M [27] datasets with significant improvements addressing mode collapse, and the ability to work with different resolutions, albeit being computationally demanding the use of at least 4 parallel GPUs. Furthermore, the introduction of the CelebA-HQ dataset in the Progressive Growing of GANs paper [28] and further implementation of this technique in StyleGAN [29] became the turning point, providing a new method to deal with high-resolution images in GANs. Additional modifications of this process were presented subsequently in StyleGAN2 [30] and StyelGAN2-ada [9]. While StyleGAN and StyleGAN2 were mainly focused on the quality of the results, there were a few datasets large enough to provide good results, the solution to this shortage came with the last model released, StyleGAN2-ada, which provides a data augmentation pipeline to avoid the discriminator over-fitting when working with little data [9], even resulting into a lower FID score, to solve the limitation caused by the number of images on which the network was trained, some techniques can be applied such as image embedding [31] to expand the latent space.

4 Datasets and Models

GANs create a latent space that can be freely explored after training to create a new variety of images different from the original data, allowing for flexibility and randomness in the output. To take advantage of both randomness and fidelity, we propose two consecutive pipelines shown in Fig. 1 and Fig. 2, while the first is targeting a basic silhouette output to jump-start the design process, the second one is employed to generate colored and textured alternatives for the silhouette, setting broader directions for designers on possible outcomes.

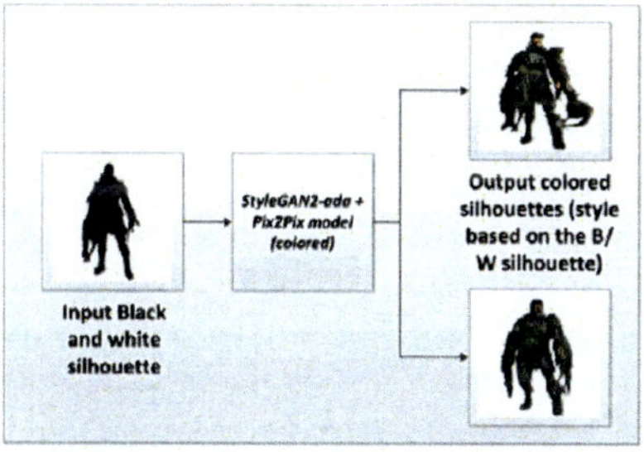

Fig. 1. Randomly generated character by a noise vector.

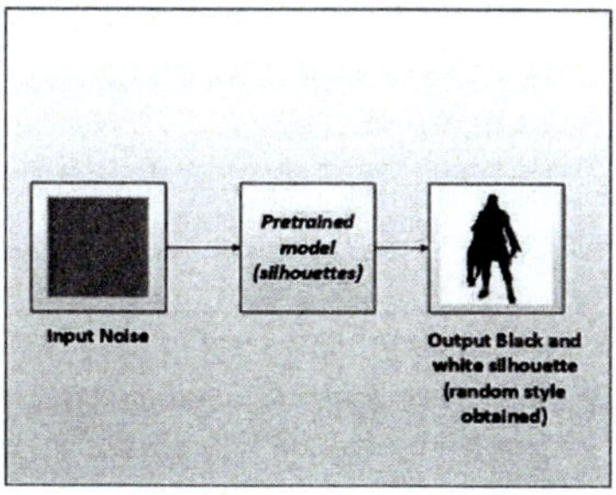

Fig. 2. Colored generated character based on a silhouette.

As a human-centered approach, we allow designers to evaluate the perceptual value of the generated silhouettes before proceeding to generate colored variations, this approach will be further extended in future work to a wider group of designers using a web application that allows interactions with the generative model.

A. The Datasets

To optimize the outcomes of the selected GANs for the creative context here, a new dataset was developed and deployed for this work [32]. This was deemed necessary as the results presented in previous GANs were limited to common datasets such as CIFAR10, MNIST, LSUN, or ImageNET. While offering wide varieties, common datasets do not share enough features with our dataset in terms of context, resolution, and style. The dataset used here included two main categories. The first one is **Character silhouettes** required to train the models for the first stage in the proposed pipeline (Fig. 1), allowing the generation of silhouettes from random noise. The output of this stage is carried as an input for the second stage (Fig. 2), during which GANs models were trained using the second category of the dataset called **Characters colored**, to generate colored/textured versions of the black/white silhouettes. Further details on the two sup-sets are provided next.

Characters Silhouettes

Shape and Resolution: Squared images, resolution of 512 × 512. The original resolution of the images was no lower than 128 × 128 and they were up-sampled using a bicubic filter. *The number of images and labeling:* The set consists of 10k images, and they are split into 3 different classes called: man, monster, and Woman. Some of the evaluated GANs required a unified class, hence, the images were merged into a single class.

Characters Colored

Shape and resolution: Squared images, resolution of 512 × 512. All images in this dataset were initially of a resolution of 512 × 512 or higher, they were downsampled when necessary. *The number of images and labeling:* The set consists of 8.7k colored images and their respective silhouette version in black and white. Similar classes were used as per the first dataset.

B. The Evaluated Models

As introduced at the beginning of this work, the proposed pipeline included two consecutive stages. The first one generates silhouettes from random noise (as shown in Fig. 1). Since this task is not as demanding as generating colored images, we explore the performance of different models trained on Characters' silhouettes. The models we tested for this first stage are: Deep Convolutional GAN (DCGAN) [19], Wasserstein GAN (WGAN) [21], WGAN with Gradient Penalty (WGAN-GP) [22], Large Scale GAN (BigGAN-deep) [26], StyleGAN2 with Adaptive Discriminator Augmentation (StyleGAN2-ada) [9]. Early GANs (DCGAN, WGAN, and WGAN-GP) share a general architecture for the generator and the discriminator, which is shown in Table 1. Other parameters and information related to optimizers, initializers, and the number of epochs are further detailed below. The size of the original images was also reduced to 64 × 64 to improve the performance of the models, since most of them are not suitable for images with higher resolutions; no other transformations were applied.

Some important parameters modified for the models are listed below:

- DCGAN (normal and conditional): *Optimizer*: Adam ($\alpha = 0.0002$, $\beta_1 = 0.5$, $\beta_2 = 0.999$), *Loss function:* Binary Cross Entropy, Leaky ReLU slopes: 0.02, *Batch size*: 64, *Epochs*: 100, *Weight/Bias initialization type*: Uniform.
- WGAN (normal and conditional): *Optimizer:* RMSprop ($\alpha = 0.00005$), $c = 0.01$, $n_{critic} = 5$, *Leaky ReLU slopes:* 0.02,
- Batch size: 64, Epochs: 100, Weight/Bias initialization type: Uniform.
- WGAN-GP (normal and conditional): Optimizer: Adam ($\alpha = 0.0002$, $\beta_1 = 0$, $\beta_2 = 0.9$), $\lambda = 10$, $n_{critic} = 5$, Leaky ReLU slopes: 0.02, Batch size: 64, Epochs: 100, Weight/Bias initialization type: Uniform.
- BIGGAN-deep: Optimizer: Adam ($\alpha = 0.0002$, $\beta_1 = 0.5$, $\beta_2 = 0.999$), Batch size: 16, Epochs: 70, Weight/Bias initialization type: Orthogonal.

Table 1. Model for non-conditional generators and discriminators (DCGAN, WGAN, WGAN-GP).

Operation	Kernel	Strides/Padding	Feature Maps	Batch Norm	Non-linearity
Generator Input: $G(z) - 100 \times 1 \times 1$, $\boldsymbol{z}$**:** Input noise					
T. Convolution	4 × 4	1/0	64 × 8	Yes	ReLU
T. Convolution	4 × 4	2/1	64 × 4	Yes	ReLU
T. Convolution	4 × 4	2/1	64 × 2	Yes	ReLU
T. Convolution	4 × 4	2/1	64	Yes	ReLU
T. Convolution	4 × 4	2/1	3	No	Tanh
Discriminator Input: $D(x) - 64 \times 64 \times 3$, $\boldsymbol{x}$**:** Real or fake image					
Convolution	4 × 4	2/1	64	No	LeakyReLU
Convolution	4 × 4	2/1	64 × 2	Yes	LeakyReLU
Convolution	4 × 4	2/1	64 × 4	Yes	LeakyReLU
Convolution	4 × 4	2/1	64 × 8	Yes	LeakyReLU
Convolution	4 × 4	2/1	1	No	Sigmoid

For the second stage of the proposed pipeline (Fig. 2), we combined the functionalities of Pix2Pix [33] and StyleGAN2-ada [9] to color the silhouettes obtained from the previous step as well as enhance the details of the image. Both models were trained using the **Characters colored** set that was built using pairs of images of silhouettes and their respective colored versions with an original resolution of (512 × 512). StyleGAN2-ada was trained on the colored images only, while Pix2Pix used the colored and silhouette pairs of the set. Due to copyright limitations, we cannot share the colored images set used initially for this work. We alternatively shared a collection of 6k pairs of colored images and their respective silhouettes. The pairs were generated by using the process described here.

5 Experiments and Results

The main objective of this section is to present an overview of the general performance of the models introduced in the previous section. To measure the performance of these models, we calculated the FID score, followed by a human expert review for the general perceptual quality of the outcome. GANs are difficult to train due to stability issues and hardware requirements. While commonly used platforms such as Google Colab offer a wide variety of GPUs for free, these are usually randomly assigned and we could not control such allocation, so we opt for our own single GPU machines. The details of both configurations are shown below.

- CPU: Intel(R) Xeon(R) @ 2.20GHz,
- GPU: K80 or T4 or P100,
- RAM: 12 GB.

  The specs of the machines used for StyleGAN-ada are:
- CPU: Intel(R) Core (TM) i7-10700K @ 3.80 GHz,
- GPU: RTX 3080Ti,
- RAM: 32 GB.

CPU: Intel(R) Xeon(R) Gold 5120T CPU @ 2.20 GHz, GPU: Quadro GV100 (32 GB), RAM: 128 GB (only 32 GB required for FID)

The software used differed according to the model. StyleGAN2-ada used Tensorflow while the others were Pytorch implementations. The requirements for DCGAN, WGAN, WGAN-GP, and BIGGAN-deep are Pytorch 1.7.1, Torchvision 0.8.2, and CUDA 11.1.

The software packages used for StyleGAN2-ada: Tensorflow 1.14, CUDA 10.0, cuDNN 7.5, Visual Studio 2015, and the VC Tools library are also required for StyleGAN2-ada. The results for DCGAN (Fig. 3), WGAN (Fig. 4), and WGAN-GP (Fig. 5) are shown below.

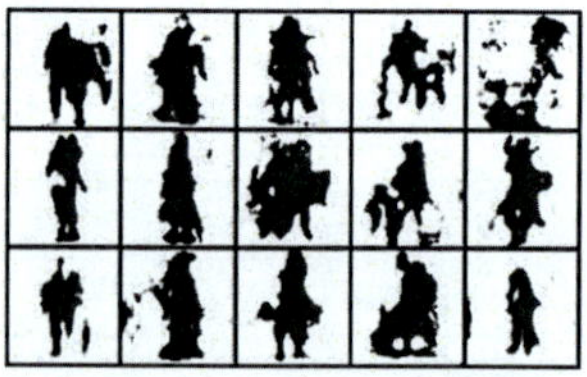

Fig. 3. Randomly generated character by a noise vector using DCGAN.

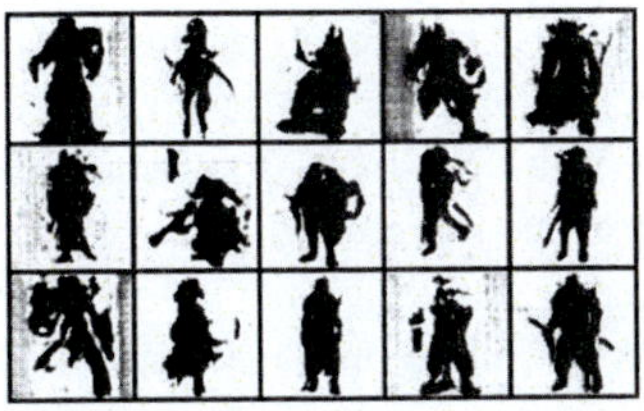

Fig. 4. Randomly generated character by a noise vector using WGAN.

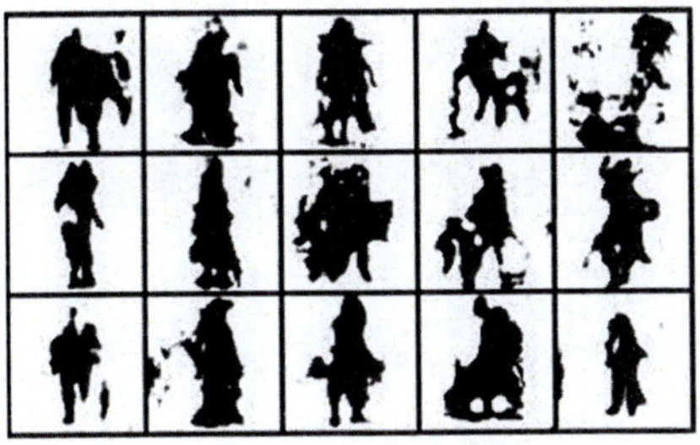

Fig. 5. Randomly generated character by a noise vector using WGAN-GP.

The results of the first models were obtained after a couple of hours of training, which is not comparable to the extended time required by BIGGAN-deep and StyleGAN2-ada whose generated images can be seen below in Figs. 5, 6, 7, 8 and 9.

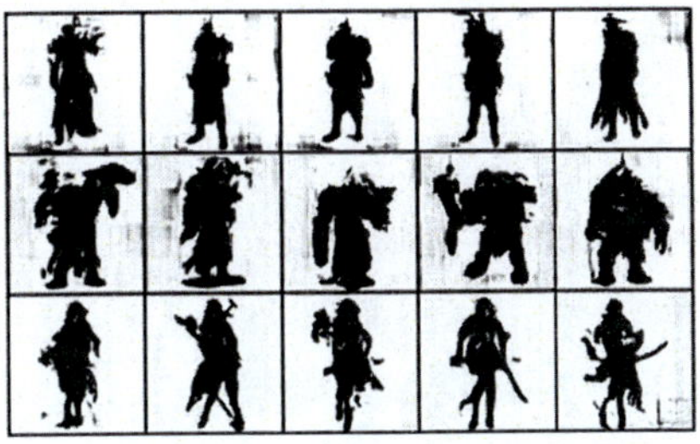

Fig. 6. Conditional results for BIGGAN-deep.

The generated samples for StyleGAN2-ada are split into three cases, one is for the model trained from scratch as shown in Fig. 7, while Fig. 8 and Fig. 9 demonstrate the obtained results while using transfer learning from the tenth snap offered by NVIDIA for the FFHQ dataset. Since BIGGAN-deep was developed as a conditional architecture, we kept this feature to evaluate the results that improved significantly when compared to the previous models. Despite the shallow details, the three classes (Men, Monster, and Women) are visually distinct, with an output resolution of 128×128 pixels. On the other hand, StyleGAN2-ada results came below expectations when trained from scratch. The classes are barely distinguishable with apparent feature similarities between the generated outcomes. Hence, the use of transfer learning was crucial to reduce processing time and improving outcome results. For the case of the exhibited outcome in Fig. 8, we directly used snap 10 from the pre-trained networks for FFHQ dataset. As for the results shown in Fig. 9, we apply different modifications to the model, such as truncation (trunc = 0.75) as well as all the available augmentation techniques (–augpipe = bgcfnc), eventually, the improvements are subtle but of considerable visual value.

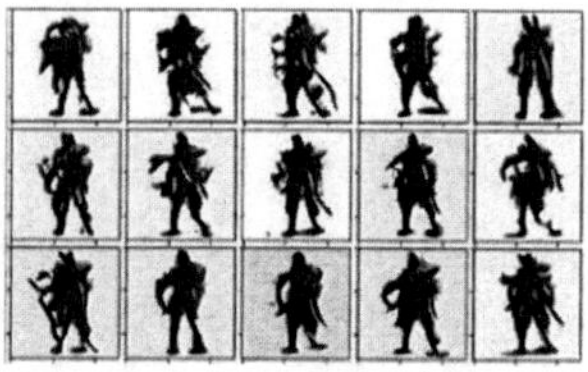

Fig. 7. Generated images obtained with StyleGAN2-ada trained from scratch

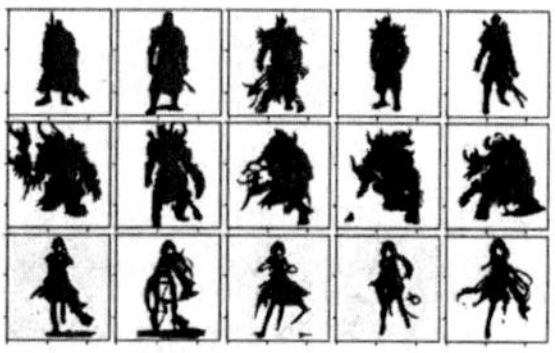

Fig. 8. Generated images obtained with pre-trained StyleGAN2-ad.

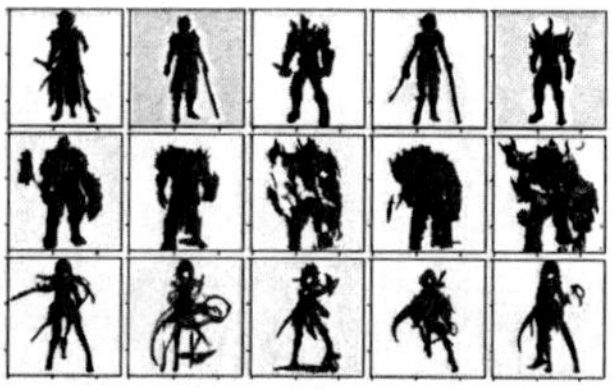

Fig. 9. Generated images obtained with a modified pre-trained StyleGAN2-ad.

Finally, we present the FID score for all the explored models with our dataset. The score was calculated based on 50K generated images per model. In the case of BIGGAN-deep, 16.6K images per class were generated and merged to reach 50K. The code used to calculate the FID score is a Pytorch implementation, and the obtained results are listed in Table 2.

A. Designers Produced Samples

We invited character designers to review the perceptual value of the generated concepts as experts in this domain. The participating designers came with different levels of

Table 2. FID scores for the models.

GAN type	FID score
DCGAN	176.92
WGAN	71.25
WGAN-GP	112.59
BIGGAN-deep	47.58
StyleGAN2-ada (Fig. 7)	105.69
StyleGAN2-ada (Fig. 8)	17.60
StyleGAN2-ada (Fig. 9)	17.53

expertise, from Novice to Expert [34]. Their qualitative review of the generated concepts was critical to evaluate the value indicated by FID scores, as it also helped fine-tune the models toward the desired balance between vagueness and fidelity. The boundaries of a scope expressed in a design brief influence the perceived permissible actions, which, in this case, are depicted as a visually suggestive cognitive stimulus to entice, intrigue, and inspire.

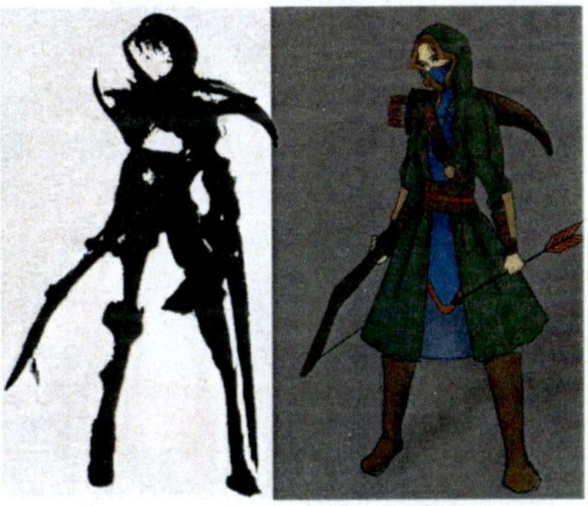

Fig. 10. Sample 1. Designed concept based on GANs-generated silhouettes.

A pool of selected silhouettes was made available for participants to be further developed into new concepts. The samples in Fig. 10 and Fig. 11 demonstrate some of the created work based on the proposed approach. Participants were asked to record their design process digitally, along with spoken narrative [35] to externalize their mental processes. The initial analysis of the collected data affirms the validity of the approach in assisting designers in creating new character concepts inspired by initial silhouettes, but novel in form, structure, and style.

Character designers described different ways of employing the generated silhouettes, from a visual design brief to metaphorical representation, inciting new directions [36]. Designers demonstrated a complex dialectical interactions [18] with the provided visuals with a verbal consensus on the uniqueness of the approach. Further analysis in future

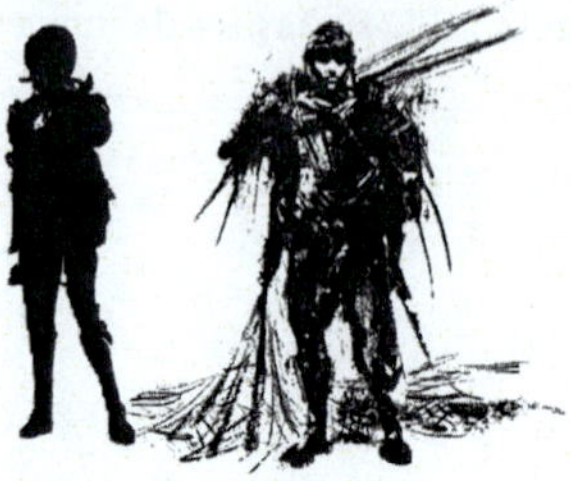

Fig. 11. Sample 2. Designed concept based on GANs-generated silhouettes.

work is necessary to clarify how and where in the design process these visual cognitive elements are of the most influence, and whether such interactions will be similar for designers with different levels of expertise.

6 Conclusion

The advancement of GANs witnessed over the last few years has extended their value and integration to a wide range of domains and purposes. Adapting GANs output into the creative domain, this work presented the implementations of different GANs to evaluate and compare their performance when deployed with limited computational resources on a new dataset created to address the contextual need of the domain. We also explored the use of transfer learning to accelerate and ameliorate the generation process. The early GAN models, such as DCGAN, WGAN, and WGAN-GP did not perform well considering the characteristics of the dataset and the random assignments in Google Colab GPU resources. BIGGAN-deep offered much-improved results under the same conditions. Nevertheless, the best results were obtained using StyleGAN2-ada with transfer learning, as indicated by FID scores and human expert evaluation. While recent generative models can produce highly realistic concepts of characters, as noted for diffusion models, such output is being challenged ethically and legally as being re-syntheses of human-designed concepts. Recently, the generated concepts are denied copyright [37] claimed by their "*Engineering*" authors. Hence, we believe a co-creative design process using machine intelligence to augment human creativity sets the path to move forward. Furthermore, we observe a positive correlation between FID scores obtained for each model with human expert evaluation, both of which are used here to ensure the developed concept will act upon their anchored value as visual cognitive elements to influence the design process. Additionally, the early work created by character designers integrating the proposed approach into their design process affirms the anticipated value of the proposed. Hence, this work not only sets a new direction for GANs applications into a unique creative domain and context, but the deployment of which is defining a novel co-design process between humans and machines. An extension of this work will further investigate the how and where of such cognitive interactions.

References

1. Goodfellow, I., et al.: Generative adversarial nets, **27**, 2672–2680 (2014)

2. Borji, A.: Generated faces in the wild: quantitative comparison of stable diffusion, midjourney and dall-e 2, arXiv preprint arXiv:2210.00586 (2022)
3. Heusel, M., Ramsauer, H., Unterthiner, T., Nessler, B., Hochreiter, S.: GANs trained by a two time-scale update rule converge to a local nash equilibrium. In: Guyon, I., et al. (eds.) Advances in Neural Information Processing Systems, vol. 30. Curran Associates, Inc. (2017)
4. Krizhevsky, A., Nair, V., Hinton, G.: Cifar-10 (Canadian Institute for Advanced Research). http://www.cs.toronto.edu/kriz/cifar.html
5. Deng, J., Dong, W., Socher, R., Li, L.-J., Li, K., Fei-Fei, L.: Imagenet: a large-scale hierarchical image database. In: 2009 IEEE Conference on Computer Vision and Pattern Recognition, pp. 248–255. IEEE (2009)
6. Yu, F., Zhang, Y., Song, S., Seff, A., Xiao, J.: LSUN: construction of a large-scale image dataset using deep learning with humans in the loop. CoRR, abs/1506.03365 (2015). http://arxiv.org/abs/1506.03365
7. Karras, T., Aila, T., Laine, S., Lehtinen, J.: Progressive growing of GANs for improved quality, stability, and variation (2018)
8. Tero Karras, T.A., Laine, S.: Flickr-faces-HQ dataset (FFHQ) (2018). https://github.com/nvlabs/ffhq-dataset
9. Karras, T., Aittala, M., Hellsten, J., Laine, S., Lehtinen, J., Aila, T.: Training generative adversarial networks with limited data. In: Larochelle, H., Ranzato, M., Hadsell, R., Balcan, M.F., Lin, H. (eds.) Advances in Neural Information Processing Systems, vol. 33, pp. 12:104–12:114. Curran Associates, Inc.(2020)
10. Tan, C., Sun, F., Kong, T., Zhang, W., Yang, C., Liu, C.: A survey on deep transfer learning. In: Kůrková, V., Manolopoulos, Y., Hammer, B., Iliadis, L., Maglogiannis, I. (eds.) ICANN 2018. LNCS, vol. 11141, pp. 270–279. Springer, Cham (2018). https://doi.org/10.1007/978-3-030-01424-7_27
11. Fregier, Y., Gouray, J.-B.: Mind2mind: transfer learning for GANs. In: Nielsen, F., Barbaresco, F. (eds.) Geometric Science of Information, pp. 851–859. Springer, Cham (2021)
12. Rombach, R., Blattmann, A., Lorenz, D., Esser, P., Ommer, B.: High-resolution image synthesis with latent diffusion models (2021)
13. Park, T., Liu, M.-Y., Wang, T.-C., Zhu, J.-Y.: Semantic image synthesis with spatially-adaptive normalization. In: 2019 IEEE/CVF Conference on Computer Vision and Pattern Recognition (CVPR). IEEE, June 2019. https://doi.org/10.1109/CVPR.2019.00244
14. Weatherbed, J.: Artstation is hiding images protesting ai art on the platform, December 2022
15. Baio, A.: Invasive diffusion: how one unwilling illustrator found herself turned into an ai model, November 2022
16. Growcoot, M.: Lawsuit filed against ai image generators stable diffusion and midjourney, January 2023
17. Fish, J., Scrivener, S.: Amplifying the mind's eye: sketching and visual cognition. Leonardo **23**, 117–126 (1990)
18. Goldschmidt, G.: The dialectics of sketching. Creat. Res. J. **4**, 123–143 (1991)
19. LeCun, Y., Bottou, L., Bengio, Y., Haffner, P.: Gradient-based learning applied to document recognition (1998)
20. Theis, L., van den Oord, A., Bethge, M.: A note on the evaluation of generative models, November 2015
21. Arjovsky, M., Chintala, S., Bottou, L.: Wasserstein generative adversarial networks. In: International Conference on Machine Learning, pp. 214–223. PMLR (2017)
22. Gulrajani, I., Ahmed, F., Arjovsky, M., Dumoulin, V., Courville, A.C.: Improved training of wasserstein GANs. In: Guyon, I., et al. (eds.) Advances in Neural Information Processing Systems, vol. 30. Curran Associates, Inc. (2017)

23. Mahdizadehaghdam, S., Panahi, A., Krim, H.: Sparse generative adversarial network. In: Proceedings - 2019 International Conference on Computer Vision Workshop, ICCVW 2019, pp. 3063–3071 (2019)
24. Hong, Y., Hwang, U., Yoo, J., Yoon, S.: How generative adversarial networks and their variants work: an overview, **52**(1), 1–43 (2019)
25. Creswell, A., White, T., Dumoulin, V., Arulkumaran, K., Sengupta, B., Bharath, A.A.: Generative adversarial networks: an overview, **35**(1), 53–65 (2018)
26. Brock, A., Donahue, J., Simonyan, K.: Large scale GAN training for high fidelity natural image synthesis. In: International Conference on Learning Representations (2019)
27. Hinton, G., Vinyals, O., Dean, J.: Distilling the knowledge in a neural network (2015). https://arxiv.org/abs/1503.02531
28. Karras, T., Aila, T., Laine, S., Lehtinen, J.: Progressive growing of GANs for improved quality, stability, and variation. abs/1710.10196 (2017)
29. Karras, T., Laine, S., Aila, T.: A style-based generator architecture for generative adversarial networks. In: 2019 IEEE/CVF Conference on Computer Vision and Pattern Recognition (CVPR), pp. 4396–4405 (2019)
30. Karras, T., Laine, S., Aittala, M., Hellsten, J., Lehtinen, J., Aila, T.: Analyzing and improving the image quality of stylegan. In: IEEE/CVF Conference on Computer Vision and Pattern Recognition (CVPR), pp. 8107–8116 (2020)
31. Abdal, R., Qin, Y., Wonka, P.: Image2StyleGAN: how to embed images into the StyleGAN latent space?, vol. Oct, pp. 4431–4440 (2019)
32. Lataifeh, M., Carrasco, X., Elnagar, A.: Diversified character dataset for creative applications (DCDCA) (2022)
33. Isola, P., Zhu, J.-Y., Zhou, T., Efros, A.A.: Image-to-image translation with conditional adversarial networks. In: Proceedings of the IEEE Conference on Computer Vision and Pattern Recognition, pp. 1125–1134 (2017)
34. Dreyfus, H.L., Dreyfus, S.E.: Peripheral vision: expertise in real world contexts. Organ. Stud. **26**(5), 779–792 (2005)
35. Payne, J.W.: Thinking aloud: insights into information processing, **5**(5), 241–248 (1994)
36. Sadowska, N., Laffy, D.: The design brief: inquiry into the starting point in a learning journey. Des. J. **20**, S1380–S1389 (2017)
37. Brittain, B.: AI-created images lose U.S. copyrights in test for new technology. Reuters (2023). https://www.reuters.com/legal/ai-created-images-lose-us-copyrights-test-new-technology. Accessed 22 Feb 2023

DCOP: Deep Learning for Road Safety System

Binod Hyoju[1], A. B. Emran Salahuddin[2](✉), Haneen Heyasat[3], Omar Hisham Rasheed Al-Sadoon[4], and Ahmed Dawoud[3]

[1] Study Group Australia, Darlinghurst, Australia
[2] Crown Institute of Higher Education, Sydney, Australia
emrans@gmail.com
[3] University of South Australia, Adelaide, Australia
haneen.heyasat@mymail.unisa.edu.au
[4] AlIraqia University, Bagdad, Iraq

Abstract. The essential component of the transportation system of the future is autonomous vehicles. Future automobiles from automotive manufacturers are being built with autonomous features. But a recent incident in Tempe, Arizona, in which an Uber driverless car killed a pedestrian, has cast severe doubt on the viability of autonomous vehicles in the near future. This paper discusses and analyses how deep learning model will make driverless cars work more intelligently in detecting objects, lanes, hazards, and preventing collisions. To improve road safety using deep learning for driverless cars, this study aims to identify and define the optimal methods in terms of accuracy and processing speed. Additionally, we have suggested a DCOP taxonomy (Data, Classifier, Object Detection, and Prediction). This taxonomy considers the categorisation of detection capabilities such as lane detection, collision detection, hazards detection, obstacles detection, and space detection by using 3D cameras and sensors that enhance the Convolution Neural Network to detect the objects in the images captured through the camera sensors to find the prediction of the steering angle for a driverless car to navigate accurately and safely. This paper introduces the DCOP taxonomy in which object detection and prediction systems can be discussed, analysed, validated, and evaluated. The driverless cars of the future transportation system can be made safer and more dependable with the aid of this DCOP taxonomy.

Keywords: Collision detection · Deep Learning · Driverless Car · Machine Learning · Neural Network · Object Detection

1 Introduction

A vehicle that is driven by a set of machine learning systems and algorithms is now possible thanks to recent technological advancements and the cleverness of computer-guided vision and applications; this type of vehicle is known as an autonomous vehicle. The development of self-driving smart machines and the internet of things is accelerating [1]. According to the research, human error is responsible for more than 90% of

K. Daimi and A. Al Sadoon (Eds.): ICR 2023, LNNS 721, pp. 93–104, 2023.
https://doi.org/10.1007/978-3-031-35308-6_8

car accidents, while just 2% are attributable to vehicle failure. This suggests that self-driving cars could provide a safer mode of transportation for people, potentially saving thousands of lives. Numerous studies have been done on the hardware and algorithms for self-driving automobiles to address various issues with putting unmanned vehicles on the road [16]. The difficulties lie in the ability of a driverless automobile to operate predictably through a variety of activities based on the application of steering, braking, and notifications, as well as the recognition of things including traffic, people, roads, lanes, obstructions, dangers, and the environment [23]. Deep learning is a group of different processing layers that enables computational prototypes to gain the illustration of data through several levels of abstraction. Many systems have been designed that use Deep Learning Technology to learn the machine and detect objects through image processing on the various models of Convolution Neural Networks (CNN), and few of the Vehicle Manufacturing companies have already implemented on their latest vehicle without being completely successful. This technology determines structure in significant informational collections by utilising the calculation on back propagation to refer how a machine would interact with its fundamental constraints through the depiction of preceding layer. The current models use Fast Convolution Neural Networks (FCNN), although a CNN called You Look Only Once (YOLO) has lately gained popularity because of its quick object identification abilities [30]. There is still a significant deficiency in object detection speed and accuracy for driverless cars. Hence, the main purpose of this study is to introduce DCOP taxonomy for deep learning that be used for driverless car in which the object detection can be conferred, examined, validated, and evaluated; and to assent the improved understanding of the most appropriate and significant components of the object detection system. The following sections of this paper are structured as follows: Sect. 2 discusses literature reviews of previous, cutting-edge publications. In Sect. 3, we introduce the major DCOP components as well as their sub-components and offer our innovative classification. Section 4 provides the classification, and evaluation of DCOP taxonomy, followed by the discussion of the components that were not well defined in selected articles in Sect. 5 and then we will address the issues and future path and guidance for the appropriate selection of algorithms and technology in terms of driverless vehicle object detection system through deep learning and conclude the paper in Sect. 6.

2 Literature Review

Deep learning technology, which uses supervised and unsupervised learning as its two sets of training methodologies, addresses these issues. To operate autonomous automobiles and guide them through urban environments, [9] suggested a model that makes use of the TensorFlow framework and Deep Learning Technique. Gallardo's work demonstrates how to apply the ideas of deep learning to the field of autonomous driving in everyday life. These approaches include CNN, supervised learning techniques, and the AlexNet framework. Similarly, [12] proposed a novel two staged architecture approach in which the first stage used a visual responsiveness model that trained the convolution network end-to-end from the captured input images to the steering angle as an output. The second stage used casual filtering that determined the influence of the output on the part of the input regions [11]. [19] investigated and proposed two methods that detect objects and guidance to the road in the real world driving by detecting the road lanes through polynomial regression. Using YOLO and a road lane detector, which could be found in the video frames that were taken, the self-driving automobile could use this information to make decisions in real time. Similar to this, [26] proposed a method for obstacle and object detection on roads for self-driving cars which was taken as an experimental platform. While on the experiment it showed that the autonomous car loses control when the accuracy rate was less than 90% for once. In context to the moving object detection, [25] approached by using datasets on CIFAR 10 through inputs being used as VGA images the accuracy enhancement using the Convolution Neural Network was figured. Similarly, [8] proposed a novel architecture using two methods Lenet and AlexNet to detect the object through Video Stream from the cameras utilizing ImageNet datasets into Support Vector Machine, the vehicle detection based on Cityscape was resulted to 0.39 precision and 0.58 in the recall. To locate and recognise signs such as road lanes, stop lines, and markings on the roadways, [12] suggested a novel approach of road and lane recognition using stereo cameras. By using CNN and Max Pooling Positions (MPP) as a discriminative feature to anticipate class labels, [21] proposed a traffic sign identification system. According to [4, 5], a Collision Prediction model based on GA-optimized Neural Network (CPGN) was suggested. This model was utilised to make decisions on rear-end collisions and the likelihood of accidents and coincidences in smart vehicles. To determine boundaries on the road that indicated the possibility for tasks using cameras, [3] developed Cognitive Map-Based Neural Network employing images from the camera as input, Road Vehicle Dataset (RVD), and Support Vector Machine (SVM). [22] proposed a different deep learning-based obstacle detection framework where a full convolution network is also used to forecast the labelling such as open space, unanticipated obstacles on road, and background. This is in relation to hazard detection on the roads and small object detection on the way to prevent unexpected accidents. The report had the advantage of increasing performance by 27.4 and the detection rate for areas up to 50 m by more than 90%. Furthermore, there is a need of fast handling of uninterrupted video data using implanted devices for which [29] proposed a disseminated embedded platform put up with NVIDIA Jetson TX1 using deep-learning techniques for real-time video processing primarily for object recognition. The model completes the same dispensation speed with much lower consumption of power. [7] proposed a method to detect the moving vehicle on the roads and the issues were addressed through using of Deep Neural Network (DDN) framework. Extensive testing was executed that produced promising results. The images are pre-processed into the CNN to find the computation part of the image where the object lies. In generating improved prediction precision there is a need to search for good context vector that is defined as the blend of convolution feature vectors.

3 DCOP Taxonomy for Object Detection in Driverless Cars

For the DCOP taxonomy to have successfully operated in the real-world context, the taxonomy should have the capabilities to detect the vital information of the road such as traffic signs, lanes, people, and other vehicles on the road, navigation map, objects, hazards etc. Several classifications have been suggested for the prediction and object classification and for prediction for the steering angle for navigating the driverless vehicle. The proposed DCOP taxonomy is based on four factors: Data, which includes capturing images, processing those images, and multimedia; Classifiers, which relate to pre-processing the input image through models; Object Detection, which defines algorithms to classify the objects present in the image to predict the class; and Prediction. The development of DCOP component classification and the object detection technique has been established based on previous and present deep learning navigation and object detection techniques for driverless cars. The proposed taxonomy is shown in Fig. 1. Through past findings and related articles, we have refined the proposed system into four different categories of components in our classification which befitted for most vital reasons for systems' expansion, validation, and development.

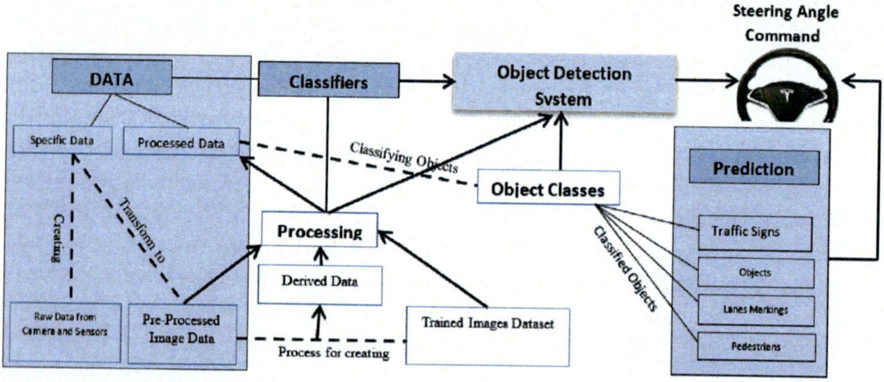

Fig. 1. The figure demonstrates four components of our DCOP classification (i.e., data, classifiers, object detection and prediction).

Data: Data undergo one or more convolution network for machine learning to become the processed image for object detection through the applied dataset. The main objective of images or videos is to classify and formulate the pixel in the images to predict the object by using datasets that are pre-trained in the deep network so that the images are matched pixel by pixel to predict and define the object in the image. The sensor data is useful to analyse the location information and make navigational decisions. The deep learning method will be used to extract the data from the camera and the sensors and identify the objects that lie on the periphery of the vehicle. The object specific data can be raw sensor data, LIDAR, RADAR, and camera data. Other types of data, such as signals from sensors and RADAR, are also taken into the count as inputs to calculate the vehicle's location, distance, and peripheral area during learning. These data are transformed into an analysed dataset to combine with the results of prior learning to form object classes during detection. Pre-processed trained data analysed datasets that are defined, and generated data can all be included in the processed data. The processed data comprises their qualities, dimensions, positions, and other characteristics that can also be referred to as previous knowledge data. The data that was analysed is picture data that underwent conversion to produce accurate data entities. Prior knowledge data, on the other hand, come from fundamental models that have previously been established and integrated. Maps, prior knowledge datasets, object detection datasets, supervised data, etc. are some examples of various sorts of data's features. **Classifier:** Various classifier models are being assessed to match the training dataset with the raw photos that were recorded using cameras and sensors to identify and categorise the items in the images. Decision tree classifiers, nave Bayes, and support vector machines are some of the top classifiers (SVM). The pre-processed images are fed into the CNN to locate the compute region of the image that contains the object. The issues associated with this classifier are the same as those associated with the DCOP data class, where the accuracy of identifying objects in photos is inversely correlated with the processing of the image data for clarity, visibility, and size. To train the convolution network for machine learning to provide an output of object detection, the goal is to select the best model algorithm to process the image as a feature extraction and produce with the result of the item categorised in the image. **Object Detection:** To deliver the post-processing of the photos, we use object detection as a component of our categorisation. The model must be able to recognise key elements of the road, such as traffic signs, lanes, people, and other vehicles on the road, as well as navigational markers, objects, and potential hazards, to function successfully in a real-world setting. The third key element of DCOP classification is object detection, which uses an algorithm to classify the things that are discovered throughout the sequencing process from the multimedia data that are used as input. Various tools and approaches are utilised for these procedures, including object detectors, classifiers, and extractors. To detect an object, various tools and algorithms are used, such as CNN, which was later replaced by R-CNN with better processing for object detection processes in the image by slicing the images that were divided into the pixels to identify the object in the image and formulate the output. The images are separated into grids of 13×13 cells, each of which is responsible for forecasting five bounding boxes and are then recognised using a completely different CNN approach called YOLO. The steering angle predictor and the object detector both share extraction layers. To produce the output for the operability of the autonomous car, they each process the photos separately. Making sure that the algorithm performs effectively in forwards object detection and backwards rear detection are the object detection challenges. **Prediction:** The system must result in a command to the steering to rotate as per the needs while the hazards on the roads are detected. The car should be able to apply the rotation of the steering or apply brakes to find safe free space to move or to avoid colliding. Safety on roads should be the priority on roads as roads are shared with others. Deep learning-based object tracking is the architecture which defines the mechanism that we could use to track the things objects around the driverless car. The purpose of prediction is termed to have improved prediction precision. For this, there is a need to search for good context vector that is defined as the blend of convolution feature vectors. For this, the architecture operates a deterministic soft responsiveness mechanism that can be trained by typical back-propagation approaches, from which it has benefits over an inflexible responsiveness appliance that necessitates reinforcement learning. The network is trained according to the detection of distortions that are above the ground level such as people, cars, buildings, objects etc. The traffic signs and lanes and the classes of detected objects are through pre-learned datasets such as traffic signs datasets, road maps, and object classes' datasets.

4 DCOP Taxonomy Classification and Evaluation

To endorse DCOP classification, this paper considered numbers of previous publications based on system component that defined and concentrated on deep learning technology for driverless vehicles specific to object detection and road safety systems on vehicles. [27] proposed a system that could detect objects on the vehicle's periphery by taking the image as raw data from the camera and processing it to form an RGB image that could be used as an input to the system. [2] used sensor raw data, HD images as an input and further pre-processed using entropies and extraction to make the image feasible for the system. However, [19] proposed a Lane Detection system where images and videos taken from the front camera were extracted and resized to match the score of the analyzed data within the pre-defined dataset. Similarly, [6] proposed an object detection method that used LIDAR bird eye view image that had go through preprocessing to form analyzed and derived image data which had a score to detect an object that was above the ground level and the classification was met. [12] used Support Vector Machine (SVM) as a classifier where the components take an input, relates a function to it and then permits the result to the following layer. The first basic process is the input to the system and after that, the feature is extracted to match and classify the object. Similarly, [6] use Shannon entropy with Bayesian Neural networks that undertake the existence of a precise feature in a class is distinct to the occurrence of any new feature. It is very simple to form and predominantly beneficial for huge datasets like the one related to the datasets of KITTI (Karlsruhe Institute of Technology and Toyota Technological Institute), TORCS (The Open Racing Car Simulator) and Udacity in the driverless Vehicle domain. The CNN are used to forecast the constraint of bounding box in terms of width, height, size etc. passes through multiple hidden layers to match the layers, pixel by pixel, in the image and calculation is done until the meaningful class is developed [23]. According to [24, 29], most articles have implemented their own set of algorithms whereas some used more than one. [1, 12] have written articles on analyzing images or videos to detect moving objects by certain sets of classifiers namely SVM and AlexNet to give the class of the object through sets of CNN and gives a mechanical actuator signal to rotate the steering into desired position. The prediction as an output has been described in only five of the selected papers whereas as other only worked on detection and classification of objects. While considering the most appropriate aspects of object detection and navigation.

The system's accuracy is provided by validation, and the evaluation is demonstrated by the system's output and usability. Some papers focused on the accuracy of the navigation system and object detection, while others focused on the speed processing of images to detect the system to reduce system loading time, and still others looked at speed and feasibility. [12] contrasted traffic sign detections in which the inputs were taken from cameras and compared to traffic sign datasets to detect the signs in the images that performed with the implementation of SVM. Similarly, [17] examined derived data that should be pre-processed and found an accuracy rate of 82%, which was higher than that of previous publications research. [22] concentrated on the part of the evaluation

Table 1. DCOP Classification of Object Detection in Driverless Car Publications

Publications		Data		Classifiers		Object Detection		Prediction	
SN	Authors and Dates	Raw (Images, Videos, Signals)	Processed (Derived, Pre-processed, Analyzed Data)	Attributes (Models)	Instances	Attributes (Algorithms)	Instances	Attribute (Object Type Prediction)	Instances
Ki	Kim, et al. (2018)	Video Clips. Images	Traffic Signs. Lane markings	Support Vector Machine (SVM)	Classification, resizing Images, feature extraction.	5 layered Convolution Neural Network (CNN)	Road Lane Detection, Sign Detection	Steering Angle	Navigation and casualty check
2	Li et al. (2017)	Video	Caltech Pedestrian Detection Benchmark	RPN+BF	Video Pre-processing, transforming to grey style images	MS-CNN	Object Detection	Object Detection	Classifying Object
3	Gallardo et al. (2016)	Image	Tensorflow	AlexNet	Analyzing images, resizing images	R-CNN	Obstacle Detection	Steering Angle	Navigation
4	Chen, et al. (2018)	Image	VISSIM	CGPN	Feature extraction, Cropping images	BP Neural Network	Vehicle and Object detection	Processing Speed	Navigation
5	Ramos et al. (2017)	Video	Lost and Found Data	GoogLeNet +UON	Classification, Feature extraction, pixel calculation	FCNN	Object Detection	Detection	Classifying Object
6	Ali et al. (2016)	VGA Image	PASCAL VOC + KITTI	AlexNet	Analyzing images, resizing images	R-CNN	Obstacle Detection	Steering Angle	Navigation
7	Atallah et al. (2018)	Sensor Data, HD Images and Speech	Lost and Found Data	GoogLeNet +UON	Classification, Feature extraction, pixel calculation	FCNN+ Deep Q Network	Hazard and Unidentified Obstacles Detection	Detection and Delay	Classifying Object
8	K, Li et al. (2022)	Image	KITTI + Cityscapes + Lost and Found data	CODA (Corner case dataset for autonomous driving)	Extraction and Classification	RCNN	Corner case Object Detection	Detection	Classifying Object
9	Shi et al, (2016)	Image	CIFAR-10 + Udacity	SSD + SVM + CGPN	Extraction and Classification	R-CNN + YOLO	Hazard Detection	Object Detection	Classifying Objects
10	Nugraha et al. (2017)	Image and Videos	Imagenet	SSD+ SVM	NS	YOLO+GoogLeNet	Pedestrian Detection	Moving Object Detection	Classifying Objects
11	(Zhang et al., 2018)	Video	KITTI and PASCAL VOC Datasets	Alexnet	Image Pre-processing and Extraction	Deep –CNN + Fast Neural Network	Speed Tracking and Accuracy	Moving Object Detection	Classifying Objects
12	Qian et al. (2016)	Image	GTSRB	SVM +TSR	Classification and Image resizing	D-CNN + MLP+MPP	Sign Detection	Traffic and Road Signs	Classifying Objects
13	Rausch et al. (2017)	Image	SGD + 3D Maps	SVM + MATLAB	Classify and feature extraction+ pre-processing	Deep CNN + YOLO	Lane Detection	Steering Angle	Prediction of Angle on Steering
14	Kim et al (2017)	Image	KITTI + VGA Image + CIFAR 10 + TORCS	SVM + ROI	Extraction+ Decomposition	RCNN + AlexNet	Object Detection	Road Detection	Classify Objects
15	Gupta, et al (2021)	LIDAR, RADAR, RGB camera data	Traffic Signs. Lane markings	SVM	Classify and feature extraction+ pre-processing	CNN+RNN+LSTM	Object Detection	Traffic and Road Signs	Object detection in bad weather condition
16	Sharma et. al (2022)	Image, video	Traffic lights, vehicle, and pedestrians.	SSD+SVM	Classify and feature extraction+ pre-processing	CNN+RNN+YOLOv5	Object Detection	Traffic Signal, Vehicle and pedestrian detection	Object detection in good and bad weather conditions

ANN: Artificial Neural Network
BF: Bayesian Filter
CNN: Convolution Neural Network
CMNN: Cognitive Map-based Neural Network
DDN: Deep Neural Network
DPM: Deep Pyramid Maps
FCNN: Fast Convolution Neural Network
LIDAR: Light Detection and Ranging
GSTRB: German Traffic Sign Rec Benchmark
MAP: Mean Average Precision
MI: Mutual Information
MPP: Max Pooling Position
MLP: Max Layer Perception
NS: Not Specified
RPN: Regional Proposal Network
R-CNN: Regional Convolution Neural Network
ROI: Region of Interest
RVD: Road Vehicle Dataset
SE: Shannon Entropy
SGD: Scholastic Gradient Descent
SHDP: Supervised Deep hashing framework
SVM: Support Vector Machine
SSD: Single Shot Multibox Detector
TSR: Traffic Sign Recognition
UON: Unexpected Obstacle Network
VOC: Visual Object Challenge
VGA: Video Graphics Array

Table 2. Validation and/or Evaluation of Object Detection and Prediction System in Driverless Cars

S N	Author and Dates	Field of study	Data Type	Component Validation and Evaluation	Criteria of Study	Validation Evaluation Methods and Datasets	Results
1	Kim, et al. 18)	Lane Detection and Casualty check	RGB Image Video Clips	Object Detection	Accuracy ate and Speed.	Traffic Signs, Road Lanes,Udacity, Comma.ai	The model could produce more accuracy in Comma.ai as Casual Blobs = 38% and whereas Surplus Blobs = 62% which showed that attention did not degrade control accuracy.
2	Li et al. 17)	Pedestrian Detection	Video	Moving Object ection	Accuracy ate	Caltech Pedestrian Detection Benchmark	The model had a result on 2 subfactors while detecting accuracy that came around 42% and Surplus Blobs = 58%
3	Gallardo et (2016)	Object Detection and Navigation Prediction	Image	Whole System	Steering ngle Prediction	Tensorflow	The steering angle prediction came after object detection while using Tensor Flow came to result in the following Occ Num = 7.68% Occ Partia = 24.3%
4	Chen, et (2018)	Traffic Signs Detection	Image	Object Detection	Accuracy	VISSIM	The system outputted the result based on VISSIM dataset while the value of object detection is as follows Precision: 83% Result: 82 %
5	Ramos et (2017)	Moving Object Detection	Video	Object Detection	Accuracy	Lost and Found Data	In accordance with the Lost and found data while moving object detection came resultant to the following Precision: 75% Result: 74%
6	Ali et al. 16)	Lane Detection	VGA Image	Pedestrian ection	Detection ate	PASCAL VOC + KITTI	While simulating on the PASCAL VOC the detection accuracy on lanes was 83% where are KITTI dataset produced 85% accuracy.
7	Atallah et (2018)	Hazard Detection	HD Video Images	Vehicle Detection Life Time	Accuracy, etection	Lost and Found Data	The model outperforms In completed request on complete request percentage (10-25%) And a lifetime of the network (55 – 65%)
8	K. Li et al, 22)	Corner case Object Detection	Image	Corner case object ection	Accuracy, ompleteness	KITTI, Lost and Found Data	Standard object detection drops no more than 12.8% on real world corner cases.
9	Shi et al, 16)	Hazard Detection	Image	Unexpected ard Object ection	Accuracy	CIFAR-10 + Udacity	The improvement in preceding time by the system is resulted time by 13% and conversion rate by 0.52.
10	Nugraha et (2017)	Pedestrian Detection	Image and eos	Moving Object ection	Detection ate	Imagenet	The system is accurate in highway region. The system seems to be confused in urban areas not distancing on sand and road.
11	Zhang et (2018)	Visual Tracking and Detection	Video	Moving Object ection	Speed acking and ccuracy	KITTI and PASCAL VOC	The model shows the improving result in a sequence of the image through the variation of data. The system shows the effective result in challenging image sequence by minimizing intra-class variation and maximizing inter-class variation
12	Qian et al. 16)	Traffic Signs Detection	Images from gle Camera	Sign and Lanes ection	Accuracy, onsistency	3D Maps + SGD	MPP demonstrated outstanding performance recognition rate = 96.95 %
13	Rausch et (2017)	Steering Angle	Images from era	Object and dmarks detection	Accuracy and ompleteness	Imagenet+ SGD + 3D Maps	Resulting in better Stability on end-to-end steering controls.
14	Kim et al. (2017)	Object Detection	Image	Object Detection	Accuracy eed and alidation	KITTI + TORCS+GTA5 + Citiscapes	While using Citiscaps the result showed Precision 0.30 and Recall= 0.58
15	Gupta, et (2021)	Object ection	LIDAR, DAR, RGB era data	Object Detection	Accuracy and mpleteness	CNN+RNN+LST	Resulting in better object detection bad weather condition such as fog,, adverse weather event, snow etc.
16	Sharma et 2022)	Object ection	Image and eo	Object Detection	Accuracy and sistency	CNN+RNN+YO v5	Resulting in better object detection bad weather condition such as rain, adverse weather event, snow etc.

of lost and found data that resulted in an object detection accuracy of 74%. Regarding the validation part, [3] examined detection systems that used the VISSIM (Traffic in cities – simulation model) datasets, and the results showed that by combining images from the vehicle's right-center and left cameras, it could combine images to a convolution network to match the trained data set to find the accuracy in detection of objects by 82%, which was recorded as an improvement over any detection in previous studies. These classification and evaluations are summarized in Table 1 and Table 2.

The qualitative and quantitative methods both are recommended for analyzing and calculating that included the domain expert's finding and views based on reliability, accuracy, sensitivity and consistency and completeness. Additionally, [9] projected a tool for ontology assessment and evaluation which is termed as "System completeness and acceptance" under which the whole system has been evaluated that resulted to the value for steering angle using TensorFlow. [29] suggested the need for fast processing of continuous video data mainly for object detection through much lower power consumption. To evaluate DCOP classification, we have looked over the intersection and combination within the classification and literature. This study precisely scrutinized the overlap of relationships between the occurrences and that can be featured and found in the study of the chosen articles that are projected in Table 1 and Table 2.

5 Discussion

This paper foresees and diversifies the information of the components of DCOP classifications which were not explained precisely in the publications that were mentioned above. We sketch on the illustrations and samples from the literature to reveal and validate those DCOP components that exist in object detection navigation systems for driverless vehicles. **Data:** The object specific data were clearly projected in the selected journal articles but rarely specified clear concept on analyzed and derived data. This paper considered various images captured by the vehicle camera and the raw sensor data as an input for the processes. The main objective of the image or video is to classify and formulate the pixel in the images to predict the object by using datasets that are pre-trained in the deep network so that the images are tallied pixel by pixel to predict and define the object in the image. Sensor based data is useful to analyze the location information and decide where to navigate. The deep learning method will be used to extract the data from the camera and the sensors to identify the objects that lie on the periphery of the vehicle. Most of the publications have included raw data but very few research had indications on derived data. To name some of the publications that described the derived data [13, 14] that used RGB images on 24 bits for the input in the system in conjunction with classifiers Support Vector Machine. **Object Detection:** Many papers have focused on object detection because this very component is vital for the self-driving domain. As the process completely depends on the images quality, dimension, and lighting, so that the system can visualize the objects accurately. For example, the pictures that are taken on different conditions on the same day might be different in visibility; this is because of differentiation in light conditions at those times. So, to solve this issue a lot of other techniques should be applied to make images on defined lighting condition so that the system accepts the pictures in different sets of time with consistency. For this very phenomenon [20, 28] reflected different tools and algorithms are being enforced to detect the object such as which later came in force with R-CNN with better processing for object detection processes in the image by slicing the images that were divided into the pixel to pixel to determine the object in the image and formulate the output. [18] later added on his publication on the search of completely different approach YOLO where the images are looked at once and detect where the images are divided into grids of 13 × 13 cells each of these cells are responsible for predicting 5 bounding boxes. YOLO is termed to be the state of art architecture for object detection.

6 Conclusion

Object identification and navigation in a driverless car are both critical and delicate tasks. It is necessary for the system to be tolerant of a high degree of precision in navigation and detection to meet the standards of road safety measures. The research presented in this work has been conducted in line with the recommended field of deep learning for use in autonomous automobiles, with the goal of enhancing road safety. The goal of this research is to eliminate the tragic consequences of human mistakes behind the wheel. The papers used to investigate the case, which included several different architectural styles and analytical approaches, were discussed. This work tried to merge the concepts of two innovative architectures, each of which uses a different detection approach implemented in two stages. Data, Classifiers, Object Detection, and Steering Prediction are the four pillars of our unique classification system, DCOP, which we suggested. Journal articles that are like our DCOP classification have been analysed in this paper. We found that some of these articles failed to provide a full picture of the system because they ignored important details about the underlying data and instead concentrated solely on detection and classification. We found the missing content by quickly reviewing their current projects. Because of this, we built a comprehensive taxonomy that incorporated all the key parts of the system and was based on our own understanding of its significance. As a result, we argue that DOCP is an improved taxonomy for researching autonomous vehicles and may be used moving forwards. We hope that DOCP taxonomy can influence further research in accurate and faster object detection for driver less vehicles.

References

1. Ali, A., Olaleye, O.G., Bayoumi, M.: Fast region based DPM object detection for autonomous vehicles. In: 2016 IEEE 59th International Midwest Symposium on Circuits and Systems (MWSCAS), pp. 1–4 (2016). https://doi.org/10.1109/mwscas.2016.7870113
2. Atallah, R.F., Assi, C.M., Khabbaz, M.J.: Scheduling the operation of a connected vehicular network using deep reinforcement learning. IEEE Trans. Intell. Transp. Syst. **20**, 1–14 (2018). https://doi.org/10.1109/TITS.2018.2832219
3. Chen, C., Xiang, H., Qiu, T., Wang, C., Zhou, Y., Chang, V.: A rear-end collision prediction scheme based on deep learning in the internet of vehicles. J. Parallel Distrib. Comput. **117**, 192–204 (2018). https://doi.org/10.1016/j.jpdc.2017.08.014
4. Chen, S., Shang, J., Zhang, S., Zheng, N.: Cognitive map-based model: toward a developmental framework for self-driving cars. In: 2017 IEEE 20th International Conference on Intelligent Transportation Systems (ITSC), pp. 1–8 (2017). https://doi.org/10.1109/itsc.2017.8317627
5. Chen, S., Zhang, S., Shang, J., Chen, B., Zheng, N.: Brain-inspired cognitive model with attention for self-driving cars. IEEE Trans. Cogn. Dev. Syst. **11**, 1 (2017). https://doi.org/10.1109/tcds.2017.2717451

6. Ess, A., Schindler, K., Leibe, B., Van Gool, L.: Object detection and tracking for autonomous navigation in dynamic environments. Int. J. Robot. Res. **29**(14), 1707–1725 (2010). https://doi.org/10.1177/0278364910365417
7. Feng, D., Rosenbaum, L., Dietmayer, K.: Towards safe autonomous driving: capture uncertainty in the deep neural network for Lidar 3D vehicle detection. arXiv preprint arXiv:1804.05132, https://arxiv.org/pdf/1804.05132.pdf (2018)
8. Forczmański, P., Nowosielski, A.: Deep learning approach to detection of preceding vehicle in advanced driver assistance. In: Mikulski, J. (ed.) TST 2016. CCIS, vol. 640, pp. 293–304. Springer, Cham (2016). https://doi.org/10.1007/978-3-319-49646-7_25
9. Gallardo, N., Gamez, N., Rad, P., Jamshidi, M.: Autonomous decision making for a driver-less car. In: 2017 12th System of Systems Engineering Conference (SoSE), pp. 1–6. IEEE, June 2017. https://doi.org/10.1109/SYSOSE.2017.7994953
10. Jeong, Y., Son, S., Jeong, E., Lee, B.: An Integrated self-diagnosis system for an autonomous vehicle based on an IoT gateway and deep learning. Appl. Sci. **8**(7), 1164–1188 (2018). https://doi.org/10.3390/app8071164
11. Johnson, J., Karpathy, A., Fei-Fei, L.: DenseCap: fully convolutional localization networks for dense captioning. In: 2016 IEEE Conference on Computer Vision and Pattern Recognition (CVPR), pp. 4565–4574 (2016). https://doi.org/10.1109/cvpr.2016.494
12. Kim, J.G., Yoo, J.H., Koo, J.C.: Road and lane detection using stereo camera. In: 2018 IEEE International Conference on Big Data and Smart Computing (BigComp), pp. 649–652. IEEE, January 2018. https://doi.org/10.1109/BigComp.2018.00117
13. Kim, J., Canny, J.F.: Interpretable learning for self-driving cars by visualizing causal attention. In: ICCV, pp. 2961–2969, October 2017. http://openaccess.thecvf.com/content_ICCV_2017/papers/Kim_Interpretable_Learning_for_ICCV_2017_paper.pdf
14. Kim, J., Park, C.: End-to-end ego lane estimation based on sequential transfer learning for self-driving cars. In: 2017 IEEE Conference on Computer Vision and Pattern Recognition Workshops (CVPRW), pp. 1194–1202 (2017). https://doi.org/10.1109/cvprw.2017.158
15. Kim, J., Yoo, J., Koo, J.: Road and lane detection using stereo camera. In: 2018 IEEE International Conference on Big Data and Smart Computing (BigComp), pp. 649–652 (2018). https://doi.org/10.1109/bigcomp.2018.00117
16. Kong, T., Yao, A., Chen, Y., Sun, F.: HyperNet: towards accurate region proposal generation and joint object detection. In: 2016 IEEE Conference on Computer Vision and Pattern (2016)
17. Li, J., Wu, Y., Zhao, J., Guan, L., Ye, C., Yang, T.: Pedestrian detection with dilated convolution, region proposal network and boosted decision trees. In: 2017 International Joint Conference on Neural Networks (IJCNN), pp. 4052–4057 (2017). https://doi.org/10.1109/ijcnn.2017.7966367
18. Miller, D., Nicholson, L., Dayoub, F., Sünderhauf, N.: Dropout sampling for robust object detection in open-set conditions. arXiv preprint arXiv:1710.06677. https://arxiv.org/pdf/1710.06677.pdf (2017)
19. Nugraha, B.T., Su, S., Fahmizal: Towards self-driving car using convolutional neural network and road lane detector. In: 2017 2nd International Conference on Automation, Cognitive Science, Optics, Micro Electro-Mechanical System, and Information Technology (ICACOMIT), pp. 65–69 (2017). https://doi.org/10.1109/icacomit.2017.8253388
20. Pham, C.C., Jeon, J.W.: Robust object proposals re-ranking for object detection in autonomous driving using convolutional neural networks. Sig. Process. Image Commun. **53**, 110–122 (2017). https://doi.org/10.1016/j.image.2017.02.007
21. Qian, R., Yue, Y., Coenen, F., Zhang, B.: Traffic sign recognition with convolutional neural network based on max pooling positions. In: 2016 12th International Conference on Natural Computation, Fuzzy Systems and Knowledge Discovery (ICNC-FSKD), pp. 578–582 (2016). https://doi.org/10.1109/fskd.2016.7603237

22. Ramos, S., Gehrig, S., Pinggera, P., Franke, U., Rother, C.: Detecting unexpected obstacles for self-driving cars: fusing deep learning and geometric modeling. In: 2017 IEEE Intelligent Vehicles Symposium (IV), pp. 1025–1032 (2017). https://doi.org/10.1109/ivs.2017.7995849
23. Rausch, V., Hansen, A., Solowjow, E., Liu, C., Kreuzer, E., Hedrick, J.K.: Learning a deep neural net policy for end-to-end control of autonomous vehicles. In: 2017 American Control Conference (ACC), pp. 4914–4919 (2017). https://doi.org/10.23919/acc.2017.7963716
24. Shi, S., Wang, Q., Xu, P., Chu, X.: Benchmarking state-of-the-art deep learning software tools. In: 2016 7th International Conference on Cloud Computing and Big Data (CCBD), pp. 1–14 (2016). https://doi.org/10.1109/ccbd.2016.029
25. Soin, A., Chahande, M.: Moving vehicle detection using deep neural network. In: 2017 International Conference on Emerging Trends in Computing and Communication Technologies (ICETCCT), pp. 1–4 (2017). https://doi.org/10.1109/icetcct.2017.8280336
26. Song, X., Du, Y.: Obstacle tracking based on millimeter wave radar. In: 2016 3rd International Conference on Systems and Informatics (ICSAI), pp. 531–535 (2016). https://doi.org/10.1109/icsai.2016.7811012
27. Yan, C., Xie, H., Yang, D., Yin, J., Zhang, Y., Dai, Q.: Supervised hash coding with deep neural network for environment perception of intelligent vehicles. IEEE Trans. Intell. Transp. Syst. **19**(1), 284–295 (2018). https://doi.org/10.1109/tits.2017.2749965
28. Yang, S., Cao, Y., Peng, Z., Wen, G., Guo, K.: Distributed formation control of nonholonomic autonomous vehicle via RBF neural network. Mech. Syst. Sig. Process. **87**, 81–95 (2017). https://doi.org/10.1016/j.ymssp.2016.04.015
29. Zhang, W., Dehai Zhao, Xu, L., Li, Z., Wenjuan Gong, Zhou, J.: Distributed embedded deep learning based real-time video processing. In: 2016 IEEE International Conference on Systems, Man, and Cybernetics (SMC), pp. 001945–001950 (2016). https://doi.org/10.1109/smc.2016.7844524
30. Gupta, A., Anpalagan, A., Guan, L., Khwaja, A.S.: Deep learning for object detection and scene perception in self-driving cars: Survey, challenges, and open issues. Array **10**, 100057 (2021)
31. Sharma, T., Debaque, B., Duclos, N., Chehri, A., Kinder, B., Fortier, P.: Deep learning-based object detection and scene perception under bad weather conditions. Electronics **11**(4), 563 (2022)
32. Li, K., et al.: CODA: a real-world road corner case dataset for object detection in autonomous driving. arXiv preprint arXiv:2203.07724 (2022)

The Effect of Sleep Disturbances on the Quality of Sleep: An Adaptive Computational Network Model

Quentin Lee Hee, Lorenzo Hogendorp, Daan Warnaars, and Jan Treur(✉)

Athena Institute and Social AI Group, Vrije Universiteit Amsterdam, Amsterdam, The Netherlands
{q.leehee,l.g.r.hogendorp,d.p.warnaars}@student.vu.nl, j.treur@vu.nl

Abstract. In this paper, an adaptive temporal-causal network model is presented for a normal night's sleep and for how disturbances and their timing interfere with such a normal night of sleep. The goal of this computational model is to explore the area of how sleep disturbances influence a person's health. This was achieved by simulating single and multiple sleep disturbances during sleep episodes and measuring the effect on light, deep, and REM sleep. The main finding from the simulated scenarios in this study is that disturbances, depending on their timing, can cause a lack of deep and/or REM sleep. This implies that sleep disturbances might lead to insufficient physical and/or emotional recovery.

Keywords: Sleep model · Sleep disturbances · Recovery · Sleep stages · Sleep quality · Hypnogram

1 Introduction

Sleep is like food, water, and air a requisite for human life (Grandner 2017). A good night's sleep for an adult lasts between 7 and 9 h and consists of 4 to 5 sleep cycles (Hirshkowitz et al. 2015; Chien et al. 2010). Such normal sleep has a basic structural organization, a sleep architecture. Two types of sleep can be differentiated within each of the sleep cycles: non-rapid eye-movement (NREM) sleep and rapid-eye-movement (REM) sleep (Colten and Altevogt 2015). NREM sleep can be subdivided into two stages; light sleep (N1 & N2) and deepest non-rem sleep (N3) (Patel and Araujo 2018). In a "normal" night's sleep, approximately 50% of the total sleep time is spent in the light sleep stage which is associated with memory consolidation (Gandhi and Emmady 2022). This stage lasts around 25 min in the first sleep cycle and gets longer with each subsequent cycle. The successive stage is the deepest non-rem sleep (N3) and is accountable for the physical recovery of the body, which includes building bone and muscle, (re)growing tissue and strengthening the immune system. This stage takes up approximately 25% of the total time slept. The final stage of each sleep cycle is the REM stage which is associated with emotion regulation and takes up the remaining 25% of

K. Daimi and A. Al Sadoon (Eds.): ICR 2023, LNNS 721, pp. 105–117, 2023.
https://doi.org/10.1007/978-3-031-35308-6_9

the total time slept (Vandekerckhove and Wang 2017). During the first sleep cycle, the REM stage lasts around 10 min and in the final cycle up to an hour (Della Monica et al. 2018).

Even though the importance of a good night's sleep for a person's health is widely emphasized, a third of American adults are not getting enough sleep on a regular basis (Center for Disease Control and Prevention CDC 2016). Various studies indicated that a consistent lack of sleep, the medical term sleep deprivation, is associated with a higher risk for cardiovascular diseases, metabolic syndrome, cancer, and depression (Irwin 2015; Jennings et al. 2007; Ko et al. 2012). Sleeping deprivation is caused by a coalescence of reasons including medical and physiological conditions and societal factors such as urbanization (Hanson and Huecker 2022; Martins et al. 2020).

Despite the risks of sleep deprivation being clearly indicated in the literature, it is still unclear how disturbances (caused by any reason) influence someone's sleep pattern. In this paper, an adaptive temporal-causal network model is presented in which both a "normal night's sleep" is addressed and how disturbances and their timing interfere with this normal night of sleep. The goal of this study is to illuminate the uncharted area of how sleep disturbances influence the health benefits of sleep.

2 Methods

First, a conceptual model was made using information and data from literature studies (Fig. 1). During sleep, the simulated person transitions from light sleep to deep sleep to REM sleep. Light sleep was defined as the NREM 1 and 2 sleep stages, deep sleep as NREM 3 stage, and REM sleep as the REM stage (Patel et al. 2022). Due to the scarcity of literature about the influence of disturbances during sleep, we concluded from an interview with a neurophysiologist at the Vrije Universiteit Amsterdam that disturbances during a sleep stage, make the sleep cycle start all over again. The model also aimed to simulate this principle. Therefore, when a disturbance is introduced, the simulated person will then move back to awake and immediately transition back to light sleep. Literature was consulted to determine outcome measures. It was found that light, deep, and REM sleep were respectively linked with memory, physical, and emotional recovery (Patel et al. 2022; Moldofsky and Scarisbrick 1976). The outcome measures reflect the time spent in the different sleep stadia.

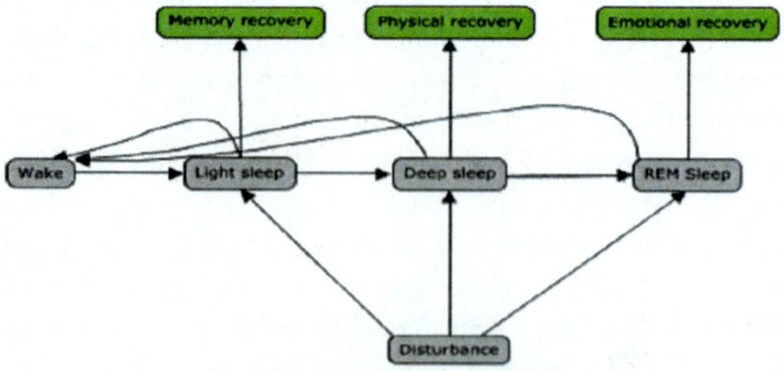

Fig. 1. Basic conceptual model

In order to translate the conceptual framework to a graphical representation of the model, the network-oriented modeling approach described in (Treur 2020) was used. A main reason for this is that using this method and its software environment, the steps from conceptual representation to numerical representation to implementation are rather small. Moreover, this method is at least as general as any method to model adaptive dynamical systems as has been proven in (Treur 2021). This network-oriented modeling approach is based on a temporal-causal network as the network is dynamic and a temporal dimension is taken into account. A temporal-causal network is described by (X and Y denote nodes/states of the network):

Connectivity Characteristics
Connections from a state X to a state Y and their *weights* $\boldsymbol{\omega}_{X,Y}$

Aggregation Characteristics
For any state Y, *combination function* $\mathbf{c}_Y(..)$ defines the aggregation of the single impacts $\boldsymbol{\omega}_{X_i,Y}X_i(t)$ on Y from its incoming connections from states X_i

Timing Characteristics
Each state Y has a *speed factor* $\boldsymbol{\eta}_Y$ defining how fast it changes for the given aggregated impact.

Aggregation characteristics can use different combination functions. In our model, we used four basic combination functions shown in Table 1.

Table 1. Combination functions used

Name	Notation	Value
identity	$\mathbf{id}(V_1, ..., V_k)$	V_1
step-once	$\mathbf{steponce}_{\alpha,\beta}(V_1, ..., V_k)$	1 if $\alpha \leq t \leq \beta$, 0 else (where t = current time)
scaled sum	$\mathbf{ssum}_{\lambda}(V_1, ..., V_k)$	$(V_1 + ... + V_k)/\lambda$
scaled maximum	$\mathbf{smax}_{\lambda}(V_1, ..., V_k)$	$\mathbf{max}(V_1, ..., V_k)\ /\lambda$

Adaptive networks are networks in which some of the network characteristics change over time, for example, changing connection weights to model forms of synaptic plasticity or adaptive excitability thresholds to model forms of non-synaptic plasticity from neuroscience. To model adaptive networks, the self-modeling network modelling approach (also called network reification) from (Treur 2020) is used. This works by adding extra states (called self-model states or reification states) to the network for the adaptive network characteristics. For example, a self-model state $\mathbf{W}_{X,Y}$ can be added to represent an adaptive connection weight $\boldsymbol{\omega}_{X,Y}$ and a self-model state $\mathbf{T}_Y$ can be added to represent an adaptive excitability threshold $\boldsymbol{\tau}_Y$. In this paper, this is applied in particular to model adaptive parameters $\boldsymbol{\alpha}$ and $\boldsymbol{\beta}$ for the step-once function used. For example, if for state Y in the network, the step-once function is used, then by adding states $\mathbf{A}_Y$ and $\mathbf{B}_Y$ to represent its parameters $\boldsymbol{\alpha}$ and $\boldsymbol{\beta}$, they can be made adaptive.

3 The Designed Adaptive Mental Network Model

A graphical representation of the model is shown in Fig. 2. In Table 2 the states and explanation are shown.

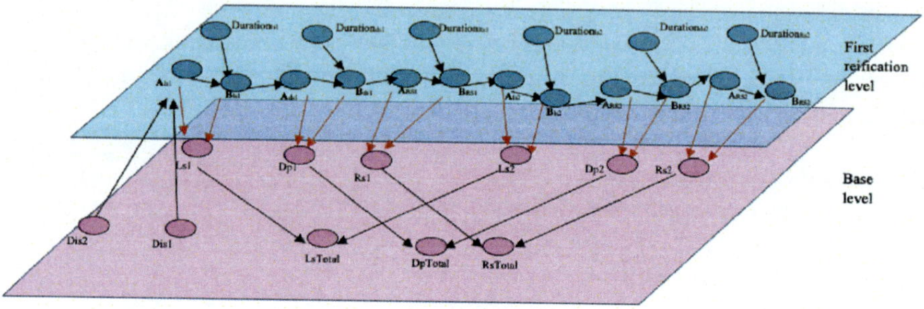

Fig. 2. Graphical representation of the connectivity of the adaptive network model

Table 2. Used states

State nr	State name	Explanation	Level
X_1	Ls1	Light Sleep cycle 1	
X_2	Ds1	Deep Sleep cycle 1	
X_3	RS1	REM Sleep cycle 1	
X_{13}	Ls2	Light sleep cycle 2	
X_{14}	Ds2	Deep Sleep cycle 2	
X_{15}	Rs2	REM Sleep cycle 2	Base level
X_{25}	Dis1	Disturbance 1	
X_{26}	LsTot	Light sleep Total	
X_{27}	DsTot	Deep sleep Total	
X_{28}	RsTot	REM sleep Total	
X_{29}	Dis2	Disturbance 2	
X_4	Als1	A state light sleep cycle 1	
X_5	Bls1	B state light sleep cycle 1	
X_6	Durationls1	Duration light sleep cycle 1	
X_7	Ads1	A state deep sleep cycle 1	
X_8	Bds1	B state deep sleep cycle 1	
X9	Durationds1	Duration deep sleep cycle 1	
X_{10}	Ars1	A state REM sleep cycle 1	
X_{11}	Brs1	B state REM sleep cycle 1	
X_{12}	Durationrs1	Duration REM sleep cycle 1	First reification level
X_{16}	Als2	A state light sleep cycle 2	
X_{17}	Bls2	B state light sleep cycle 2	
X_{18}	Durationls2	Duration Light sleep cycle 2	
X_{19}	A2ds2	A state deep sleep cycle 2	
X_{20}	Bds2	B state deep sleep cycle 2	
X_{21}	Durationds2	Duration deep sleep cycle 2	
X_{22}	Ars2	A state REM sleep cycle 2	
X_{23}	Brs2	B state REM sleep cycle 2	
X_{24}	Durationrs2	Duration REM sleep cycle 2	

This computational model was designed by first developing a basic model which consisted of only the sleep stages, thereafter, adding new states which would reflect the outcomes and disturbances. Timings of the stages in the model were determined by using the scale of a hypnogram. The model consists of a basic state level and a (first) reification level.

In the base level, two sleep cycles are shown. Each sleep cycle is split into three different sleep stages: light sleep, deep sleep, and REM sleep. These are connected to the sleep stage Total states which sum up the time spent in the concerning sleep stages in both cycles. The timings of the sleep stages are determined by the step-once combination function. The parameter values inserted in the step-once are adaptively determined by the self-model **A**- and **B**-states in the first reification level. The **A**-state of a sleep stage defines the beginning of the sleep stage determined by identity functions, and the **B**-states of a sleep stage define the ending of the sleep stage. This is determined by the scaled sum function applied to the duration state and the **A**-state. To explore the effect of disturbances, two disturbance states were added to the model. These were set with a step-once combination function, depicting a value of 1 at a certain time point. A disturbance state is connected to the **A**-state of the light sleep cycle 1, thus resetting the sleep cycle, i.e., starting at the beginning again. More details can be found as Linked Supplementary Data at https://www.researchgate.net/publication/367022940.

4 Simulation Results

Figure 3 shows a simulation outcome for all states of the simulation. The states that take off at the beginning of the figure and stabilize to an equilibrium with a value of a maximum of 180 min are the parameter values for the step-once functions. The total time spent in a sleep stage is visible in the states that take off orderly, stabilize, and increase again.

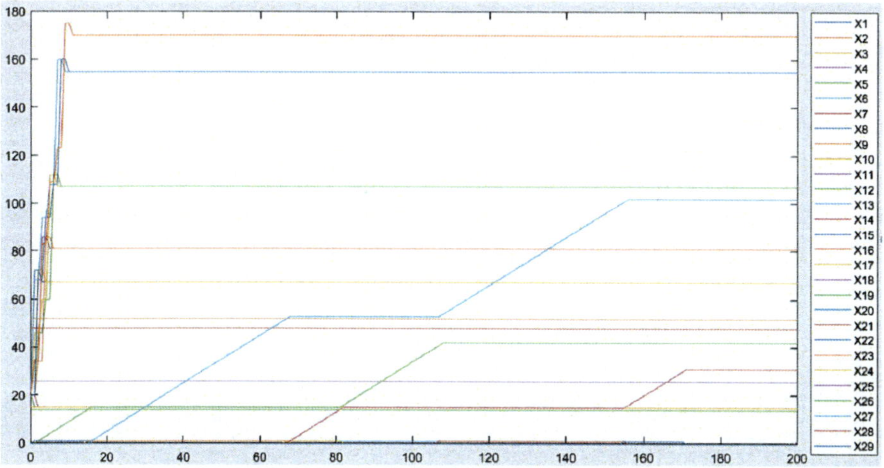

Fig. 3. Overall view: graph of all states of the model

Due to the scale, a lot of information is hard to analyze in this graph. Therefore, in Fig. 4 only the sleep stage transitions are shown in detail. In later figures, this is repeated but with the influence of the disturbance. In this figure, the progression through the sleep phases, which are controlled by the self-model **A**- and **B**-states of the step-once function, are clearly visible. It should be noted that the subsequent phase in this figure is activated before the one earlier sleep phase ends.

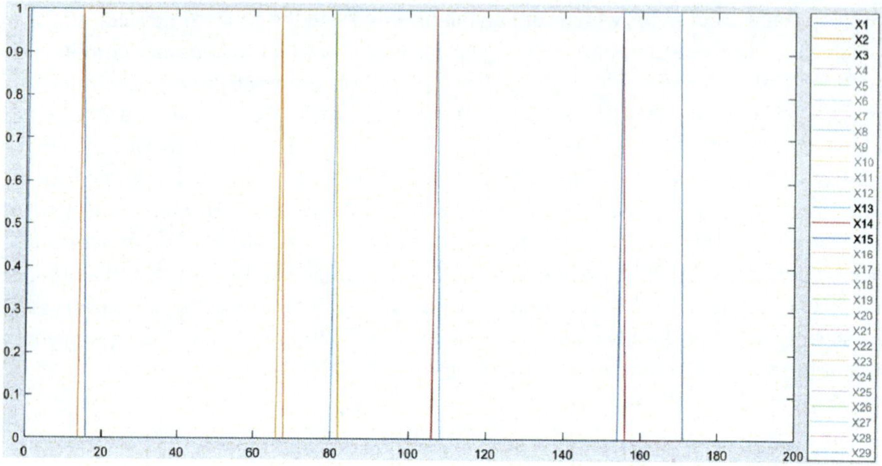

Fig. 4. The progression through the sleep stages in the first two cycles of a normal night's sleep.

Figure 5 gives a general overview of the cumulative time (in minutes) of a certain phase in the first two sleep cycles. The blue line depicts the total time spent in light sleep, the red/orange line corresponds to deep sleep and the yellow line to REM sleep. Just as in reality, it can be seen that light sleep is followed by deep sleep and consequently REM sleep. After 170 min, all stages remain stationary as two cycles have fully passed. We can observe that at the beginning of the night, i.e., the first two sleep cycles, the time spent in light sleep, and deep sleep is much longer than REM sleep, respectively 42, 102, and 31 min.

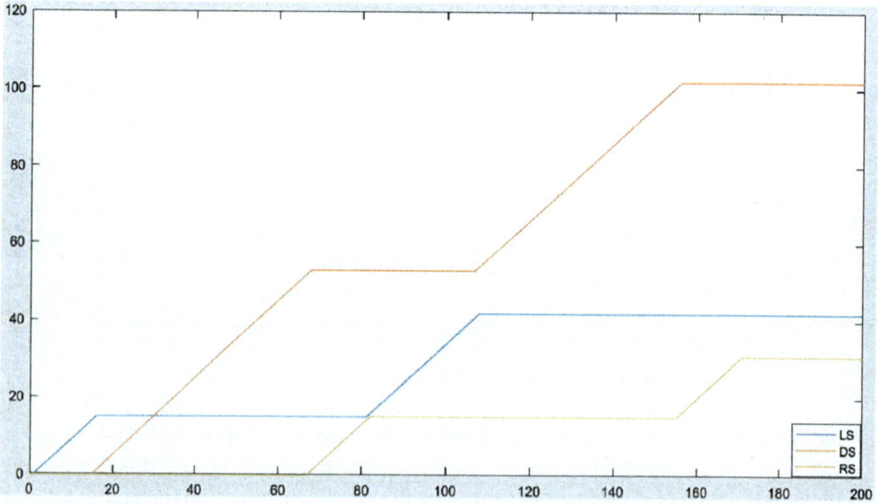

Fig. 5. Graph of time spent in different sleep stages; blue = Light Sleep; red/orange = deep sleep, yellow = REM sleep.

After the basic model was made, disturbances were introduced in the model. The timing of these disturbances were chosen to see a variety of effects in the time ultimately spent in each sleep stage. Disturbances close at the beginning and end of the simulation were not included as these would have little impact in that domain. In Fig. 6, a disturbance is added to the system at $t = 67$. This resets the cycles during the simulation. Resulting in not two but three time periods spent in light sleep and deep sleep compared to the graph without disturbance. Compared with the graph of the undisturbed model not all lines are stationary towards the end of the simulation. This is due to the reset by the disturbance and the characteristic of the model to only stop adding until the two cycles have fully passed. Therefore, at the end of the simulation ($t = 170$), in this model, a person would still be in their deep sleep. The time spent in light, deep, and REM sleep was respectively 50, 105, and 21 min for this simulation.

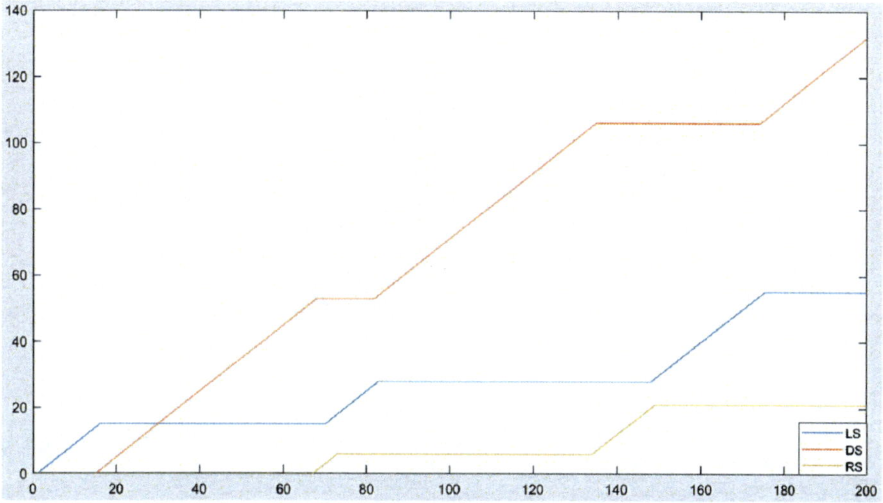

Fig. 6. Graph of time spent in sleep stages with a disturbance at time $t = 67$

In Fig. 7, the onset and impact of a disturbance at $t = 67$ are shown. After the onset of the disturbance, a reset of other states can be seen. The line representing REM sleep 1 (X_3), can also be seen changing to zero, however, the turning on was not seen of REM sleep 1. This is probably because of the line being behind the blue line, which represents the turning off of light sleep 1. Additionally, REM sleep 1 turns off after the stimulus of the disturbance was on. This is probably because of the delay in our model.

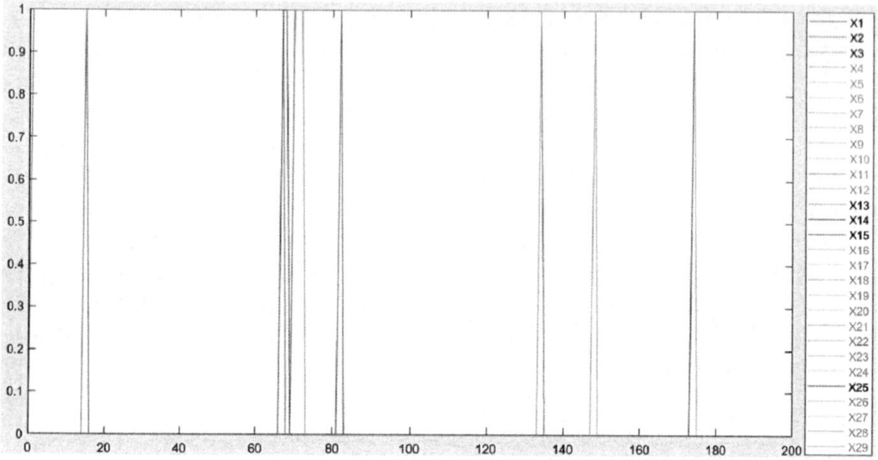

Fig. 7. Graph of onset and impact of disturbance $t = 67$

In addition, a disturbance was also set at $t = 90$, during the second light sleep period. A steeper rise in that light sleep period can be observed. This might be caused due to a delay in the information that the light sleep 2 state needs to receive to be shut off. Resulting in a five time-steps double count in light sleep (also shown in Table 3). With disturbances set at this time point, the model shows relatively more light sleep, than in a model with a disturbance set during a different sleep stage. Time spent in light, deep, and REM sleep was respectively 45, 106, and 28 min for this simulation (Fig. 8).

Table 3. Five time-steps double count of total LS

	$t = 93$	$t = 94$	$t = 95$	$t = 96$	$t = 97$	$t = 98$	$t = 99$	$t = 100$
X_{26} Total LS	26	27	29	31	33	35	37	38

Furthermore, a disturbance was set at $t = 140$, during the second Deep Sleep state. This results in an absence of the second REM sleep stage. Additionally, during the two cycles, the amount of deep sleep is larger than in the undisturbed sleep cycles. Time spent in light, deep, and REM sleep was respectively 55, 111, and 15 min for this simulation (Fig. 9).

In addition, multiple disturbances were added to the model. In Fig. 10, disturbances were added at $t = 40$ and $t = 130$. A delay in the onset of REM sleep can be observed due to resetting back to light sleep. The second disturbance cuts the second REM sleep stage short, reverting the model back to light sleep. The second disturbance in REM shows the same double counting as in the figure with a singular disturbance at $t = 90$. Time spent in light, deep, and REM sleep was respectively 58, 107, and 15 min for this simulation.

In Fig. 11, different time points for disturbances are set. Here, the first disturbance is set in during REM sleep stage cycle one. It can be observed that in the first cycle, the

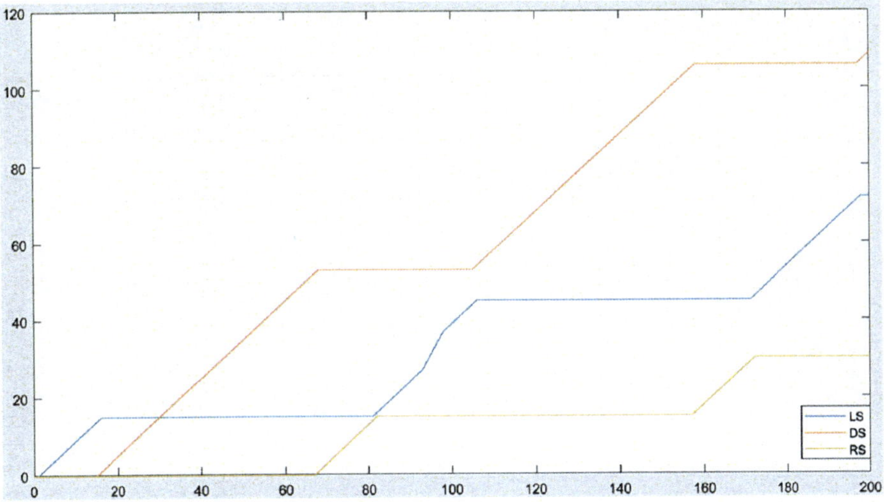

Fig. 8. Graph of simulation with disturbances at $t = 90$

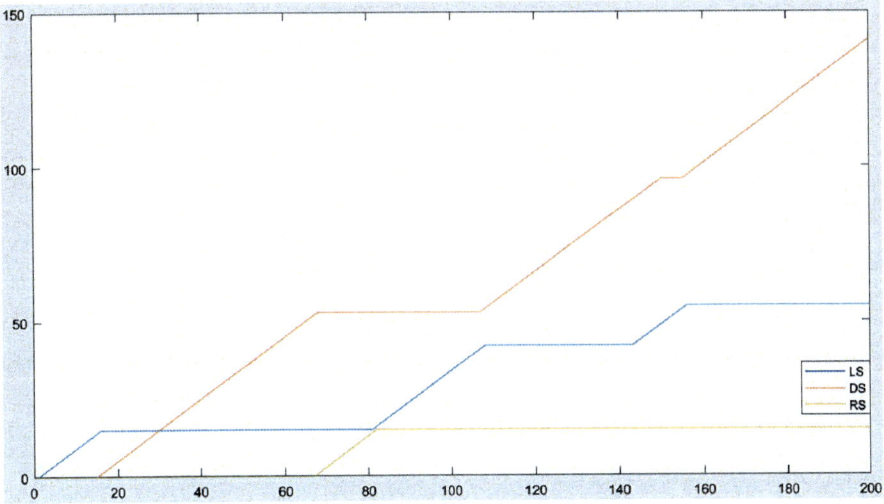

Fig. 9. Graph of simulation with a disturbance at $t = 140$

model still gets REM sleep. Whereas, in the previous simulation, the first cycle of REM sleep was completely disregarded. The second disturbance also cut the REM stage in the second cycle short. Time spent in light, deep, and REM sleep was respectively 41, 127, and 9 min in this simulation.

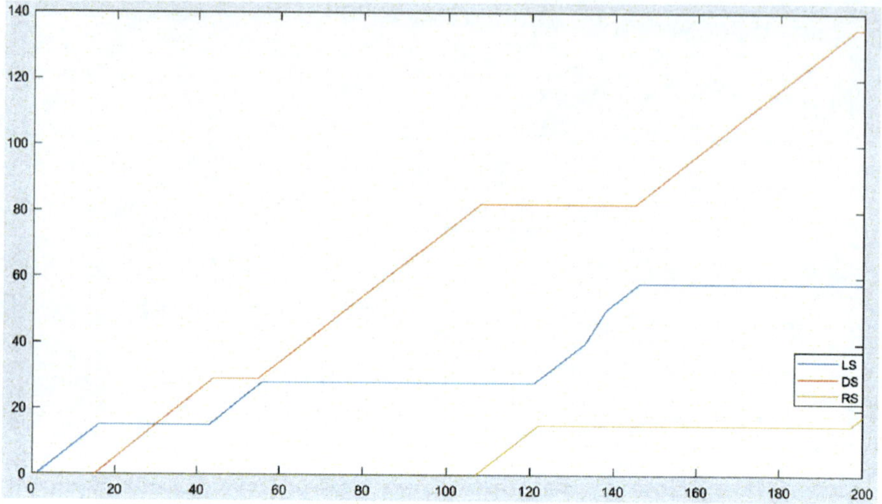

Fig. 10. Graph of sleep stages with disturbances at $t = 40$ and $t = 130$

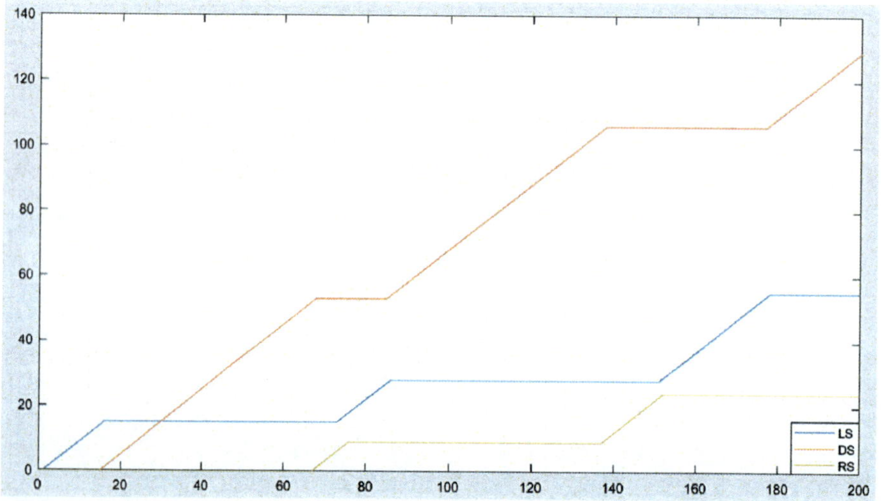

Fig. 11. Graph of sleep stages and disturbance at $t = 70$ and $t = 130$

5 Discussion

In this section, the findings are discussed. Subsequently, the strengths and limitations and their implications are presented. Finally, recommendations for future research are suggested and a conclusion is stated.

The main finding from the simulated scenarios in this study is that disturbance(s) depending on their timing can cause a lack of deep and/or REM sleep which implies getting insufficient physical and or emotional recovery. This can be linked to studies by other scholars that associate sleep deprivation with for example anger (Saghir et al.

2018) and a study that links sleep deprivation to impairing physical recovery from sports training (Rae et al. 2017).

Timings were important for our sleep model. Instead of choosing the percentages found in the literature for the timings of the sleep stages, empirical data from a hypnogram was used to determine the timings in our model. This was chosen as the percentages of the total sleep stages in the literature did not show how the proportion of the amount of sleep progressed during the night. Data was extracted by using the scale of the hypnogram. This implies that this model is a personalized model. However, with only minor adjustments, this model can be adapted to the sleep architecture of any individual or even the sleep of the average in a certain population or circumstance. This flexibility to adjust the model to make it fit for purpose is one of its strengths.

In this paper sleep and corresponding sleeping stages are objectively measured with the outcome measures of emotional, physical and memory recovery (Gandhi and Emmady 2022; Patel and Araujo 2018). However, in literature, there is an ongoing debate on if sleep should be evaluated subjectively or objectively (Jackowska et al 2011; Landry et al. 2015). The availability of empirical data on the sleeping stages in this study was limited to extracting data from hypnograms by hand because most literature uses inconclusive data for this. Moreover, scholars argue that sleep should be evaluated by combining both subjective and objective measures as it for example enhances the classification accuracy of sleeping disorders (Tahmasian et al. 2017). Therefore, it is important to acknowledge that one of the weaknesses of the model developed in this study is that it cannot define sleep quality by itself and could benefit from external data such as some subjective measures.

The model can be personalised to specific persons by using different values for its network characteristics, for example by using lower values for excitability thresholds or higher values for connection weights to model persons that are more sensitive and stronger in their responses.

With the model that is developed in this paper disturbances and their effects can be simulated in a normal night's sleep. However, this model can be refined by tackling imperfections that came to light when running the simulations. To exemplify, when the model transitions from one phase into another, a small inaccuracy occurs as for 1 or 2 min it seems both phases are counted. Similar counting inaccuracy occurred when disturbances were introduced at a later stage in sleep cycles. Besides tackling these minor issues of the model, the model could become more comprehensive by incorporating the remaining three sleep cycles of a night's sleep. Accordingly, additional measures, as explained in the previous paragraph, could be introduced so that the model gives a more holistic view of sleep quality.

6 Conclusion

In conclusion, the aim of this paper was to design an adaptive temporal-causal network model to demonstrate how disturbances influence a normal night's sleep. It became clear that depending on the timing of disturbances, people might not get deep or REM sleep. This may result in not getting (enough) physical and emotional recovery. Future research may focus on extending the model and incorporating other aspects and measures, such as, for example, discussed in (Georgiev, 2020).

References

Centre for Disease Control and prevention retrieved, 4 January 2023. https://www.cdc.gov/media/releases/2016/p0215-enough-sleep.html

Chien, K.L., et al.: Habitual sleep duration and insomnia and the risk of cardiovascular events and all-cause death: report from a community-based cohort. Sleep **33**(2), 177–184 (2010)

Colten, H.R., Altevogt, B.M.: Sleep Physiology. Nih.gov; National Academies Press (US) (2015). https://www.ncbi.nlm.nih.gov/books/NBK19956/

Della Monica, C., Johnsen, S., Atzori, G., Groeger, J.A., Dijk, D.J.: Rapid eye movement sleep, sleep continuity and slow wave sleep as predictors of cognition, mood, and subjective sleep quality in healthy men and women, aged 20–84 years. Front. Psych. **9**, 255 (2018). https://doi.org/10.3389/fpsyt.2018.00255

Gandhi, M.H., Emmady, P.D.: Physiology, K Complex. In: StatPearls. StatPearls Publishing (2022)

Georgiev, I.: Neurophysiological control of sleep with special emphasis on melatonin. Trakia J. Sci. **18**, 355–376 (2020). https://doi.org/10.15547/tjs.2020.04.011

Grandner, M.A.: Sleep, health, and society. Sleep Med. Clin. **12**(1), 1–22 (2017). https://doi.org/10.1016/j.jsmc.2016.10.012

Hanson, J.A., Huecker, M.R. Sleep deprivation. In: StatPearls. StatPearls Publishing (2022)

Hirshkowitz, M., et al.: National sleep foundation's sleep time duration recommendations: methodology and results summary. Sleep Health **1**(1), 40–43 (2015). https://doi.org/10.1016/j.sleh.2014.12.010

Irwin, M.R.: Why sleep is important for health: a psychoneuroimmunology perspective. Annu. Rev. Psychol. **66**, 143–172 (2015). https://doi.org/10.1146/annurev-psych-010213-115205

Jackowska, M., Dockray, S., Hendrickx, H., Steptoe, A.: Psychosocial factors and sleep efficiency: discrepancies between subjective and objective evaluations of sleep. Psychosom. Med. **73**(9), 810–816 (2011)

Jennings, J.R., Muldoon, M.F., Hall, M., Buysse, D.J., Manuck, S.B.: Self-reported sleep quality is associated with the metabolic syndrome. Sleep **30**(2), 219–223 (2007)

Ko, Y.J., et al.: High-sensitivity C-reactive protein levels and cancer mortality. Cancer Epidemiol. Biomarkers Prevent. Public. Am. Assoc. Cancer Res. Cosponsored Am. Soc. Prevent. Oncol. **21**(11), 2076–2086 (2012). https://doi.org/10.1158/1055-9965.EPI-12-0611

Landry, G.J., Best, J.R., Liu-Ambrose, T.: Measuring sleep quality in older adults: a comparison using subjective and objective methods. Front. Aging Neurosci. **7**, 166 (2015). https://doi.org/10.3389/fnagi.2015.00166

Martins, A.J., Isherwood, C.M., Vasconcelos, S.P., Lowden, A., Skene, D.J., Moreno, C.R.C.: The effect of urbanization on sleep, sleep/wake routine, and metabolic health of residents in the Amazon region of Brazil. Chronobiol. Int. **37**(9–10), 1335–1343 (2020). https://doi.org/10.1080/07420528.2020.1802287

Moldofsky, H., Scarisbrick, P.: Induction of neurasthenic musculoskeletal pain syndrome by selective sleep stage deprivation. Psychosom. Med. **38**(1), 35–44 (1976)

Patel, A.K., Araujo, J.F.: Physiology, Sleep Stages. Nih.gov;StatPearls Publishing, 27 October 2018. https://www.ncbi.nlm.nih.gov/books/NBK526132/

Patel, A.K., Reddy, V., Araujo, J.F.: Physiology, sleep stages. In: StatPearls [Internet]. StatPearls Publishing (2022). https://www.ncbi.nlm.nih.gov/books/NBK526132/

Rae, D.E., et al.: One night of partial sleep deprivation impairs recovery from a single exercise training session. Eur. J. Appl. Physiol. **117**(4), 699–712 (2017). https://doi.org/10.1007/s00421-017-3565-5

Saghir, Z., Syeda, J.N., Muhammad, A.S., Balla Abdalla, T.H.: The amygdala, sleep debt, sleep deprivation, and the emotion of anger: a possible connection?. Cureus **10**(7), e2912 (2018). https://doi.org/10.7759/cureus.2912

Tahmasian, M., et al.: Differentiation chronic post traumatic stress disorder patients from healthy subjects using objective and subjective sleep-related parameters. Neurosci. Lett. **650**, 174–179 (2017). https://doi.org/10.1016/j.neulet.2017.04.042

Treur, J.: Network-Oriented Modeling for Adaptive Networks: Designing Higher-Order Adaptive Biological, Mental and Social Network Models. Springer Nature, Cham (2020). https://doi.org/10.1007/978-3-030-31445-3

Treur, J.: On the dynamics and adaptivity of mental processes: relating adaptive dynamical systems and self-modeling network models by mathematical analysis. Cogn. Syst. Res. **70**, 93–100 (2021)

Vandekerckhove, M., Wang, Y.L.: Emotion, emotion regulation and sleep: an intimate relationship. AIMS Neurosci. **5**(1), 1–17 (2017). https://doi.org/10.3934/Neuroscience.2018.1.1

Deep Learning Based Path-Planning Using CRNN and A* for Mobile Robots

Muhammad Aatif(✉), Umar Adeel, Amin Basiri, Valerio Mariani, Luigi Iannelli, and Luigi Glielmo

University of Sannio, Benevento, Italy
{maatif,umadeel,basiri,vmariani,luigi.iannelli, glielmo}@unisannio.it

Abstract. We present a novel approach for solving path-planning problems using a state-of-the-art data-driven deep learning technique. Although machine learning has been previously utilized for path planning, it has proven to be challenging due to the discrete nature of search algorithms. In this study, we propose a deep learning-based algorithm for path planning, which incorporates a Convolutional Recurrent Neural Network (CRNN) to create an end-to-end trainable neural network planner. This planner is then combined with the A* algorithm through an adaptive autonomy concept to autonomously select the best path planning strategy for increasing time efficiency and completeness. To train the CRNN, a labeled data set is generated autonomously from various maps by changing the starting and endpoints. The trained CRNN can find the shortest path from the starting point to the goal point by evaluating map images in one go. Additionally, the CRNN can predict way-points on image inputs. Our simulation results demonstrate that our proposed strategy is capable of finding the shortest path much faster than the A* algorithm in sparse environments, achieving a speed-up of up to 831 in some cases, which is exceptional.

Keywords: Machine learning · Deep learning · A* · Adaptive Autonomy · CRNN (Convolutional Recurrent Neural Network) · data-driven-based · Path Planning

1 Introduction

Path planning algorithms are integral to many mobile robotics applications, particularly those aimed at accomplishing complex user-defined missions. In essence, Path planning can be defined as a process that breaks down a desired path into a series of iterative steps, allowing for discrete movements that optimize various factors [1]. In recent years, significant progress has been made in the field of path planning algorithms. Some of the well-researched algorithms include search based planning, A* search [2], and dual arm manipulation for humans, among others. To enable mobile robots to navigate, a variety of algorithms have been employed, such as Artificial Neural Networks, Genetic Algorithms, and the A* algorithm [4]. The robots identify the minimum grid cells to reach the destination by operating on the workspace grids. Four main motion planning

K. Daimi and A. Al Sadoon (Eds.): ICR 2023, LNNS 721, pp. 118–128, 2023.
https://doi.org/10.1007/978-3-031-35308-6_10

algorithms, including graph search, and sample-based, have been compared based on planning based reasoning, such as policies for reinforcement learning [5, 13]. It has been observed that sampling-based planning has provided the optimal solution for path planning. Expert demonstrations have become increasingly popular in the field of path planning, surpassing the traditional heuristic-based approach. Recent research has identified the superiority of data-driven path planning, which can be categorized into two types: (1) Shortest path search problems from one point to another point, which are more systematic than classical heuristic plan ners [7]. (2) Path planning utilizing convolutional neural networks on images, which has demonstrated superior effectiveness compared to classical planners.

Search-based planning has limitations due to its incremental search steps and discrete nature, which makes it challenging to study using backpropagation. While heuristic cost functions can be trained using oracle planners [7] and ex haustive pre-computation of heuristic functions [9], a labor-intensive manual an notation process [11] can limit availability and scalability. To address this issue, , which allows for learning from both combinational algorithms and search-based algorithms. However, the use of black-box functions makes training difficult as it can lose track of internal steps. To overcome the challenge of computing the optimal path from one point to another within a reasonable amount of time, we propose a deep learning-based approach using CRNN with adaptive auton omy for optimal path planning, which generates the path way-points for the mobile robot. In this study, we compared the sample-based search algorithms with the proposed deep learning-based CRNN approach in terms of computation time. The simulation results demonstrate that the computation time of the deep learning-based CRNN approach has the edge over sample-based search algorithms for finding the shortest path.

2 Deep Learning-Based Path Planner Using CRNN

In this section, a deep learning-based approach to path planning is discussed. To achieve completeness in path planning, adaptive autonomy is required that can select the best path-planning algorithm according to the situation. Adaptive autonomy is the property of an autonomous system in which the distribution of autonomy is changed dynamically to optimize overall system performance [16]. Here we are particularly using the A* search algorithm, which is widely used for discovering a solution path by exploring free space while minimizing the total cost, usually represented by the path length. When an obstacle creates a dead-end between the start and the goal, leading to unnecessary exploration of free space. Additionally, while humans can detect such obstacles and find a way to bypass them easily using past experiences, the full algorithm search for a given problem often falls short of our ability to perceive problem structures and plan more intelligently. Therefore, training in the deep learning-based approach is a critical step in path planning and the labeled data set is required for the training. Section 2.1 will discuss the creation of a labeled data set and our proposed approach to increase the time efficiency in path planning.

2.1 Data Labeling and Experimentation

The availability of labeled data[15] set is of utmost importance for the deep learning-based algorithmic development and evaluation of the algorithm. The first step towards the development of a comprehensive labeled data set is data collection. In our study on deep learning-based path planning, data refers to the collection of maps. For the data and experimentation, we have taken nine different maps M0, M1, M2, M3, M4, M5, M6, M7 and M8 as summarized in Fig. 2. Map M0 is a most simple case, it has no obstacle. M_1 is a map with one obstacle with a plus sign. M_3 and M_9 with two obstacles of different sizes. M4 has four obstacles with low density. M_5 has four obstacles with high density. However to check the robustness of the algorithm of the proposed approach take concave obstacles with different complexity levels in maps M2, M6, and M7. Maps M1, M2, M3 and M4 maps are inspired from the previous approaches [17]. A simulation setup 1 is developed in python to automate the labeling process. We have created multiple scenarios of the maps. Algorithm 1 is an Autonomous Ground Truth Labeling algorithm for generating labeled data for training ma chine learning models. The algorithm generates a dataset of waypoints and maps by following these steps:

1. For each iteration from 1 to N, select a map randomly from a set of 9 available maps.
2. Randomly select a starting position until a valid starting position inside the map is found. If the randomly selected starting position is inside an obstacle, the algorithm continues to select a new position until a valid starting position is found.
3. Similarly, randomly select an end position until a valid position inside the map is found.
4. Compute the optimal waypoints using the $A*$ algorithm, which finds the shortest path between the starting and ending positions on the map. 5. Save the generated waypoints and map image, which together form a labeled data point.

By repeating the above steps for N iterations, the algorithm generates a dataset of labeled data points, where each data point consists of a map image and the corresponding set of optimal waypoints for traversing that map. The purpose of this algorithm is to generate ground truth labels for a dataset of images containing obstacles and corresponding paths, which can be used to train the deep learning models for obstacle detection and path planning. By generating ground truth labels automatically, the algorithm eliminates the need for manual labeling, which can be time-consuming and error-prone. A simulation setup is developed in python with pytorch. The operating system is 64-bit window 10 with Intel(R) Core(TM) i5-9300H CPU @ 2.40 GHz and RAmM 8 GB.

Algorithm 1 Autonomous Ground Truth Labeling

```
for Iteration = 1, 2, . . . , N do
    Randomly select the map among 9 maps
    Randomly select the starting position while The starting position Inside the ob stacle do
        Randomly select the starting position
    end
    Randomly select the end position while The end position Inside the obstacle do
        Randomly select the end position
    end
    Calculate the way-points using A* algorithm
    Save the way-points and map image
end
```

All maps are created at a resolution of 80 × 80. For algorithmic development and preliminary evaluation, we target a set of the 9 maps as you can see in Fig. 2. Subsequently, once the system has been developed, it can be employed to find the shortest path between two points. From the viewpoint of the shortest path, each map needs to be labeled therefore way-points of the shortest path are associated with each map. To evaluate the performance of the system, waypoints must be identified and stored. In the following sections, we discuss in detail about the path planner module.

2.2 Reliability of Autonomous Ground Truth Labeling

The accuracy and reliability of the ground truth labels are essential for training machine learning models that can use for finding the path. Autonomous ground truth labeling is an efficient way of developing and validating the deep learning based path-planning algorithm.

Table 1. Autonomous data labeling performance.

number of Maps	number of scenarios	completeness
9	30000	100%

To verify the reliability of autonomous ground truth labeling we used the A* algorithm for training the deep learning-based path planning algorithm. The A* algorithm is a widely used path-finding algorithm commonly used to find a path. It is based on a heuristic search and is particularly useful for finding the shortest path between two points in a graph. This approach was chosen due to the completeness and shortest path guarantees provided by the A* algorithm [20]. We tested this approach on 30000 scenarios spread across 9 maps. A high degree of reliability ensures that the deep learning-based path planning algorithm can accurately identify obstacles and make informed decisions about the best route to take in a given scenario. By verifying the reliability of autonomous ground truth labeling using the A* algorithm for training a deep learning-based path planning algorithm, with 100% accuracy with respect to the completeness and shortest path in the 30000 scenarios across 9 different maps as shown in Table 1, we can be confident that the system will perform accurately and reliably in a wide range of real-world scenarios. This level of accuracy and completeness is essential for using Autonomous ground truth labeling, which has the potential to revolutionize the way we create labeled data sets for training the machine learning-based model. In conclusion, the reliability of autonomous ground truth labeling using the A* algorithm is an efficient way for training deep learning-based path planning algorithms.

2.3 Deep Learning-Base Path-Planning Module

The Deep learning-based path-planning module relies on a C-RNN (Convolutional Recurrent Neural Network). Map images along with the way-points generated by A*, are extracted from CSV. A data preparation step is employed that converts the raw data into CSV format, which is fed to train the C-RNN model. Once the model is trained, a query unknown map can be presented to the system which, outputs the predicted way-points. A summary of these steps is presented in Fig. 1 The C-RNN model consists of a combination of CNN and RNN. CNNs are state-of-the-art feature extractors/classifiers. It is, however important to mention that finding the way-points for the shortest path requires the prediction of a sequence rather than a single class label. The number of way points also varies. CNNs, on the other hand, require a fixed input (fixed number of neurons in the input and output layers). Consequently, CNNs cannot be directly applied for way-point generation and are employed in combination with RNNs. RNNs represent a special type of artificial neural network where units are connected in the form of a directed graph with a sequence. RNN uses memory or internal state for handling the sequence of inputs. RNNs have been successfully employed for problems like speech and handwriting recognition. RNNs exploit the time series information where the previous step affects the next step. There are cycles that provide short memory to the network as illustrated Prior to training the model, a prepossessing step is required that converts the given input into a sequence of features that can be fed for training.

C-RNN (Convolutional Recurrent Neural Network) is the combination of Convolutional Neural Network (CNN) and Recurrent Neural Network (RNN). The combination is known to outperform the performance of individual CNNs or RNNs when it comes to modeling sequential data. In our implementation, we feed the images along with ground truth way-points of the shortest path to the C-RNN. The convolutional layers in the CNN act as feature extractors and the resulting activation sequences are fed to the recurrent layers. Sequence labeling is carried out in the recurrent layers implemented using the Long Short Term Memory (LSTM) units. LSTM represents a special type of recurrent unit with three gates, input, output and forget. For storing contexts for a long time, we use the input and output gates, while forget gate is used for clearing a memory. We combine the forward and backward LSTM resulting in a bidirectional LSTM. It converts the feature map into feature sequences that are fed back to the convolutional layers. Figure 1 illustrates the model training using C-RNN. Once the model is trained, a query map with starting and end locations is presented to the system. To study the effectiveness of the C-RNN model in deep learning-based path planning, we trained the system using 9 different maps. The map dataset comprises more than 30000 different scenarios of the maps. The idea of using scenarios of 9 different maps in the training set is to capture as much variation in data as possible. Following are the results. Table 2 shows the results of a classification task performed on a dataset, which has been divided into two subsets: a training set and a testing set.

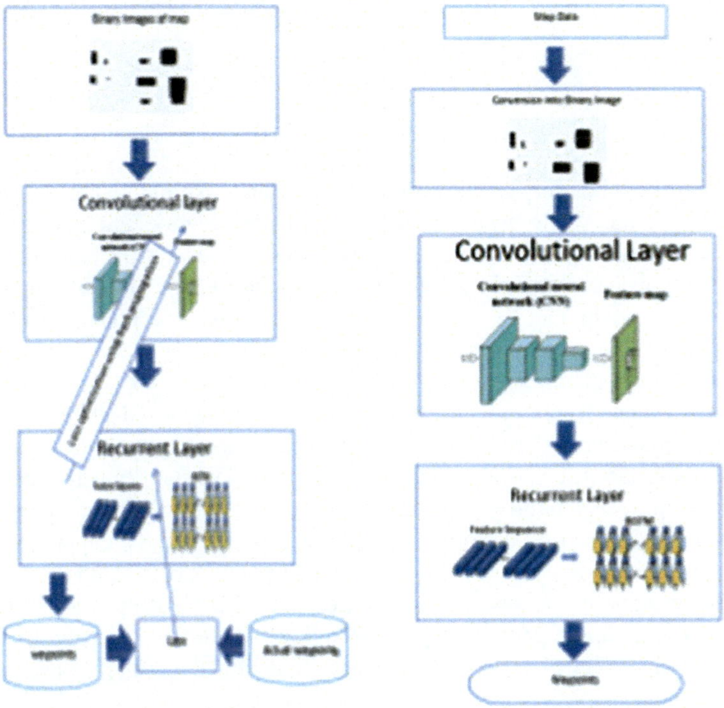

((a)) Training for deep learning-based path-planning module

((b)) Testing for deep learning-based path-planning module

Fig. 1. Deep learning-based path-planning module

The first row of the table corresponds to the training set, which contains 27,000 scenarios. The classification model has been trained on this set, and its performance on this data is summarized in the second column. The accuracy achieved on the training set is 92.5%, which means that the model correctly classified 92.5% of the scenarios in the training set. The second row of the table corresponds to the testing set, which contains 3,000 scenarios that were not used during the training phase. The model's performance on this set is summarized in the third column. The accuracy achieved on the testing set is 61%, which means that the model correctly classified 61% of the scenarios in the testing set. In order to meet the completeness criteria in path planning, we will present the concept of adaptive autonomy in Sect. 2.3.

Table 2. Classification table for training and testing.

Group	number of scenarios	Accuracy
Training	27000	92.5%
Testing	3000	61%

2.4 Introducing Adaptive Autonomy

Introducing adaptive autonomy can be a valuable addition to path-planning algorithms that use deep learning. While deep learning can provide accurate and efficient path planning, it may not always be able to find the path. In such cases, if the deep learning-based path planning algorithm fails to generate a complete path, an alternate approach, such as the A* algorithm, can be used to generate a path. A* is a popular algorithm used for finding the shortest and complete path between two points in the map, and it is widely used in for path planning.

The given algorithm 2 represents an approach called "Introducing adaptive autonomy to path planning algorithm". The algorithm iterates N times and each time takes an input map with a list of obstacles, a starting point, and an endpoint. The algorithm then attempts to find a path using a deep learning-based model. If the deep learning-based model fails to find a path, the algorithm then uses the A* algorithm to find a path. This approach is an example of adaptive autonomy, where the algorithm adapts its level of autonomy based on the success or failure of the deep learning based model. If the deep learning-based model succeeds in finding a path, the algorithm relies on it for subsequent iterations, but if it fails, the algorithm switches to the A* algorithm, which is a more conventional approach for path planning.

Algorithm 2 Introducing adaptive autonomy to path planning algorithm

```
for Iteration = 1, 2, . . . , N do
    Input map with a list of obstacles, a starting point, and an endpoint Find path using
    deep learning-based model if The deep learning-based model failed then
        Find path using A*
    end
end
```

To introduce adaptive autonomy into this scenario, the robot can be programmed to switch from the deep learning-based path planning algorithm to the A* algorithm if the former fails to generate a complete path. The robot can also adjust its level of autonomy as it switches to the A* algorithm. For example, the robot can be given a higher level of autonomy to navigate through the environment using A* and a lower level of autonomy once it has found a complete path. By introducing adaptive autonomy in this way, the robot can increase its chances of finding a complete path to its goal, even in cases where the deep learning-based path planning algorithm fails. This approach can help make path-planning algorithms more robust and adaptable to changes in the environment.

3 Results

Predicted way-points and output using deep learning-based path planning are shown in Fig. 2. This shows it is able to find the shortest path between two points by avoiding the obstacle. The table presents a comparison of the time efficiency in milliseconds of two path-planning algorithms, A* and a deep learning-based algorithm, for different maps with varying obstacle types and areas. The table consists of five columns:

1. "Map" denotes the label given to each map for reference.
2. "Obstacles type" describes the type of obstacle present on the map.
3. "Area of Obstacles (percentage)" represents the percentage of the total map area covered by obstacles.
4. "A*" denotes the time taken by the A* algorithm to plan a path on the given map.
5. "Deep learning-based path-planning algorithm" represents the time taken by the deep learning-based algorithm to plan a path on the given map.

Overall, the table demonstrates that the deep learning-based algorithm is more efficient than A* in terms of time for planning paths on maps with various obstacles. The deep learning-based algorithm consistently takes around 10 ms, while A* takes longer and its time efficiency varies significantly depending on the complexity and size of the obstacles. Table 3 shows deep learning-based path-planning algorithm outperforms the sample-based algorithm concerning time efficiency in every map containing obstacles. For map M0 has no obstacle, A* has more computational time than CRNN as A* always

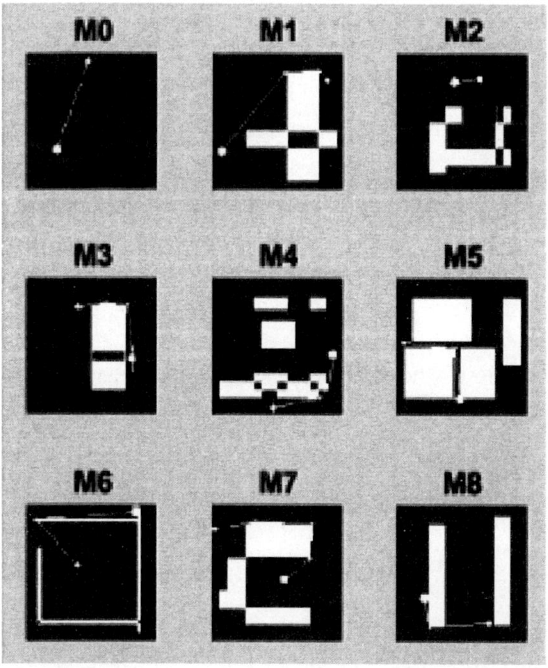

Fig. 2. Results of vision based path-planning module

explores the path in the direction of the goal point. In contrast, a deep learning-based model has a neural network that can find waypoints from full map images in a single evaluation. As a result, the computation time for a deep learning-based path planner remains consistent across various maps, while it varies for A*.

Table 3 results also demonstrate that, in comparison to A*, the deep learning-based path planner exhibits significantly greater time efficiency for M_1 through M_8. Additionally, our findings indicate that A* requires more time to identify a path for maps with larger concave obstacles. This is evident from the computation time for M_8, which is greater than that of other maps.

Table 3. Performance comparison between A* and Deep learning-based path planning algorithm.

Map	Obstacles type	Area of Obstacles (percentage)	A* Time (ms)	Deep learning-based path-planning algorithm Time (ms)
M0	No Obstacle	0	.11	10
M1	One plus sign	29	1612	10
M2	One big concave Obstacle	17	3500	10
M3	one vertical Obstacle	17	1603	10
M4	4 different sizes of rectangular obstacle	21	5722	10
M5	4 big rectangular obstacle	43	2011	11
M6	1 very big concave	7	8315	10
M7	One big concave Obstacle	24	5323	10
M8	2 vertical Obstacle	20	2063	11

3.1 Limitation

When faced with situations where the deep learning-based path planner cannot ensure completeness, we have opted for a sample-based method using adaptive autonomy. Although the current implementation of the deep learning-based path planner displays impressive time efficiency, it relies on the assumption of grid world environments with rectangular shapes and unit node costs.

4 Conclusion

Our proposal involves a novel approach to address path-planning issues through the utilization of a CRNN-based deep learning model, trained with labeled data produced by the A* Algorithm. Moreover, introducing adaptive autonomy to path-planning algorithms that use CRNN-based deep learning and A* can be an effective way to ensure completeness and reliability in robot path-planning tasks. Additionally, we have designed software to generate the labeled data and introduced the concept of adaptive autonomy to ensure path completeness. Our experimentation has demonstrated that this algorithm significantly enhances efficiency in terms of time. In the future, reinforcement learning (RL)techniques will be introduced to improve the completeness of generated paths instead of relying solely on deep learning-based path-planning algorithms. By incorporating RL into the path generation process, the system could learn to make adjustments to the paths based on feedback from the environment, such as obstacles or other unexpected obstacles. This could potentially result in more robust and complete paths, capable of handling a wider range of environments and scenario

References

1. Guruji, A.K., Agarwal, H.,Parsediya, D.K.: Time-efficient A* algorithm for robot path planning. Procedia Technol. **23**, 144–149 (2016). 3rd International Conference on Innovations in Automation and Mechatronics Engineering 2016, ICIAME 2016 05–06 February 2016. ISSN 2212-0173
2. Hart, P.E., Nilsson, N.J., Raphael, B.: A formal basis for the heuristic determination of minimum cost paths. IEEE Trans. Syst. Sci. Cybern. **4**(2), 100–107 (1968). Publisher: IEEE
3. Algfoor, Z.A., Sunar, M.S., Kolivand, H.: A comprehensive study on pathfinding techniques for robotics and video games. Int. J. Comput. Games Technol. (2015)
4. Kala, R., Shukla, A., Tiwari, R., Rungta, S., Janghel, R.R.: Mobile robot navigation control in moving obstacle environment using genetic algorithm, artificial neural networks and A* algorithm. In: 2009 WRI World Congress on Computer Science and Information Engineering, vol. 4, pp. 705–713, IEEE (2009)
5. Tamar, A., Wu, Y., Thomas, G., Levine, S.,Abbeel, P.: Value iteration networks. arXiv preprint arXiv:1602.02867 (2016)
6. Smith, T.F., Waterman, M.S.: Identification of common molecular subsequences. J. Mol. Biol. **147**, 195–197 (1981)
7. Choudhury, S., et al.: Data-driven planning via imitation learning. Int. J. Robot. Res. **37**(13–14), 1632–1672 (2018)
8. Qureshi, A.H.,Simeonov, A., Bency, M.J., Yip, M.C.: Motion planning networks. In: 2019 International Conference on Robotics and Automation (ICRA), pp. 2118–2124. IEEE(2019)
9. Takahashi, T., Sun, H., Tian, D., Wang, Y.: Learning heuristic functions for mobile robot path planning using deep neural networks. In: Proceedings of the International Conference on Automated Planning and Scheduling, vol. 29, pp. 764–772 (2019)
10. Ichter, B., Schmerling, E., Lee, T.W.E., Faust, A.: Learned critical probabilistic roadmaps for robotic motion planning. In: 2020 IEEE International Conference on Robotics and Automation (ICRA), pp. 9535–9541. IEEE (2020)
11. Kim, B., Pineau, J.: Socially adaptive path planning in human environments using inverse reinforcement learning. Int. J. Soc. Robot. **8**(1), 51–66 (2016)
12. Kretzschmar, H., Spies, M., Sprunk, C., Burgard, W.: Socially compliant mobile robot navigation via inverse reinforcement learning. Int. J. Robot. Res. **35**(11), 1289–1307 (2016)
13. Lee, L.,Parisotto, E., Chaplot, D.S., Xing, E., Salakhutdinov, R.: Gated path planning networks. In: International Conference on Machine Learning, pp. 2947–2955. PMLR (2018)
14. Pol, R.S., Murugan, M.: A review on indoor human aware autonomous mobile robot navigation through a dynamic environment survey of different path planning algorithmand methods. In: 2015 International Conference on Industrial Instrumentation and Control (ICIC), pp. 1339–1344. IEEE (2015)

15. Yonetani, R., Taniai, T., Barekatain, M., Nishimura, M., Kanezaki, A.: Path planning using neural A* search. In: International Conference on Machine Learning, pp. 12029–12039 (2021)
16. Scerri, P., Reed, N.: Designing agents for systems with adjustable autonomy. Citeseer (2001)
17. Tang, S.H., Yeong, C.F., Su, E.L.M.: Comparison between normal waveform and modified wavefront path planning algorithm for mobile robot. Appl. Mech. Mater. **607**, 778–781. Trans. Tech. Publ. (2014)
18. Noreen, I., Khan, A., Habib, Z.: Optimal path planning for mobile robots using memory efficient A. In: 2016 International Conference on Frontiers of Information Technology (FIT), pp. 142–146. IEEE (2016)
19. Botea, A., Müller, M., Schaeffer, J.: Near optimal hierarchical path finding. J. Game Dev. 1(1), 1–30. Citeseer (2004)
20. Benders, S., Schopferer, S.: A line-graph path planner for performanceconstrained fixed-wing UAVs in wind fields. In: 2017 International Conference on Unmanned Aircraft Systems (ICUAS), pp. 79–86. IEEE (2017)

An Implementation of Vehicle Data Collection and Analysis

Aaron Liske and Xiangdong Che(✉)

Eastern Michigan University, Ypsilanti, MI, USA
{aliske1,xche}@emich.edu

Abstract. In this work, a prototype for vehicle data collection and analysis based on OBDII protocol is built with only using consumer grade hardware and open-source software. Real-time data via the OBDII port on most any modern vehicle can be retrieved and stored for use later. Potential uses of this data are general data logging and tracking, machine learning, vehicle diagnostics, and fine tuning in performance driving tasks. The data may also be used to compare multiple driver's performances in the same vehicle. This work focuses on vehicles pre-2008 when the modern CAN-Bus was not mandatory in the United States.

Keywords: Data Collection · Driver Behavior Analysis · Driver-Vehicle Systems · Data Processing · OBDII

1 Introduction

While operating a vehicle, could it be an 18-wheeler, a household car, or a performance Formula 1, the drivers usually do not have access to the essential internal vehicle performance readings and parameters, such as oil pressure, oil temperature and current gear, beyond what the dashboard could provide. While an ordinary driver probably does not care, it is critical for a performance driver to know those details and benefit from the analysis of those data. The primary goal of our work is to explore the feasibility of real time data logging and monitoring while the vehicle is in operation. The prototype could be used to assess the driver and the vehicle performance under various driving circumstances. Additionally, the system could be used to monitor and diagnose vehicle issues in real time. The universal On-Board Diagnostics (OBD) has been a vehicle standard in the United States since 1996 [1]. The OBDII port on modern vehicles, and the protocols that the Engine Control Unit (ECU) use to communicate with it, are generally only used by vehicle service professionals. Vehicle service centers have used the OBD interface mainly to retrieve vehicle trouble codes and to perform other diagnostics. This technology has only recently come into the consumer market with USB or Bluetooth scanners and closed software. While there are options available for the consumer, very few of them are capable to collect real time information about driving status and events when a vehicle is in motion. There are also packages that run on iOS or Android devices, but any data is generally stored in a proprietary format and is unavailable for outside analysis [2]. To achieve more open and customizable real-time vehicle data collection and

K. Daimi and A. Al Sadoon (Eds.): ICR 2023, LNNS 721, pp. 129–141, 2023.
https://doi.org/10.1007/978-3-031-35308-6_11

analysis, we adopt OBD port as our data source to build a proof-of-concept experimental framework.

The modern vehicle Controller Area Network ("CAN") Bus was made mandatory for new vehicles in 2008. This is a network between the ECU, driver systems, sensors, and other manufacturer specific items. This network runs about 100 times faster than previously used On Board Diagnostics protocols [3]. While the CAN Bus is a superior network for data transmission in a vehicle, between components, it is often not available on older models of vehicles, and a more primitive method of data acquisition must be utilized. This work will work on newer CAN Bus era vehicles, but there are better alternatives that can directly read that network data.

2 Related Work

There has been other previous work done in this field, ranging from expensive manufacturer-dependent tools to apps for the phone. One such studies was done in 2012, using a Bluetooth OBDII reader and an Android application [4]. This has the benefit of being portable and being able to be moved between different vehicles easily, but the downsides are that it is not expandable, and this solution uses a closed-source application over the phone. Using Bluetooth communications also has the downside of communications latency between the vehicle and device. This solution also saves the data to a flat CSV file on the device.

Some commercial options include the Cobb AccessPort, however these have the disadvantage of being specific to a certain vehicle's make and model. These devices are primarily used for tuning the ECU for performance or economy, but they can also do data recording. These range in price from several hundred to a few thousand dollars, several times more expensive than an open-source solution that can be used by multiple vehicles. Devices such as these also lack expandability and any wireless connectivity for accessing the data stored on them.

3 Materials and Methods

Figure 1 illustrates an overview of the system, including the hardware and data flow in communication, processing, and storage. While there are differences in the implementation of OBD ports by different vendors, the OBDII protocols and regulations standardize the parameters and services used for polling data [5]. The OBDII scanning device runs on the ELM327 chipset, which emulates an RS-232 serial interface on the host system. We use a Raspberry Pi 3B as the main computer which is connected to the OBDII port scanner via USB or Bluetooth. The ELM327 uses a baud rate of 38400, 1 stop bit and 8 data bits, with no parity [5, 6]. In this implementation, it utilizes the ttyUSB0 entry in the /dev Raspberry Pi filesystem. The retrieved data is stored locally on a MySQL server, and then uploaded to a remote data store when uplink with Wi-Fi/cellular network is available.

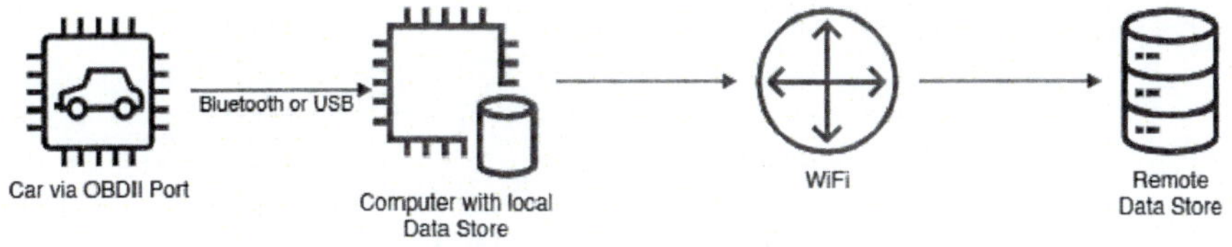

Fig. 1. An Overview of the Prototype System

3.1 Experimental Framework Setup

The wiring of the prototype to integrate into the vehicle electronics is shown in Fig. 2. The on-board TP-Link wireless router and the Raspberry Pi devices are wired into the vehicle power and are protected with a 10-amp fuse. A 12–5 v step-down transformer is used to connect the Raspberry Pi to prevent over-voltage. Instead of using Bluetooth and Wi-Fi, we use USB and 100Base-T to lower power consumption on the Raspberry Pi device during the test. Power should either be run through a switch, or attached to a relay, powered by the ignition switch wire, which prevents the system from being a constant power draw on the vehicle when not in use. A second 12–5 VDC step down transformer with switch was implemented and connected to GPIO01 on the J8 GPIO header on the Raspberry Pi so that the data recording can be toggled on/off while the system was in operation.

When dealing with vehicle operations, safety is paramount. The Sports Car Club of America ("SCCA") rules states that "All loose items, inside and outside the car, must be removed" and "Pedal operation must not be impeded." [6] Thus, the OBDII port device must not have a cord loose or hanging, as that can interfere with the pedal function or get tangled up around the driver's legs in the case of an emergency. We mount the main computer behind the radio head unit, utilizing the existing cable channels through the vehicle firewall. We also make sure all cords are routed behind the dashboard panels, and firmly secured. This prototype is also permitted in the aforementioned rules by the statement "Data acquisition systems (including video cameras) and the accompanying sensors are allowed but may serve no other purpose during a run than real-time display and data recording." [7] In summary, this prototype system falls well within the realm of the aforementioned rules, which also allows for additional sensors to be included in future implementations.

3.2 Sending and Receiving Data

The OBDII port, with the ELM327 bridge, communicates through the serial protocols. The ELM327 settings are commonly notated as "8N1" [5], which is 8 bits, no parity bit, and 1 stop bit. The ELM327 chipset operates on a basic AT-style command structure used for modems. All commands are processed when the carriage return character (hex #0A) is received. The commands give basic control over the function and data formatting of the ELM327. For the purposes of this implementation, echo is set to off, and the line feeds are enabled to ensure data uniformity. When the ELM327 is ready to receive commands, it sends the " >" prompt character. The commands sent are not case sensitive and white spaces are ignored. For example, "AT Z" is the same as "atz", and "01 5C" is the same

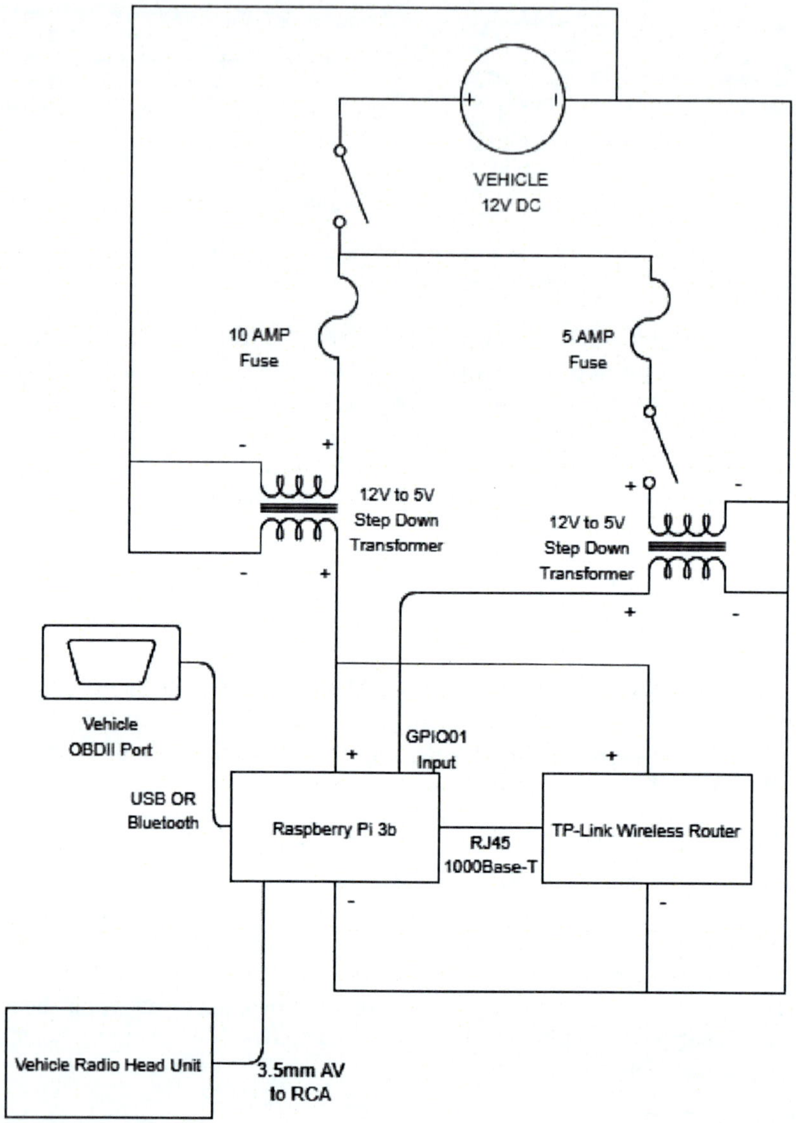

Fig. 2. Shows the vehicle wiring and vehicle integration with the experiment framework.

as "015C" [5]. The ECU operates on a query/response command structure. As shown in Fig. 3, to receive values from the ECU, the "Service" and the "Parameter ID" (PID) must be specified. If a PID is requested that the vehicle is unable to support, it sends either "NO DATA" when it was sent alone, or it is omitted entirely from the return query when it is sent with other PIDs simultaneously. Any number of PIDs can be requested in a single query if they are on the same service.

The response returned from the ECU is predictable and can be interpreted easily with software. Each PID has a set number of bytes that are expected from it, and a formula to turn the returned hex values into a human-readable value, which changes per PID. The commands are sent in the structure of <Service> {PID #1}[{PID #2}...]. When only a carriage return character is sent, the previous command is repeated. The Service number and the first PID is required, then up to six PIDs can be added to the query. The response comes in on multiple lines, first with the length of the response in bytes and written in a three-digit hex number with leading zeroes, then the response starting with the responding responder's identifier, then the listing of each PID and the response for that, in sequence. Sometimes, the order received is not the same order sent, which cannot be hard coded for interpretation. With the responses being a predictable length, the interpreter software was written to verify data integrity. The encoding used for the responses is UTF-8 text [5]. Figure 3 demonstrates the ECU processing of queries and commands and building the output string to be sent through the ELM327 chipset, back to the user.

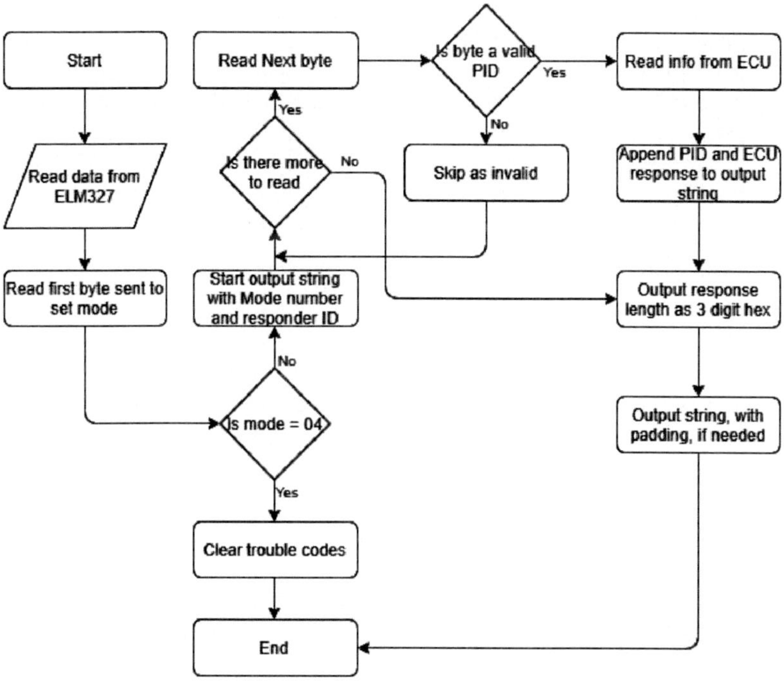

Fig. 3. ECU Processing

Once the settings are set in the software, the device can be connected, and data retrieved. According to the ELM327 data sheet, the device itself is controlled via a basic AT style command set, which simplifies and standardizes the commands on different devices that use the same chipset. Table 1 outlines a list of commonly used commands to set up the data output as well as verify communication with the vehicle's Engine Control Unit.

Table 1. Common AT style Commands

Z	Hard reset the device
WS	Soft reset the device
E0, E1	Turn command echoing off or on
L0, L1	Turn line feed off or on
@1	Display the device identifier
DP	Display the vehicle protocol used
RV	Display the voltage on the battery pin

The vehicle ECU uses various "services" number as memory banks for various purposes. Each of these have various Parameter IDs (PIDs) that return the values, in a predictable length and format. Table 2 lists the different standard services offered by the protocol, keeping in mind that some vehicles may not include all of them [8].

Table 2. Standard ECU Service List

Service Number	Name
01	General Data
02	Saved Data
03	Requests Trouble Codes
04	Resets Trouble Codes
05	02 Sensor Bank Data
09	Vehicle Information

All of the services have PIDs that are used to query the data. The exception of this is Service 04, which is used to clear the trouble codes from the vehicle, without a PID. Each PID returns a set number of bytes [9], and using a conversion formula, this can be made human-readable for interpretation and storage. Table 3 shows some of the PIDs used in the software developed and the formula to decode it. All of the values are sent in UTF-8 encoded hex values [5]. When data is returned for each PID, each set of two bytes in the response is one segment of the overall response, with the first being denoted as "A" in the formula, second is "B", and so on, until the next PID response.

Table 3. PIDs used in the Prototype

PID	Name	Response Length	Formula
45	Throttle Position	2 Bytes	(100 * A)/255
05	Coolant Temperature	2 Bytes	A-40
0C	Engine RPM	4 Bytes	((256 * A) + B)/4
0D	Vehicle Speed	2 Bytes	A

Once we are able to query and interpret the responses, we use the jSerialComm library in Java to achieve bi-directional serial communications. Because of the nature of serial port communications, without sequencing control, it cannot be guaranteed that the entirety of the response will be received in a single polling cycle. The window for listening for a response begins when the ELM327 chipset receives the carriage return character (hex #0A) and ends when the prompt character (" >") is received. All the spaces and new line characters are stripped out so that the response turns into a single string before it is parsed.

The first three characters in the response from the ELM327 is the response length in bytes with leading zeroes. Following that, the data is split on multiple lines with line numbers. The line number is a single digit from 0-F (repeating) followed by a colon. The standard response has 12 bytes in the first line (line 0), then 14 bits in the following lines. In the final line, the full 14 bits is filled with zeroes as padding if they are not used. For most PIDs or in the case of bit encoded values, the data is parsed using a formula, looked up from an enumeration table, e.g. the Available PID Query (Service 1, PID 00, 20, 30 and 40).

Once the data is interpreted into a human readable format, it is available to be stored, displayed, or otherwise used. In this implementation, the data is displayed on a Graphical User Interface (GUI) and updated as new data becomes available from the software interpreter. Data can also be stored to a database, along with the timestamps of the data interpretation. Data can either be stored as raw values, or the parsed values. By using a cellular router with 3G or 4G capabilities, the software should be able to connect to a database directly. If that is not available, then the database server can be installed locally on the computer used. The data can be uploaded at a later date, over Wi-Fi or wired ethernet.

Due to safety requirements, the prototype system must be mounted in the vehicle while the vehicle's radio head unit is used as the monitor using the A/V connection. Because the head unit does not support any input thought the A/V connection, we need to develop an automatic polling process with GUI. When the vehicle starts and the OBDII port scanner is ready to accept commands, the automatic process will poll available ports, set the baud rate, and send the appropriate reset and formatting commands periodically. Generally speaking, the vehicle responds to commands after the vehicle is turned on or in "Accessory" mode, although different years, makes, and models might respond differently. The GUI also must gracefully display status report when data is unavailable for the various values.

3.3 Proof of Concept

As displayed in Fig. 4, we use the "screen" command to query the device identifier, vehicle protocol, and all of the available Service 1 PIDs. Figure 5 shows the device is reset, echo and line feeds are turned on, and a few PIDs in Service 01 are queried, including 5C, which is not supported by the vehicle's ECU. We successfully establish the communication by using consumer grade equipment and free software in the built-in repositories of Raspbian OS. This is the proof of concept that our design of the prototype is valid and can support further development to query and interpret the data from modern vehicles that employ the OBDII standard protocols.

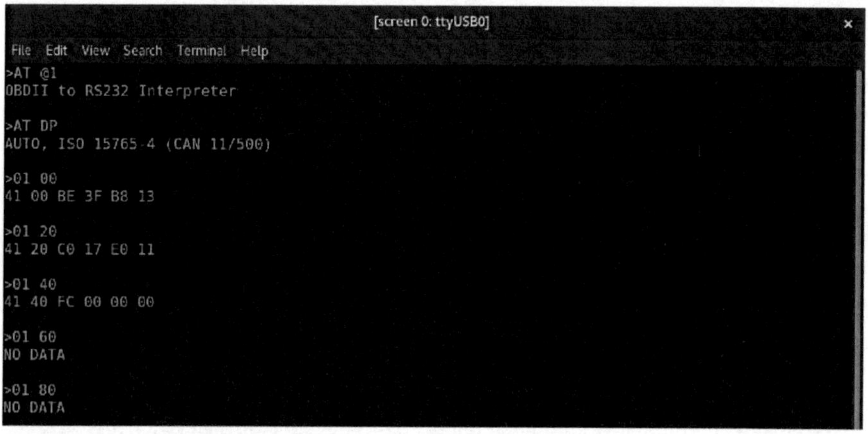

Fig. 4. The "screen" terminal command output Part 1

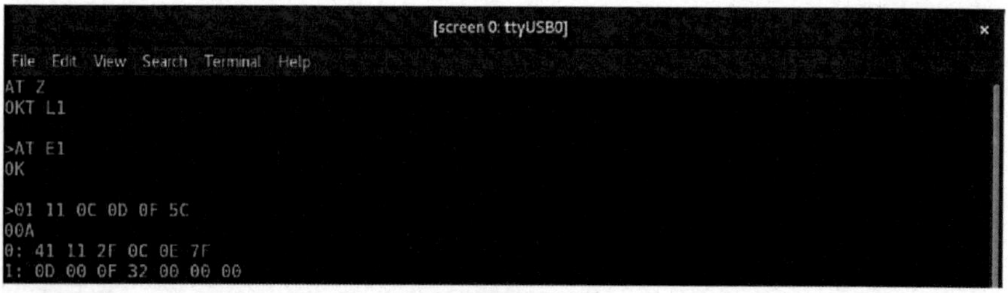

Fig. 5. The "screen" terminal command output Part 2

3.4 Software Development

Following the validation step by the proof of concept using the terminal emulation, we develop the stand-alone software. We use Java 8 and Java AWT Swing for the GUI design, and the jSerialComm library for reading and writing to the serial port, as the Java Virtual Machine does not have native support for serial or parallel communications. Figure 6 shows a screenshot of the GUI interface displaying the various live data collected from a connected vehicle in motion. The readings are displayed in metric because the formulas for value converting are based on metric system. Data not valid for the vehicle or not being retrieved for any reason is shown as "N/A".

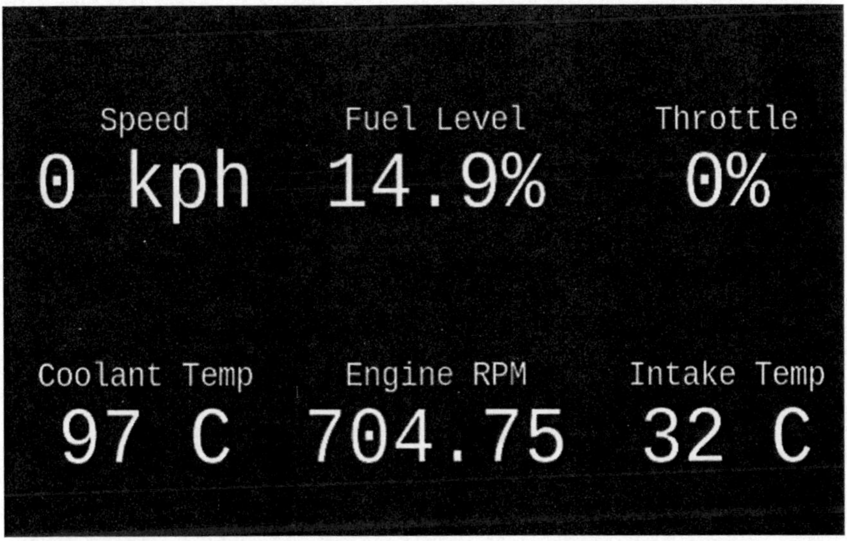

Fig. 6. A Display of Live Data Collected from a Vehicle in Motion

Once the responses were able to be queried and interpreted, the next step was writing the software for automating the polling and recording process. Using open-source software and libraries, the software itself can be written relatively cheaply and quickly. For this purpose, Java was used as the base programming language, which had the added issue of not having serial or parallel communications standard in the Java Virtual Machine because of the differences in how operating systems handle communications differently, so it has never been fully natively supported. This was achieved, using the jSerialComm library, which was freely available. Once bi-directional serial communications were achieved, the data could be freely retrieved and parsed from the vehicle.

Because of the nature of serial port communications, without sequencing control, it cannot be guaranteed that the entirety of the response will be received in a single polling cycle. The window for listening for a response begins when the ELM327 chipset receives the carriage return character (hex #0A), and it ends when the prompt character (" >") is received. All of that data can be stored in a single string, then parsed. The way that this was done in the software written for this was that all the spaces and new line characters were stripped out, so the response was a single string, and then it was parsed.

The settings of the application are saved and loaded from a configuration file upon startup. When the software starts, it gives the user a set amount of time to change a value, or the screen times out and attempts to start with the pre-loaded values from the configuration file. This file can be edited in any standard text editor, remotely. By implementing the configuration file and the screen timeout, it mitigates the need for user input devices to be utilized, other than initial setup. This is ideal, so that the user does not need to always have a keyboard and mouse in the vehicle.

Table 4 shows the table schema used for data storage in a local MySQL database during an active data collection. A Redis database was used as a caching intermediary location due to the write limitations of the Raspberry Pi that was being used. This stored data can be parsed by an external parser for analysis and use. We use the system time in milliseconds for timestamp. The response is the raw data output from the OBDII port. This universal table format allows for any dataset to be collected and stored. The entire response is stored as a single string so that it can be extracted and parsed directly with the R programming studio and analyzed as a CSV data source, but in the database form, it can be queried based on the timestamps, since the only source of data is the individual vehicle. Another reason to store the entire string was that parsing the string only amplified the data write bottlenecks that were being experienced on the hardware given.

Table 4. A universal table schema used for data storage.

Field	Type	Null	Key	Extra
id	int(11)	NO	PRI	auto_increment
timestamp	bigint(20)	YES		
response	varchar(1000)	YES		

After the data collection, we can run the data through a parser to retrieve the "Human Readable" values. Table 5 shows the outcome in terms of collected PIDs. These values were saved to a CSV file for charting and analysis in this implementation.

Table 5. Service 1 PIDs used in this implementation.

PID	Description
45	Relative Throttle (%)
05	Coolant Temperature (C)
0C	Engine Revolutions Per Minute
0D	Vehicle Speed (KPM)
0F	Intake Air Temperature (C)
2F	Fuel Tank Level (%)

4 Results

This implementation makes it evident that data logging on vehicles is possible. Using this data, even without the aid of GPS, it is possible to evaluate and compare the drivers against each other. By integrating the speed over time, the distance can be calculated, and used as a possible metric. Figure 13 displays the speed over distance graph. This shows areas where one driver braked or accelerated more efficiently than the other, and it demonstrates the distance length between the two attempts on the course. This allows the course elements to be lined up and evaluated, with a slight margin of error, due to the different lines a driver might take, to negotiate the course, relative to the elements in the course.

With this prototype system, we can extract, store, and parse the data from the OBD port. The goal of this implementation is to analyze the data that the car generates and use it as a foundation to establish further research on vehicle monitoring, safety control. Figure 12 and Fig. 13 shows a demonstration of using the data collected by the prototype for driving performance analysis. In Fig. 7, the time-series of vehicle speed, throttle, coolant temperature and engine RPMs are displayed while the date was collected from a single attempt drive by a single driver on a driving course of approximately 1 km in length. The coolant temperature and engine RPMs are merely demonstrative data points, but we can potentially observe how performance related data correlated with all other vehicle status data from this diagram. Since the data was based on a single attempt at the course, it did not show where the driver improved or regressed over time, in terms of performance.

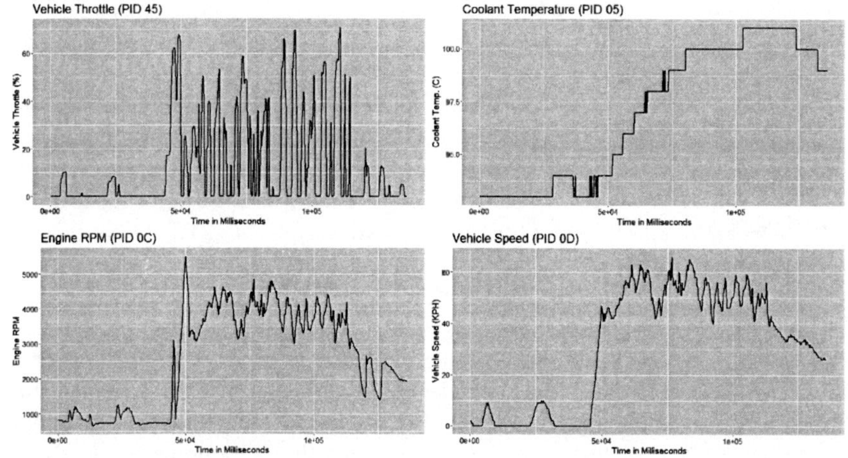

Fig. 7. Vehicle Data over 1 km driving course. The horizontal axis indicates elapsed time since the recording

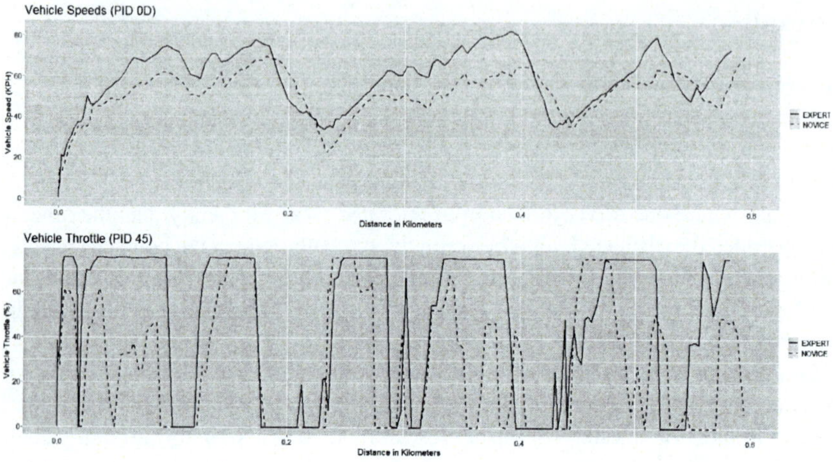

Fig. 8. Performance comparison of two drivers

Figure 8 displays, side by side, the performance of two drivers with different experience navigating the same course in the same vehicle. Comparing and contrast the relevant datasets collected will provide the "Novice" driver insight into where performance could be improved using the expert driver's results as a baseline.

For example, the experienced driver finished the course 5.512 s ahead of the novice driver, as shown in the figure. This is due to a difference in the lines taken through the course, demonstrated by the differences in distance. The total distance for the novice driver was 0.5943 km, and the total distance for the experienced driver was 0.5813 km, for a difference of 0.013 km. It should be noted that due to the vehicle configuration, the maximum throttle possible was ~ 75.19%. Due to this, a scaling was applied to each data point in the "Vehicle Throttle (PID 45)" chart, to accurately display the maximum as 100%. The mean speed of the novice was 47.866 km per hour, with an adjusted mean throttle use of 39.407% ($n = 179$), and a raw mean throttle use of 29.669%. The mean speed of the experienced driver was 53.446 km per hour, with an adjusted mean throttle use of 59.084% ($n = 157$), and a raw mean throttle use of 44.484%. Of a set of five attempts per driver, the fastest attempt for each were used.

While the data is gathered, as a function of time, it is difficult to make assumptions on the faults of the novice driver because each driver reached each element of the course at a different time. Figure 8 also demonstrates how this was overcome by calculating the integral of speed over time, as actual GPS data was unavailable for this implementation. The course in this example was approximately 0.58 km in length. This allows the braking and acceleration points of each driver to be shown and allows for proper comparison.

With the data polling, there was variation in the time between each data record, the delta time. The delta time minimum was 210 ms, maximum was 340, with a mean delta time of 250.89 ms, where $n = 336$. This is likely due to the software polling speed and may be able to be improved up in future iterations with optimization in processing.

5 Conclusions and Future Work

In conclusion, it is feasible to extract, interpret and process live vehicle data from the OBDII port on modern vehicles using low-cost consumer grade hardware and open-source software. With proper design, our prototype can be integrated in a vehicle in a manner that is safe for the driver. Since we use Raspberry Pi as the main computing platform, the system is highly modular and expandable with additional function modules and sensors. Evaluation and comparison between different drivers in similar vehicles have practical applications in performance driving analysis, vehicle diagnostics. The prototype system shall have a broad scope of applications, stretching from simple vehicle diagnostics to performance-based settings and control. In the future, we will integrate the prototype with the growing Vehicular Ad hoc Network, for vehicle-to-vehicle communications systems. This would allow the vehicles on the network to "see" the other vehicle's speed, locations, and direction of travel, to reduce collisions [10]. With the on-board wireless network installed, a mobile interface may also be implemented to display the data to anyone who connects to it, and not just available to the driver. Future versions of this implementation may include GPS data, live charting of the data, and an inclusion of an accelerometer to calculate g-forces on the vehicle. The UI can also be optimized for more radio head units that can support touch interfaces with attached devices. This would allow for a better user interface and further customization for the user. The data gathered from an implementation such as this can be used for general data logging, driver training, and vehicle tuning.

References

1. OBDII: Past, Present & Future (2012). www.autotap.com/techlibrary/obdii_past_present_future.asp [Retrieved: April 2021]
2. Haq, A.U., Ali, S., Rehman: OBDII, Android and OpenERP Based Vehicle's 3M System. KS Omniscriptum Publishing (2015)
3. Walter, R., Walter, E.: Data Acquisition From HD Vehicles Using J1939 CAN Bus. SAE International (2016)
4. Cabala, M., Gamec, J.: Wireless real-time vehicle monitoring based on android mobile device. Acta Electrotechnica et Informatica **12**(4), 7–11 (2012). https://doi.org/10.2478/v10198-012-0039-x
5. ELM327 (2016). https://www.elmelectronics.com/wp-content/uploads/2016/07/ELM327DS.pdf [Retrieved: April 2021]
6. Anusha, et al.: RS232 Protocol – Basics. Electronics Hub, 30 July 2018. www.electronicshub.org/rs232-protocol-basics/
7. 2020 SCCA National Solo Rules. Sports Car Club of America (2020)
8. Seyfert, K.: OBD II Generic PID Diagnosis (2007). www.motor.com/magazine-summary/obd-ii-generic-pid-diagnosis-september-2007. [Retrieved: January 2021]
9. "Supported OBDII Parameters." OBD, www.obdautodoctor.com/obd-parameters. [Retrieved: March 2021]
10. Vehicle-to-Vehicle Communication. NHTSA, 18 Dec. 2019, www.nhtsa.gov/technology-innovation/vehicle-vehicle-communication

Data, Recommendation Techniques, and View (DRV) Model for Online Transaction

Abdussalam Ali[1,2](✉), Waleed Ibrahim[3,4], and Sabreena Zoha[5]

[1] Australian Catholic University, Canberra, Australia
abdussalam.ali@acu.edu.au
[2] Asia Pacific International College (APIC), Parramatta, Australia
[3] The University of Sydney, Sydney, Australia
waleed.ibrahim@sydney.edu.au
[4] Central Queensland University, Rockhampton, Australia
[5] Western Sydney University, Sydney, Australia
s.zoha@westernsydney.edu.au

Abstract. With the development of information technology, online transactions, including E-commerce, have been developed. Accordingly, recommendation systems were developed to facilitate customer preferences and increase business revenue. In this paper, our analysis shows that each of these systems was implemented to facilitate the recommendation process of a specific product or service category and applied to a dedicated context. The issue here is if the business provides more than one category of products and/or services it needs to utilize more than one approach to have an effective recommendation process. That would make it more complicated to implement and with a high cost. In addition, each of these systems was developed to overcome a specific problem. There is no guarantee that the system developed to address a dedicated problem could overcome the other problems. Examples of these problems include cold-start, data sparsity, accuracy, and diversity. In this paper, we develop Data, Recommendation Technique, and View (DRV) model. We consider this model to be a foundation for a generic framework to develop recommendation systems that overcome the issues mentioned.

Keywords: Recommendation Systems · Content Based · Collaborative Based · Hybrid · Cold Start · Accuracy

1 Introduction

Recommendation systems had become widely used and utilized by the development of information technology. E-commerce and online transaction services were emerged and developed throughout this technology. E-commerce and online transaction services are those services implemented to facilitate the selling and buying processes on the Internet [1, 2]. Accordingly, many categories of products and services are purchased throughout the Internet. Although there is a debate in differentiating between the product and service, in this paper, we consider the product as it refers to the tangible goods while the service refers to the intangible [3, 4]. Recommendation systems play the role of promoting

K. Daimi and A. Al Sadoon (Eds.): ICR 2023, LNNS 721, pp. 142–152, 2023.
https://doi.org/10.1007/978-3-031-35308-6_12

these products and services to customers on regular bases. These systems recommend products and services based on the customer's behavior and preference. One advantage of recommendation systems is personalizing the customer's preferences. That makes it easy for the user to reach the products he/she prefers. The other advantage is that these systems support businesses to establish proper marketing strategies to achieve business outcomes [5]. As per the literature each of these recommendation systems is developed to support specific categories of products or services. Also, each of these recommendation systems and models was developed to overcome specific defined problems and issues. These problems include cold-start, data sparsity, accuracy, scalability, and diversity. The question here is, how the organization or the business does choose the proper recommendation system for the products or services it sells? However, the business may sell products, services, or both.

In this paper, we explored various literature and research to investigate different recommendation systems and models. We analyzed the findings of the literature review to define the main issues and problems of these models based on the previous questions and argument.

In this paper, we present what we call Data, Recommendation Technique, and View (DRV) model based on literature analysis. The model is a taxonomy developed based on three components: the data utilized by recommendation systems, approaches used (the techniques), and the view (the way to present the data to the user). This model provides a kind of presentation on how these components are related to each other based on the models reviewed. We followed the DRV model with a discussion and how it might benefit from the model to develop a framework so the needs of the recommendation process can be customized and supported easily.

The structure of this paper starts with the introduction which provides a clear idea about the paper and its purpose. The literature review is followed and summarized in an illustrated table. The proposed model was then presented and followed by the discussion and conclusion.

2 Literature Review

The content-based (CB) approach and collaborative filtering (CF) approach are the two known approaches used to develop recommendation systems [6]. In the CB approach the information related to the items is used to generate the recommendations that match the user profile. The major issue of the CB approach is the process of learning about the preferences of the user and how to match them with the other items. CF approach relies on the relationships between users and items. The recommendations for the user are created by looking to the preferences of other users who purchased the same items. Hybrid approach is the other approach that combines both, CB, and CF approaches. The CF approach is considered the most popular [7].

Various research and literature that developed recommendation systems and models, based on the three approaches, have been reviewed.

Mezni and Abdeljaoued [8] have developed Fuzzy Formal Concept Analysis (Fuzzy FCA) model to facilitate the recommending of the cloud computing services. Two main issues have been addressed, data sparsity and cold-start. The model was developed by utilizing the lattice theory approach. The authors report that FCA organizes the links of user-service-rating in a hierarchical manner. By this way the hidden relations will be considered to find out the similarities between users for more efficient recommendation outcomes. Meznin and Abdelijaoued [8] used user profiles to match with other users.

Wei et al. [7] designed their approach to address the cold-start problem and applied their approach on Netflix movies. The authors implemented a general framework based on CF and machine learning to design recommendation systems. The model [7] showed good results over the previously implemented models. Further work is needed in terms of the techniques used for the evaluation and applying the system on other categories of products as per authors.

Hsieh et al. [9] designed the keyword-aware recommender model to overcome the cold-start problem. It acquires the data from the external domains based on the user's keywords. In addition to the user keywords and profile the model extends the search through Big Data over the Internet. The authors found that the model provided high degree of accuracy and efficiency. One of the limitations of the model that it has not been evaluated on different contexts. That is in addition to the privacy, security, and client-server issues as mentioned by the authors.

Zhang et al. [10] address the problem of recommendation in micro-blog as crowd-sensing tool for sharing information. With the increasing of such micro-blogs, it is difficult for the user to find the related topics that they search for. The authors developed their model to address such problem throughout two steps. First, building the relationships between the users. Second, utilizing specific algorithms to compute the similarities between the users according to their preferred topics. The authors report that their model is accurate and efficient with some degree. More research for future work is to be conducted in accordance to tracking, recognition and credibility issues [10].

Chai et al. [11] proposed their model of recommendation to address the diversity-accuracy problem. This problem refers to the fact that if the recommendation system focuses on the diversity that will lead to accuracy loss. The goal is to implement a model that considers the diversity without losing accuracy. Authors developed their model based on collaborative filtering by utilizing singular value decomposition (SVD) with multi-objective immune algorithm (MOIA). The authors conclude that the model provides good results by producing recommendation list with high degree of accuracy and diversity for a specific user. However, the model still needs improvements for better efficiency and accuracy [11].

Accuracy-diversity problem has been addressed by Gan and Jiang [12] as well. They have proposed their model based on what is called network-based collaborative filtering. The approach relies on the concept of filtering out the weak relationships between users. Accordingly, the similarity network is constructed, and the scores are calculated. The model has been applied on data set derived from MovieLens and Netflix. The authors mention that the model achieved excellent results as the accuracy and diversity have been improved due to removing of the weak relationships between users. Further work is needed, as per authors, to implement the system based on the items rather than the users.

Xu et al. [13] implemented their system to support the recommendation process by finding the suitable information in relation to different domains, such as proper jobs, experts, and projects. The system has been developed to address the difficulty to search within Big Data and achieving a good recommendation about the domain and topic needed. The other issue is the disconnection dilemma between the information creator and the information searcher. To overcome such issues authors developed their system based on two-stage process for R&D projects recommendation. These two stages are profiling and matching. In the profiling stage the system searches within different websites about the R&D projects. In the second stage, the similarities are discovered by utilizing a matching algorithm according to the user profile. These similarities are filtered to select the suitable list for the user. It has been verified that the requirements of the researchers can be met in an effective way compared to the other methods. The authors report that some issues are to be addressed for future development. One of these, the system does not support the processing of user feedback as a valued source of information. Also, the system is limited to a specific information service, R&D projects search.

Yun et al. [14] address the prediction accuracy problem in CF algorithm. In this paper, the authors mention that the traditional methods of gathering user data are not effective, because they aren't sufficient to find the user interest and preferences. The paper proposes the opinion mining technique to support the CF algorithm for better performance of recommendation. Opinion mining approach relies on users reviews as input data. The proposed solution has been adopted by the authors from the bases that the other approaches are more quantitative based. This approach combines both the quantitative and qualitative data. The authors conclude that by utilizing the after-sale feedback the accuracy of predictability increases. There are some issues require further work and research. One of these, is the combined words that refer to one meaning. The other problem is that not every user provides feedback.

Liu, and Wu [15] developed their model to address the cold-start and context-aware problems. To address this problem the approach utilizes what is called buffer update and sampling methods. The model focuses on large scale recommendation systems and the top N items supposed to be preferred by the user. The authors mention that the model is flexible as it can be utilized in different domains.

Ahn [16] proposed his model to address the cold-start problem when there is a small number of ratings for a specific user. The aim is to enhance the performance when the number of ratings is small but not zero. According to the authors, a new technique of similarity calculation has been implemented out of this research to replace the traditional techniques. In this approach more data is needed and less modifications in the CF methods are required.

Other approaches such as content-based (CB) and hybrid models have been utilized to implement various recommendation systems as well.

Achakulvisut et al. [17] and Wang et al. [18] developed their models based on the CB approach to facilitate the recommendation of the academic publications. The model developed by Wang et al. [18] is, however, dedicated to computer science related publications. The two models have been developed as there is a lack in facilitating the recommendation process for scientific publications [17, 18].

Ochirbat et al. [19] built occupation recommendation system that integrates both collaborative filtering and content-based filtering. Although the research successfully builds the hybrid system, the user may bias towards a specific option by different influences.

Kanavos et al. [20] developed their Supermarket model to facilitate utilizing Big Data, in addition to the user behavior, as a source of data to enhance the recommendation process outcomes. There system has been implemented in the cloud environment by utilizing cloud computing tools. The authors report that the system is dataset limited and more datasets to be added for experiment and evaluation in the future.

Scholz et al. [21] proposed the decision support system for e-commerce user, based on the hybrid system with attribute weights on items. They report that the method utilized in their system has better accuracy measures compared to the other methods.

A number of the latest literature that is based on Artificial Intelligence (AI). Systems presented in these papers using Neural Networks (NN) deep learning approach by implementing deep long-short term memory (LSTM) technique. These papers include [22, 23] and [24]. These approach utilize NN to overcome issues that are common in the traditional approaches such as the accuracy and the lack of adequate data to overcome the cold-start situation.

Based on the literature investigated we illustrate the Table 1 below to present the main attributes and related patterns to present our model later. These attributes are listed as following:

- Reference: refers to the source of the information.
- Problem addressed: the issue or the problem addressed by the source.
- Technique: the recommendation approach adopted by the source authors.
- Context: the context represents the domain that the recommendation model/system has been utilized or evaluated within.
- Deliverables: this attribute has two sub-attributes, Type and Regularity. The Type sub-attribute indicates what type of deliverable the recommendation system is used for, a product, service, or both. The Regularity sub-attribute indicates if the deliverable is rarely or regularly purchased by the customers.
- Data: this attribute indicates the sort of the data utilized by the system. This data can be implicit or explicit. The system uses one of the two types or both. Explicit data [21] is the data that generated voluntarily by the user such as the rating provided. The implicit data [21] is the data that created by using the system such as the clicks of the users in different items, their history of browsing and consuming the product or services.

Table 1. Literature Analysis (CF = Collaborative Filtering, CB = Content-Based Filtering, H = Hybrid, NN = Neural Networks)

					Deliverables				Data	
No	Reference	Problem Addressed	Technique	Context	Type		Regularity			
					Product	Service	Regular	Rare	Implicit	Explicit
1	[8]	Data sparsity and Cold-Start in cloud services	CF	Cloud computing services		✓		✓	✓	
2	[7]	Cold-Start	CF	Online shopping and social networks	✓		✓			✓
3	[9]	Cold-Start	CF	Online shopping	✓		✓		✓	✓
4	[10]	Choosing a specific topic with Big Data	CF	Topic selection		✓	✓		✓	✓
5	[11]	Accuracy-Diversity problem	CF	Purchasing items	✓		✓		✓	
6	[12]	Accuracy-Diversity problem	CF	Movies	✓		✓		✓	
7	[13]	Difficulty to search in Big Data & disconnection	CF	R&D projects		✓		✓	✓	✓
8	[15]	Context aware recommendation and Cold-Start	CF	Movies – Songs - Advertising	✓		✓			
9	[16]	Cold-Start	CF	Movies	✓		✓			✓
10	[25]	Accuracy	CF	Movies	✓		✓		✓	
11	[26]	Data sparsity and prediction accuracy	CF	Movies	✓		✓		✓	✓
12	[19]	Comparing five types of similarity finding techniques	H	Recommend major study for students		✓		✓	✓	
13	[20]	Analytics through Big Data	CB	Online Shopping	✓		✓		✓	✓
14	[21]	Attribute weights	H	Online Shopping	✓		✓		✓	✓
15	[27]	Accuracy and Cold-Start	H	Movies	✓		✓		✓	✓
16	[28]	Limitations of CB	H	Movies Database	✓		✓		✓	✓
17	[17]	The search and recommending the scientific content	CB	Scientific Publications	✓			✓	✓	✓
18	[18]	Lack of systems to recommend using author's abstract	CB	Computer science publications	✓			✓	✓	✓

(*continued*)

Table 1. (*continued*)

No	Reference	Problem Addressed	Technique	Context	Deliverables				Data	
					Type		Regularity			
					Product	Service	Regular	Rare	Implicit	Explicit
19	[22]	Choosing improper electives by the students (accuracy)	NN	Elective subjects selections		✓		✓	✓	✓
20	[23]	The lack of data about tourism locations (accuracy)	NN	Tourism		✓	✓		✓	✓
21	[24]	The fake information posted in social media (data sparsity)	NN	Social media		✓	✓			✓
22	[29]	The lack of data for better recommendation outcomes	NN	Tourism		✓	✓		✓	✓

3 Data, Recommendation Technique, and View (DRV) Model

Based on the literature review we have developed the DRV model as illustrated in Fig. 1 below. The DRV Model is based on the analysis of recommendation techniques across different contexts. The functionality of the model is categorized into three major components, which are fundamental to develop any recommendation system. These components are, data, recommendation techniques and view.

3.1 Data

Data represents the user's activities that he/she conducts throughout the system. Data is the main component that is used by the system to recommend for the user. Based on the definition stated previously data has been categorized into two types implicit and explicit. The Big Data component shown in Fig. 1 means these sorts of data could be extracted from Big Data sources as well.

3.2 Recommendation Techniques

The recommendation techniques are the core component of the recommendation system. Different techniques and approaches are utilized to extract the user characteristics and finding the similar items. The three main methods, explained previously, have been presented here as they are considered the most popular. As per our analysis, shown in Table 1, we absorb that the CF and Hybrid techniques are utilized for both, the products and services. CB technique is mostly applied on products. The other attribute is considered in the illustration is the regularity of products and services purchases. Regular deliverables are the most common purchases and mostly supported by CF as shown in the table.

3.3 View

The outcome of processing the data by the recommendation system is a personalised recommendation list. The recommendation list is generated by the recommendation technique and displayed through web-based application, mobile-based application or other.

As it is shown in Fig. 1 the data is generated by the user. This data is extracted and feed into the recommending system as an input raw data. It is based on the approach and algorithm implemented to define what kind of data to be extracted and processed by the system. Accordingly, the outcome of this process is the recommendation list to be displayed in the proper platform and viewed by the user for decision making.

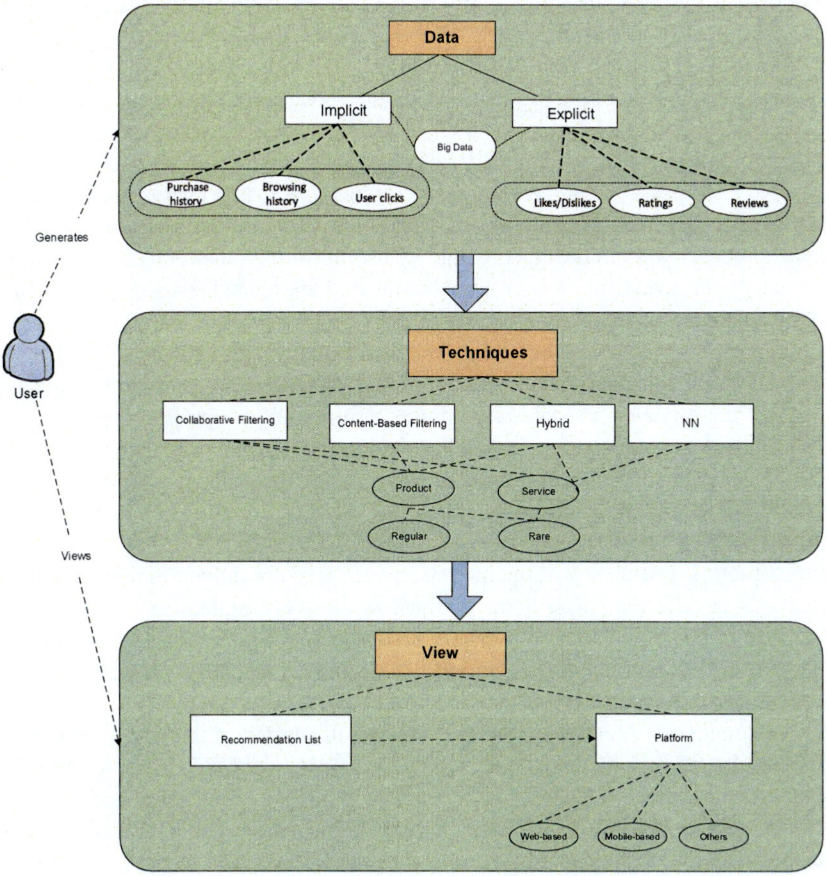

Fig. 1. Data, Recommendation Techniques and View (DRV) model

4 Discussion and Future Work

According to the literature review and the DRV model presented we state our discussion and what should be done for future work.

By referring to Table 1, all of the approaches utilize both types of data, implicit and explicit. As the models that implement NN address the problem of the lack of data, these models consider Big Data as one of the main sources to supply the required data for the learning process.

The papers reviewed are mostly focusing on the cold-start problem and data sparsity, in addition to enhancing the performance and accuracy. However, such problems have been well addressed by utilizing NN techniques. Many other issues should be considered and addressed including privacy issues.

Each of the systems presented is applied in a specific context. For example, Gan and Jiang [12], Fu et al. [25] and Liu and Wu [15] applied their models on movies related data. Wei et al. [7], Hsieh et al. [9], Chai et al. [11] and Yun et al. [14] applied their models in the online shopping process. Some others have applied their models to special services. For example, Mezni and Abdeljaoued [8] developed their model to support cloud computing services recommendations. Xu et al. [13] designed their approach to support R&D projects recommendation. The issue here is that every recommendation system is designed to be applied on a chosen context or domain. There is no adequate evidence that each system designed would be useful for the other contexts or domains.

Based on our investigation we found that most of the related research focuses on the regular purchases, either products or services. Systems based on the NN approach, as per literature, addresses the lack of data provision. As it is illustrated in Fig. 1 the NN approach is suitable to facilitate the recommendation of services that rarely purchased.

Most of the models presented rely on user ratings and user profiles. These are considered as the data sources to be utilized to recommend for the user. The question here is, what about the experience of the user when utilizing the product or service, and how to capture this experience and knowledge to be used as input to the recommendation process?.

From Table 1, it is clear that the models investigated are limited in their capabilities and features in different ways. Some of these systems are limited to support only the products (tangibles), and some others are limited to support the services (intangibles). The other question here is, how to support the businesses that deal with selling tangible and intangible deliverables?.

As we mentioned previously, the DRV model illustrated in this paper presents the outcome of the study done in this research. DRV model, is one step to comprehensively understand such systems and their issues, as the next step is to think about how to design a generic framework to address such issues and designing proper recommendation systems by customizing the components based on the business and user needs.

5 Conclusion

In this paper, we have defined the DRV model. Diverse types of data and techniques have been defined to design the model. One of the benefits of the DRV model, in our opinion, is to build a kind of foundation to design a generic framework to facilitate recommendation systems design and development in a better way. The main feature to be considered in such a framework is to overcome the issues of the recommendation systems mentioned in our previous discussion.

DRV model needs to be enhanced by investigating more literature through other disciplines to discover more patterns, features, and issues. An example of that is the literature related to knowledge management. Also, more AI literature based is to be explored as well. That leads to discover and define other sources of data and approaches in developing recommendation systems to enhance the DRV model and have a better foundation to develop the generic framework.

This analysis needs to be supported by the model evaluation process. The model is to be evaluated by defining the proper methodology.

References

1. Stanujkic, D., Karabasevic, D., Maksimovic, M., Popovic, G., Brzakovic, M.: Evaluation of the e-commerce development strategies. Quaestus **1**, 144–152 (2019)
2. Abadi, S., et al.: Design of online transaction model on traditional industry in order to increase turnover and benefits. Int. J. Eng. Technol. **7**(2.27), 231–237 (2018)
3. Khan, M.K., Nawaz, M.R., Ishaq, M.I., Tariq, M.I.: Product versus service: old myths versus new realities. J. Basic Appl. Sci. Res. **4**(1), 15–20 (2014)
4. Parry, G., Newnes, L., Huang, X.: Goods, products and services. In: Macintyre, M., Parry, G., Angelis, J. (eds.) Service Design and Delivery, pp. 19–29. Springer US, Boston, MA (2011). https://doi.org/10.1007/978-1-4419-8321-3_2
5. Isinkaye, F.O., Folajimi, Y.O., Ojokoh, B.A.: Recommendation systems: principles, methods and evaluation. Egypt. Inform. J. **16**(3), 261–273 (2015)
6. Barbosa, C.E., Oliveira, J., Maia, L., Souza, J.: MISIR: recommendation systems in a knowledge management scenario. Int. J. Continuing Eng. Educ. Life-Long Learn. **20**, 02/01 (2010)
7. Wei, J., He, J., Chen, K., Zhou, Y., Tang, Z.: Collaborative filtering and deep learning based recommendation system for cold start items. Expert Syst. Appl. **69**, 29–39 (2017)
8. Mezni, H., Abdeljaoued, T.: A cloud services recommendation system based on fuzzy formal concept analysis. Data Knowl. Eng. **116**, 100–123 (2018)
9. Hsieh, M.-Y., Weng, T.-H., Li, K.-C.: A keyword-aware recommender system using implicit feedback on Hadoop. J. Parallel Distrib. Comput. **116**, 63–73 (2018)
10. Zhang, S., Zhang, S., Yen, N.Y., Zhu, G.: The recommendation system of micro-blog topic based on user clustering. Mob. Netw. Appl. **22**(2), 228–239 (2016)
11. Chai, Z.-Y., Li, Y.-L., Han, Y.-M., Zhu, S.-F.: Recommendation system based on singular value decomposition and multi-objective immune optimization. IEEE Access **7**, 6060–6071 (2018)
12. Gan, M., Jiang, R.: Constructing a user similarity network to remove adverse influence of popular objects for personalized recommendation. Expert Syst. Appl. **40**(10), 4044–4053 (2013)
13. Xu, W., Sun, J., Ma, J., Du, W.: A personalized information recommendation system for R&D project opportunity finding in big data contexts. J. Netw. Comput. Appl. **59**, 362–369 (2016)
14. Yun, Y., Hooshyar, D., Jo, J., Lim, H.: Developing a hybrid collaborative filtering recommendation system with opinion mining on purchase review. J. Inf. Sci. **44**(3), 331–344 (2018)
15. Liu, C.-L., Wu, X.-W.: Fast recommendation on latent collaborative relations. Knowl.-Based Syst. **109**, 25–34 (2016)

16. Ahn, H.J.: A new similarity measure for collaborative filtering to alleviate the new user cold-starting problem. Inf. Sci. **178**(1), 37–51 (2008)
17. Achakulvisut, T., Acuna, D.E., Ruangrong, T., Kording, K.: Science concierge: a fast content-based recommendation system for scientific publications. PLoS ONE **11**(7), e0158423 (2016)
18. Wang, D., Liang, Y., Xu, D., Feng, X., Guan, R.: A content-based recommender system for computer science publications. Knowl.-Based Syst. **157**, 1–9 (2018)
19. Ochirbat, A., et al.: Hybrid occupation recommendation for adolescents on interest, profile, and behavior. Telematics Inform. **35**(3), 534–550 (2018)
20. Kanavos, A., Iakovou, S.A., Sioutas, S., Tampakas, V.: Large scale product recommendation of supermarket ware based on customer behaviour analysis. Big Data Cogn. Comput. **2**(2), 11 (2018)
21. Scholz, M., Dorner, V., Schryen, G., Benlian, A.: A configuration-based recommender system for supporting e-commerce decisions. Eur. J. Oper. Res. **259**(1), 205–215 (2017)
22. Mariappan, P., Viswanathan, V., Čepová, L.: Application of semantic analysis and LSTM-GRU in developing a personalized course recommendation system. Appl. Sci. **12**(21), 10792 (2022)
23. An, H.-W., Moon, N.: Design of recommendation system for tourist spot using sentiment analysis based on CNN-LSTM. J. Ambient. Intell. Humaniz. Comput. **13**(3), 1653–1663 (2019)
24. Kiruthika, N.S., Thailambal, D.G.: Dynamic light weight recommendation system for social networking analysis using a hybrid LSTM-SVM classifier algorithm. Opt. Mem. Neural Networks **31**(1), 59–75 (2022)
25. Fu, M., Qu, H., Moges, D., Lu, L.: Attention based collaborative filtering. Neurocomputing **311**, 88–98 (2018)
26. Wang, Y., Deng, J., Gao, J., Zhang, P.: A hybrid user similarity model for collaborative filtering. Inf. Sci. **418**, 102–118 (2017)
27. Khalaji, M., Dadkhah, C., Gharibshah, J.: Hybrid movie recommender system based on resource allocation. arXiv preprint arXiv:2105.11678 (2021)
28. Debnath, S., Ganguly, N., Mitra, P.: Feature weighting in content based recommendation system using social network analysis, pp. 1041–1042 (2008)
29. Shafqat, W., Byun, Y.-C.: A context-aware location recommendation system for tourists using hierarchical LSTM model. Sustainability (Basel, Switzerland) **12**(10), 4107 (2020)

Comparative Analysis: Accurate Prediction to the Future Stock Prices

Nada AlSallami[1(✉)], Razwan Mohmed Salah[2], Munir Hossain[3], Syed Altaf[4], Emran Salahuddin[4], and Jaspreet Kaur[5]

[1] CS Department, Worcester State University, Worcester, USA
nada.alsalami@yahoo.com
[2] The University of Duhok, Duhok, KRG, Iraq
[3] Western Sydney University, Sydney, Australia
munir.hossain@westernsydney.edu.au
[4] Kent Institute Australia, Melbourne, Australia
syed.altaf@kent.edu.au
[5] Study Group Australia, Darlinghurst, Australia

Abstract. Accurate stock price prediction has an increasingly prominent role in a market where rewards and risks fluctuate wildly. Market control is a technique utilized by brokers to adjust the cost of budgetary resources. Recently there has been a significant increase in the use of artificial intelligence techniques in stock markets. Reinforcement learning has become particularly important in stock market forecasting. There is a need for modern techniques to improve share analysis and to detect unfair trading. Due to the high volatility and non-stationary nature of the stock market, forecasting the trend of financial time series remains a big challenge. This research explores, compares, and analyses the different artificial intelligent techniques used in predicting stock prices. The aim of this research is to give a comparative analysis to understand how to detect and analyze unfair trading and to detect price manipulation. Also, our aim is to explain how reinforcement deep learning could avoid and analyze the risks and unfair trading in stock market. The result of this study addresses current challenges of reducing the unfair trading across the stock. A successful and accurate prediction to the future stock prices ultimately results in profit maximization. Such prediction is important for many individuals including companies, traders, market participants, and data analysts. In conclusion, Reinforcement learning in the stock market is in its early development and a lot more research is needed to make it a reliable method in this field.

Keywords: Reinforcement learning · Stock market · Computational Intelligence · Knowledge Transfer · Stock price prediction

1 Introduction

There has been an increase in the use of intelligence to perform financial trading. Which involves preprocessing raw data to extract the features and finding or recognizing patterns during the training process, then making a correct decision. This process, i.e. machine

K. Daimi and A. Al Sadoon (Eds.): ICR 2023, LNNS 721, pp. 153–164, 2023.
https://doi.org/10.1007/978-3-031-35308-6_13

learning process can be used to understand rules for buying and selling and executing them. While in Reinforcement learning process, the system is repeatedly fed new information from the available raw data in an iterative process to maximize the value of a certain predetermined reward. It is a new and interesting method to make predictions in the financial market. Deep reinforcement learning method can be used in the stock market to detect and analyze financial risk. It can improve unfair trading in the stock market by analyzing them. Stock markets can use reinforcement learning algorithms and computational intelligent to maintain risk activities [1]. It is necessary to resolve this problem in order to make the best analysis for the risk and unfair trading across the stock market, to detect the risks for the customers and therefore enhance the share predictions of the stocks using deep learning reinforcement technology [2]. The purpose of this research is to detect and analyze unfair trading and to detect price manipulation. In this paper, we have modelled two strategies, spoofing and pinging trading, from a macroscopic perspective of profit maximization. These two strategies are differing in the legal background but share the same elemental concept of market manipulation. This research is trying to answer the following questions; how can reinforcement deep learning avoid and analyze the risks and unfair trading in the stock market? How can algorithms be implemented to efficiently reduce unfair trading? How are deep learning techniques enhancing better share predictions? What are the situations faced with implementing the computational intelligence reinforcement algorithms? What could be methods for reinforcement learning technique applications? How can risks and trading be improved? In the current stock market, there is a need for modern techniques to improve share analysis and to detect unfair trading. Computational intelligence can be used to solve this problem. The proposed work is predicting the data of stocks properly to reduce the risk using the deep learning algorithms technique. The remaining sections of this paper are organized as follow: In section two, a literature review is given based on the detection of unfair trading using the reinforcement deep learning technique. In section three, model components are developed and discussed based on their subcomponents and instances. Section four includes the validation and evaluation of proposed model components. The discussion is given in section five. At last, the conclusion of the study and the future works are given in section six.

2 Literature Review

M. C. Day et al.[3] used a SECI (socialization, externalization, combination, and internalization) model where long short- term memory networks, recurrent neural networks, convolutional neural networks as deep learning algorithms and Word2Vec, GloVe, and FastText as word embedding models are evaluated and used. The paper was also successful in testing whether machine learning, and AI algorithms can find patterns in annual financial statements that indicate a fraudulent corporate culture and whether a company is committing various sorts of massive financial crime. M. Nabipour et al. [4] used adaptive learning, intelligent tutorial systems and systematic reviews, which can bump up a person's accuracy and learning motivation since it starts to feel more personal. This may also give rise to a more personalized learning system in the future. The research used multiple machine learning models (Decision Tree, Random Forest, Adaptive Boosting

(Adaboost), eXtreme Gradient Boosting (XGBoost), Support Vector Classifier (SVC), Naïve Bayes, K-Nearest Neighbours (KNN), Logistic Regression and Artificial Neural Network (ANN)) and two powerful deep learning methods, (Recurrent Neural Network (RNN) and Long short-term memory (LSTM). Unlike traditional user interfaces. The study of Q. Chen et al. [5] aims to significantly reduce the risk of predicting trends with machine learning and deep learning algorithms. R. Pathan at el. [6] worked on this issue and showed initial evidence that machine learning techniques can identify (non-linear) dependency in the stock market price sequences. However, due to the high volatility and non-stationary nature of the stock market, forecasting the trend of financial time series remains a big challenge. Falci et al. [7] conducted research regarding the forecasting of the direction of the prices, i.e., the up and down trends of the time series. Since there are too many factors such as public opinions, general economic conditions, or political events, which all have direct or indirect impacts on the evolution of financial time series, extracting these features is tedious and costly. Alivar et al. [8] proposed a novel hybrid deep learning model integrating attention mechanism (AM), MLP, and a bidirectional long-short term memory neural network (BiLSTM) to forecast the closing prices of four stock indexes due to their respective advantages. A similar approach is followed in the study of Kumari et al. [9] to achieve the optimum results. The prediction of shares offers huge chances for profit and is a major motivation for research in this area; knowledge of stock movements by a fraction of a second can lead to high profits [10, 11]. This was the first attempt to forecast the direction of the BIST 100 market using deep learning and word embedding techniques. To predict the market, most researchers use either technical or fundamental analysis. Terry et al. [13] reviewed some stock/forex trading articles that used reinforcement learning and concluded that research on reinforcement learning should focus on the possibility of comparing reinforcement learning techniques with other sophisticated models used for forecasting or trading on the financial market. Payal et al. [14] proposed a comparative study for predicting stock prices. This paper studied different algorithms like RF, KNN, SVM, Sentiment analysis, Time series analysis, and Graph-Based algorithms. The study compared results of these algorithms to predict the stock prices of various companies. Payal et al. [14] concluded that combining the sentiment analysis of stocks related information and the numeric value associated with the historical value of stocks. This combination plays an important role in predicting stock prices.

3 Future Stock Prediction Model Components

We have selected three-factor model, i.e., Input, Process, and the Prediction Model. These have further helped in selecting the major components of our research, which are Data, Detection, Image scaling, and Recognition. Table 1 lists the subclasses, attributes, and instances of the selected factors/classes. The table has three factors, eight sub factors, twelve attributes and multiple instances for each attribute.

Table 1. Future Stock Prediction Model Components

Class/factor	Attributes	Instances
Input		
Databaseman- agement systems	Data architec- ture	Data architecture; Knowledge sharing; SECI model; Value proposition; University-industry collaboration; Engineering education; Expectancy-value, Self-efficacy, Self-regulation, Learning ob- ject recommendation; Virtual learning environment optimization; Heuristics; Computational Intelligence, Decision Tree, Random Forest, Adaptive Boosting (Adaboost), eXtreme Gradient Boosting (XGBoost), Support Vector Classifier (SVC), Naïve Bayes, K-Nearest Neighbours (KNN), Logistic Regression and Artificial Neural Network (ANN)) and two powerful deep learning methods (Recurrent Neural Network (RNN)
	Research area	Personalized learning; Adaptive learning; Learning; Intelligent tutoring systems; Learning analytics; Personalized adaptive learning; Systematic review; Deep learning; Stock market trend; Feature engineering; Feature engineering, Deep learning, Stock Market Trend Prediction, textual features extraction, model stacking, stock movement direction prediction
Computational in- telligence	Approach	Virtual reality; Learner's behaviour; Logfile; Sequential pattern mining; Stock prices forecasting, attention mechanism, bidirectional long-short term memory neural network, multi-layer perceptron, deep learning

(*continued*)

Table 1. (*continued*)

Class/factor	Attributes	Instances
	Dataset name	Stock market, trends prediction, classification, machine learning, deep learning
Process		
Attribute-based keyword search	Algorithm	classical algorithms, quantum algorithms, realistic algorithms, bifurcation tools, genetic algorithms, classical algorithms, evolutionary algorithms, adaptation algorithm, SPM algorithm, sequential pattern mining algorithm, hypothesis-testing-based adaptive spline filtering (HASF) algorithm, Genetic Algorithms, K-Nearest Neighbour algorithm
	Techniques	Reinforcement learning, Value proposition, augmented technology, Dual enrolment; College readiness; Achievement goal theory; Expectancy-value theory; Self-efficacy; Self-regulation; MSLQ; Virtual learning environment optimization, low complexity Heuristics, Intelligent tutoring systems, Personalized learning, Adaptive learning
	Tools	database management systems, SECI model, OR-Tools, simulated experimental analysis tool, Individualized learning, Learning analytics tool, Learning Activity Sequence Analysis Tool, Meta Cognitive tools, Support Vector Classifier
Evaluation	learning objects	Prediction; Deep learning; Stock market trend; Feature engineering; Feature engineering, Deep learning, Stock Market Trend Prediction, textual features extraction, model stacking, stock movement direction prediction

(*continued*)

Table 1. (*continued*)

Class/factor	Attributes	Instances
	accuracy met- rics	High, medium, low
Output		
Secondary output	Model	Machine learning, model stacking, sentiment analysis, stock movement direction prediction, textual features extraction, tweets mining
	Efficiency	Expectancy-value, Self-efficacy, Self-regulation
Primary output	visualization	multi-layer perceptron, attention mechanism, Stock prices forecasting, Computational Intelli- gence, Decision Tree, Random Forest, Adaptive Boosting (Adaboost), eXtreme Gradient Boost- ing (XGBoost), Support Vector Classifier (SVC), Naïve Bayes, K-Nearest Neighbours (KNN), Lo- gistic Regression and Artificial Neural Network (ANN)) and two powerful deep learning methods (Recurrent Neural Network (RNN)

4 Future Stock Prediction Model Classification and Evaluation

Table 2 shows the classification of the system components based on the proposed model. The Input data is classified based on attributes like data source. The parameters for classification of detection are method, algorithm, and tools used in the system for detecting objects and faces and, its deployment. Figure 1 shows the flow diagram of the proposed system. We have reviewed articles based on unconventional business research using in-depth learning support. This stock is then encrypted with SSH and then stored in the database. During the last stage, the stock visualization is shown as the primary output in the output devices. These stock trends are stored in the database for future reference and testing purposes. Table 3 shows the evaluation of the overall system based on several parameters such as total input instances, number of samples, performance evaluation matrices, method for validation and evaluation, precision, system accuracy, overall performance, and result of the system. These parameters are evaluated on the given input, by selecting the most effective evaluation method as per the research. The most common methods of evaluation for the proposed system are SVM, background subtraction, and HOG. To verify the system, we have counted the number of the subcomponent terms

Table 2. Classification Table

Author	Data architecture	Research area	Approach	Dataset name	Accuracy metrics	Tools	Learning objects	Techniques	Algorithm	Model	Efficiency	Visualization
[1]	DA	LOR	deep learning	(ANN))	SPMA,	K-Nearest	L (ANN)	VRLB	CA	ML	deep learn- ing	XGBoost
[2]	Knowledge sharing;	Self- effi- cacy,	SM	SVC	AA	SFS	(SVC),	LSPM	quan- tum al- go- rithms	MS	SM	PSO
[3]	SECI model;	SR	CML	NB (KNN),	SPM	GA,	(KNN),	SPF	RA	SA	CML,	IDS
[4]	DA	LOR	deep learning	(ANN))	SPMA,	K-Nearest	L (ANN)	VRLB	CA	ML	deep learning	CNN
[5]	SECI model;	SR	CML	NB (KNN),	SPM	GA,	(KNN),	SPF	RA	SA	CML,	IoMT
[6]	DA	LOR	deep learning	(ANN))	SPMA,	K-Nearest	L (ANN)	VRLB	CA	ML	deep learning	WEFU
[7]	Expectancy value,	DA	VRLB	MLP	CA	ML	MLP	deep learning	EA	EV	VRLB	FFDNN
[8]	Self-effi cacy,	Self- efficacy,	SM	SVC	AA	SFS	(SVC),	LSPM	quan- tum al gorithms,	MS	SM	RF
[9]	Self-regu lation,	DA	VRLB	MLP	CA	ML	MLP	deep learn- ing	EA	EV	VRLB	NB
[10]	Learning object rec ommendation	Self- efficacy,	SM	SVC	AA	SFS	(SVC),	LSPM	quan- tum al gorithms,	MS	SM	SVM
[11]	VLEO	LOR	deep learning	(ANN)	SPMA,	K-Nearest	L (ANN))	VRLB	CA	ML	deep learning	HC- IBGSA SVM
[12]	Self-effi- cacy,	Self- efficacy,	SM	SVC	AA	SFS	(SVC),	LSPM	quan- tum algorithms,	MS	SM	RF

that have been used in the overall system. It is very important to analyze the components of the study and the methods used and to evaluate and validate this work properly.

The bar graph below in Figure 1, shows the percentage of the subcomponents selected from the proposed model in the system. A scale of range 0 to 1000 is selected for the measurement and further comparison of the subcomponents of the system. Table 4 depicts the frequency of subcomponents used in numbers. The most used subcomponent is computational intelligence, which is followed by database management systems. Every literature has used datasets, but the best researches conducted in Table 2 have selected a dataset for training purposes, which is also used for system testing. The least used subcomponent term is evaluation. This is because many researches have not used any evaluation method.

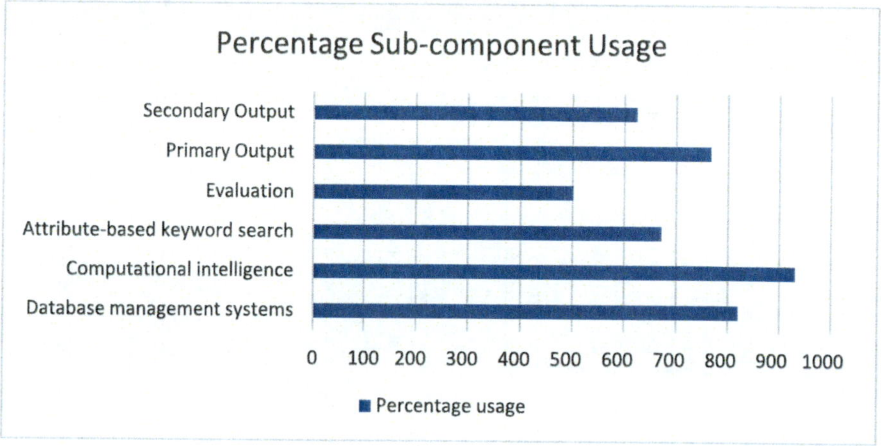

Fig. 1. Term Frequency Chart

Table 3. Evaluation Table

Refs.	Area/Domain	Input Images	Performance Evaluation Metrics	Validation and evaluation method	Recall	Precision	Accuracy	Output result
[1]	Object Detection	12289 images	Large size	SVM	56.2	95.46	45	profit
[2]	Face Detection	788	position	Frame numbering	99.02	98.7	99.41	recall, f-score, precision
[3]	Face Detection	300	scalability	HOG	88.2	60.09	57.7	execution time

(*continued*)

Table 3. *(continued)*

Refs.	Area/Domain	Input Images	Performance Evaluation Metrics	Validation and evaluation method	Recall	Precision	Accuracy	Output result
[4]	Object Detection	76	Majority Voting	Haar Classifier	63.2	78.33	73.45	Processing time
[5]	Object Detection	10 million	non-uniform illumination	Background subtraction	80.6	76	97.12	threshold of IoU
[6]	Object Detection	1000	non-maximum suppression	optical flow method	78.22	49.09	150	speed of GPU
[7]	Face tracking	5600	Gamma Correction	skin colour detection	54.09	85.91	95.46	FDR
[8]	Human segmentation	17389	Majority Voting	Single Shot Multi Box Detection	68.003	98	93.44	stock prediction
[9]	ATM Surveillance	8787	non-uniform illumination	Artificial intelligence	56.785	70	80.8	Industry advances
[10]	video surveillance	8678	Gamma Correction	SVM	56.2	95.78	250	improvement in speed
[11]	Real time OD	32000	gradient intensity	HOG	99.02	95.46	89	execution time
[12]	fire detection	74500	gradient intensity	Background subtraction	54.09	85.91	78.33	accuracy

Table 4. Frequency of sub-component used in the system

Term	Frequency
Database management systems	820
Computational intelligence	930
Attribute-based keyword search	671
Evaluation	501
Primary Output	765
Secondary Output	624

5 Discussion

The proposed factors are listed with their subclasses, attributes, and instances in Table1. For the first component, i.e. Input, in each research paper, different kinds of data architecture were used to gather the input data. However, it is difficult to explain the use of multiple sensors at single place. Some papers have used cloud as their common data store but some papers such as [1, 6, 9], and [12] have gathered their input data directly from photodetectors, underwater sensors, turbulence genera tors, seabed sensors, optical wireless sensors, charge-coupled Devices, silicon single- photon avalanche diodes, multi-pixel photon counters, etc. Many papers like [1, 2, 5] and [7] have used a Seedlings Dataset with 960 images, signals, Candida dataset of a generic type with 418 nodes, 398 edges, and 7 layers. M. Nabipour et al. [4] has used multi-valued sensors, which gather data with multiple values such as the SCADA dataset. The researchers in [8] and [9] have explained how attributes, such as location, temperature, soil stickiness, generalization error, soil conditions, atmospheric environment, canopy temperature, etc., can be useful in designing an optimal network for the agriculture fields. Jha et al. [10] has taken 345 big data instances of user activities while R. Pathan et al. [6] has taken 722 instances of computational intelligence and other factors.

Nevertheless, most of the papers have failed to explain the use of environmental factors on the users' fraud activity prediction. The work of M.Nabipour et al. [4] and Huang et al. [11] have failed to provide an overview of the biological networks in the agriculture sector and its significance. For the second component, i.e. Process, the average rate of seed and farming growth of all papers is 3.904 m/s. Those researchers have described the use of precision agriculture and exactness farming as the best techniques that are the most efficient and energy optimized techniques among all. The system proposed by E. Tzavida et al. [1] uses only 398 and 343 total number of input plant samples, with 418 and 340 total number of sensors, respectively, in the field network and offers 98% sensitivity, 95.12 F-score and 98.15% efficiency with 85% overall performance result. M.C. Day [3] and S.H. Falci et al. [7] have focused on lowering the resource utilization, energy consumption, and processing time of the algorithm in the overall system. The most optimal approach so far is precision agriculture using transfer learning adopted by [1, 4] and [5]. M. Nabi- pour et al. [4] claims to be the best network algorithm with 0.284 recall and 92% band- width improvement. Although, Argo technology technique gives 200% bandwidth improvement with 78.22 recall and 66% efficiency. Base detector, image slices, GPU fast restoration and Image Decomposition techniques are used by [5, 10] and [9] for communication and transferring the data from sensor nodes to the application and vice versa. The researchers in [1, 2, 6, 8, 11] have tested and evaluated their system on the basis of parameter like accuracy, recall, precision, node quality, computational complexity, network bandwidth, etc. Jha et al. [10] and N.Jha et al. [12] have failed to explain how Fine Tuning and Agricultural cybersecurity can be helpful in evaluating their systems. Papers like [3, 7, 11] and [12] have acquired 97.321% bandwidth performance in with 91.09% system efficiency for transferring the agricultural data. Neural Network Toolbox (NNT), Embedded video systems, Jetson Nano tool, Nvidia Profiler and Jetson TX1 are the most efficient and opt mal tools used in the research papers [1, 4, 6, 7, 10] and [11]. They also have very low computational overheads according to M.C. Day et al. [3] when used with the tools such as ANN, CNN, RNN, DCF, 3FDBS-LC, Grey scale conversion and Plant high-throughput phenotypic platform, etc. Many authors have failed to define the actual use of agile methodologies with computational intelligence. For decision-making, M.Nabipour et al. [4] used an Integer linear programming algorithm that takes 2.42 ms to process 6490 data instances. An adaptive cooperative routing algorithm is used by E. Tzavida et al. [1] and a Bandwidth Blocking Probability (BBP) algorithm is used by J.Wyrobek et al. [2] and both take 6.66 ms and 4.2 ms respectively. The last component is Output, most of the papers have divided their output into 2 categories – primary and secondary output. Primary output focuses on visualization of the proposed system. However, the secondary output incorporates different parameters to evaluate and measure the designed system. E. Tzavida et al. [1] takes 6342 instances as input and achieves horticultural area increase by 50%–60% with a RMSE value and correctness of 89.7% and 43.8% respectively. M. Nabipour et al. [4] used adopted weighted neurons with 66% reduced noise and a learning hypothesis model for transferring the prediction results using FogBus to the servers. Huang et al. [11] and Jha et al. [10] used smart office gateway to enhance cultivating measures by 200% to 400% and send an SMS notification as a graphical display to the users and banks on their smartphones, computers, laptops, etc. Smart watches, IPADs and iPhones are used by [2, 10] and [7] to display the predicted suture events for the users in smart offices. Some research like [12] showed that using motion artifacts, an alarm can be generated when an unusual object is recognized. Investors, fund managers and investment companies can use the model proposed by the research of [13] to enhance their ability to pick outperforming stock. Researcher of [14] recommended combining the sentiment analysis of stocks related information with the historical value of stocks for predicting stock prices.

6 Conclusion

A successful and accurate prediction to the future stock prices ultimately results in profit maximization and can enable the investor to anticipate a situation of their company so that they do not lose their precious money. This prediction is important for many individuals not only companies, but also traders, market participants, data analysts, researchers working in deep machine learning and artificial intelligence areas. Although there are many new and old improvements in stock market prediction, due to its volatile nature, predicting it has always been a challenge. Reinforcement learning in the stock market is in its early development and a lot more research is needed to make it a reliable method in this field. Furthermore, as a future work in this area, using a live trading platform rather than just performance on historical data with machine learning algorithms might enhance prediction accuracy.

References

1. Tzavidas, E., Enevoldsen, P., Xydis, G.: A University-industry knowledge transfer online education approach via a cloud-based database global solution. Smart Learning Environments **7**(1), 1–16 (2020). https://doi.org/10.1186/s40561-020-00128-5
2. Wyrobek, J.: Application of machine learning models and artificial intelligence to analyze annual financial statements to identify companies with unfair corporate culture. Procedia Computer Science **176**(2), 3037–3046 (2020). https://doi.org/10.1016/j.procs.2020.09.335
3. Day, M.C., Kelley, H.M., Browne, B.L., Kohn, S.J.: Assessing motivation and learning strategy usage by dually enrolled students. Smart Learning Environments **7**(1), 1–19 (2020). https://doi.org/10.1186/s40561-020-00131-w

4. Nabipour, M., Nayyeri, P., Jabani, H., S.S., Mosavi, A.: Predicting stock market trends using machine learning and deep learning algorithms via continuous and binary data; a comparative analysis. IEEE Access **8**(3), 150199–150212 (2020). https://doi.org/10.1109/access.2020.3015966
5. Chen, Q., Zhang, W., Lou, Y.: Forecasting Stock Prices Using a Hybrid Deep Learning Model Integrating Attention Mechanism, Multi-Layer Perceptron, and Bidirectional Long-Short Term Memory Neural Network. IEEE Access, vol. 8, no. 1, pp. 117365–117376 (2020). https://doi.org/10.1109/access.2020.3004284
6. Pathan, R., Rajendran, R., Murthy, S.: Mechanism to capture learner's interaction in VR-based learning environment: design and application. Smart Learning Environments **7**(1), 1–15 (2020). https://doi.org/10.1186/s40561-020-00143-6
7. Falci, S.H., Dorça, F.A., Andrade, A.V., Mourão Falci, D.H.: A low complexity heu- ristic to solve a learning objects recommendation problem. Smart Learning Environments, vol. 7, no. 1, Sep. 2020, doi: https://doi.org/10.1186/s40561-020-00133-8
8. Alivar, et al.: Smart bed based daytime behavior prediction in Children with autism spectrum disorder - A Pilot Study. Med. Eng. Phys. **83**(8), 15–25 (2020). https://doi.org/10.1016/j.medengphy.2020.07.004
9. Kumari, D.V., Gupta, R., Tanwar, S.: Redills: Deep learning-based secure data analytic framework for smart grid systems. In: 2020 IEEE International Conference on Communications Workshops (ICC Workshops), vol. 21, no. 3, Jun. 2020, doi: https://doi.org/10.1109/ic-cworkshops49005.2020.9145448
10. Jha, N., et al.: IoTSim-Edge: A simulation framework for modeling the behavior of Internet of Things and edge computing environments. Software: Practice and Experience, vol. 50, no. 6, pp. 844–867, Jan. 2020, doi: https://doi.org/10.1002/spe.2787
11. Huang, D.-Y., Chen, C.-H., Chen, T.-Y., Hu, W.-C., Guo, Z.-B., Wen, C.-K.: High-efficiency face detection and tracking method for numerous pedestrians through face candidate generation. Multimedia Tools and Applications **80**(1), 1247–1272 (2020). https://doi.org/10.1007/s11042-020-09780-y
12. Saponara, S., Elhanashi, A., Gagliardi, A.: Real-time video fire/smoke detection based on CNN in antifire surveillance systems. J. Real-Time Image Proc. **18**(3), 889–900 (2020). https://doi.org/10.1007/s11554-020-01044-0
13. Terry & Khushi, Matloob: Reinforcement Learning in Financial Markets. Data. 4. 110 (2019). https://doi.org/10.3390/data4030110
14. Soni, P., et al.: Machine Learning Approaches in Stock Price Prediction: A Systematic Review, J. Phys.: Conf. Ser. 2161 012065 (2022)

CNN-Based Handwriting Analysis for the Prediction of Autism Spectrum Disorder

Nafisa Nawer[1(✉)], Mohammad Zavid Parvez[2,3,4,5], Muhammad Iqbal Hossain[1], Prabal Datta Barua[6,8,9], Mia Rahim[7], and Subrata Chakraborty[8]

[1] Department of Computer Science and Engineering, BRAC University, Dhaka, Bangladesh
nawernafisa8@gmail.com, iqbal.hossain@bracu.ac.bd
[2] Information Technology, APIC, Melbourne, Australia
zavidparvez@gmail.com
[3] Information Technology, Torrens University, Melbourne, Australia
[4] Peter Faber Business School, Australian Catholic University, Melbourne, Australia
[5] School of Computing, Mathematics, and Engineering, Charles Sturt University, Bathurst, NSW, Australia
[6] School of Business (Information System), University of Southern Queensland, Darling Heights, QLD 4350, Australia
prabal.barua@usq.edu.au
[7] School of Law, University of New England, Armidale, Australia
mrahim@une.edu.au
[8] School of Science and Technology, Faculty of Science, Agriculture, Business and Law, University of New England, Armidale, NSW 2351, Australia
subrata.chakraborty@une.edu.au
[9] Cogninet Australia Pty Ltd, Level 5, 29-35 Bellevue St., Surry Hills, NSW 2010, Australia

Abstract. Approximately 1 in 44 children worldwide has been identified as having Autism Spectrum Disorder (ASD), according to the Centers for Disease Control and Prevention (CDC). The term 'ASD' is used to characterize a collection of repetitive sensory-motor activities with strong hereditary foundations. Children with autism have a higher-than-average rate of motor impairments, which causes them to struggle with handwriting. Therefore, they generally perform worse on handwriting tasks compared to typically developing children of the same age. As a result, the purpose of this research is to identify autistic children by a comparison of their handwriting to that of typically developing children. Consequently, we investigated state-of-the-art methods for identifying ASD and evaluated whether or not handwriting might serve as bio-markers for ASD modeling. In this context, we presented a novel dataset comprised of the handwritten texts of children aged 7 to 10. Additionally, three pre-trained Transfer Learning frameworks: InceptionV3, VGG19, Xception were applied to achieve the best level of accuracy possible. We have evaluated the models on a number of quantitative performance evaluation metrics and demonstrated that Xception shows the best outcome with an accuracy of 98%.

K. Daimi and A. Al Sadoon (Eds.): ICR 2023, LNNS 721, pp. 165–174, 2023.
https://doi.org/10.1007/978-3-031-35308-6_14

Keywords: ASD · InceptionV3 · VGG19 · Xception · ROC AUC · kappa · Confusion matrix

1 Introduction

Autism is a neuro-developmental condition that, in general, is identified by several characteristics: deficiencies in social interaction, stereotyped and repetitive behaviors, and difficulties in communication. In addition to these fundamental concepts, autism is linked to a high frequency of motor deficits and executive function impairments. Motor deficits hinder the development of skilled motor tasks, which are likely contributors to handwriting difficulties in children with autism. As a result, analyzing a child's handwriting can be very helpful in determining whether or not they have ASD at an early age. In fact, studies on handwriting focused on writing activities, such as loops, letters, handwritten texts, or signatures, with the purpose of diagnosing illnesses like Alzheimer's disease [1], Parkinson's disease [2], and depression. In spite of these, the study of ASD, which is the cornerstone of this research, has rarely made use of the assessment of handwriting tasks. Therefore, for the non-invasive and automated early identification of autism, we have presented a novel dataset in this study that consists of handwritings of autistic children along with the handwritings of normal children of similar age group.

Handwriting, being a psycho-mechanical activity, is a distinctive behavioral bio-metric trait that certifies a person's individuality. Because the handwriting of each individual is unique, it can provide insight into their backgrounds, personalities, mental health, and other aspects of their lives [3]. Hence, examining a person's handwriting has emerged as a central focus of research in a wide range of fields, including medical diagnosis, the study of psychological illnesses, forensic investigations, and a variety of other fields as well, such as e-security [4].

The act of handwriting is often narrated by specialists as a perceptual motor act. This necessitates the concurrent processing of both physical and cognitive demands. The development of a child's gross and fine motor skills, which serve as the basis for the child's ability to control precise hand-wrist movements and eye-hand coordination, plays a significant role in determining whether or not the child is ready to start writing. Studies, however, indicate that children with autism show poor outcomes in motor functions besides oral motor functions and balance coordination [5]. This results in the inability to align limbs accurately, indicating a heightened probability of handwriting difficulties among children with Autism Spectrum Disorder. As a result, the objective of this study is to develop a handwriting-based model that is capable of accurate ASD diagnosis. In this study, we look for characteristics in people's handwriting that could differentiate autistic spectrum disorder patients from healthy controls.

2 Literature Review

In the following section, a synopsis of the findings of earlier research studies pertaining to the identification of autism spectrum disorder, along with the most current findings concerning handwriting analysis has been presented.

2.1 Autism Spectrum Disorder

A study incorporated several classifiers: Random Forest, SVM, Decision Tree, KNN, Logistic Regression and Naive Bayes to detect ASD precisely at an early age [6]. In [7], authors utilized seven distinct machine learning techniques to predict autism and obtained 97% accuracy on the test cases. However, decision tree provided the maximum accuracy in another study of early ASD screening in children [8]. Again, researchers have investigated state-of-the-art classification and feature selection strategies to identify the most effective classifier along with feature set utilizing four datasets containing information on people of all ages with ASD, from toddlers to teenagers [9]. Their experiments reveal that the multilayer perceptron (MLP) classifier is superior to other benchmark classification models, accomplishing full accuracy with a small amount of characteristics across all age groups. Another research introduced a flexible and modular framework for the diagnosis of ASD and evaluated with unsupervised ML techniques [10]. A current study demonstrated that facial characteristics can be used to recognize ASD using DenseNet [11]. Furthermore, authors in [12] followed a different approach by analyzing fMRI in order to detect autism since fMRI captures better brain activities than EEG. Besides, a recent research suggested a deep learning model of assessing the resting-state functional near-infrared spectroscopy (fNIRS) signals to predict ASD [13]. To decrease the number of optical channels while obtaining high precision, the research employed the SHapley Additive exPlanations (SHAP) approach.

2.2 Handwriting Analysis

In [3], the authors have analyzed handwriting signature to assess Neurological Disorder, i.e. Alzheimer's Disease and Parkinsonism using three classifiers: KNN, Decision Tree and SVM. They preprocessed the image dataset by filtering, smoothing and reducing noise. Another study narrates the usage of handwriting to identify personality by utilizing AlexNet architecture with 5 convolution layer and 1 fully-connected layer [14]. The authors incorporated vertical segmentation to identify the features of curves and final strokes and horizontal segmentation to identify the features of upper and middle stroke. Another paper suggested using biGRUs to detect Parkinsonism from hanwriting [15]. Authors in [16] used SVM classifier along with AutoML to analyze handwriting and detected depression with 82.5% accuracy. Additionally, researchers used BiLSTM to identify anxiety and stress states from handwriting and obtained improvement upto 8.9% compared to the baseline approaches [17]. In another research, authors have mentioned the significance of subtle changes in fine motor control to detect early dementia [18]. Their handwriting kinetics and quantitative EEG analysis based classification model achieved 96.3% accuracy using SVM with RBF kernel as the base classifier.

3 Methodology

The suggested four-stage structure consists of data collection, data parsing, classification models, and accuracy testing.

3.1 Data Acquisition

Raw handwritten samples have been captured for further analysis. 17 participants were enrolled for the experiment. In detail, the participants were composed of 11 subjects with ASD (9 males, 2 females, age: 7 to 10 years) and 6 healthy ones (2 males, 4 females, age: 7 to 10 years). Each participant was asked to complete the handwriting task on a blank piece of white A4 paper using pencil. Further, the papers have been scanned. All information obtained has been treated as strictly confidential and used exclusively for research purpose. Sample images from the dataset are depicted in Fig. 1.

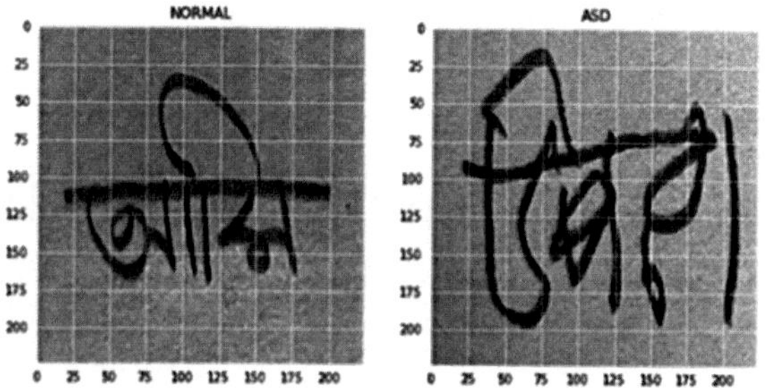

Fig. 1. Illustrations from the dataset. The image on the left represents the handwriting of a healthy child. The image on the right represent the handwriting of a child with ASD.

3.2 Dataset Preprocessing

In a ratio of 8:2, the dataset was divided into training and testing sets. In addition, the training set was subdivided into a validation set and a training set at a 9:1 ratio. The images have been downsized to 224×224 pixels in size for a better architectural efficiency. Images were scaled down to 299×299 pixels to train InceptionV3 and Xception. Nearest-Neighbor Interpolation was utilized for uniform image resizing. Data augmentation has been employed to improve the generalizability of an over-fitted data model as well as to resolve the class imbalance issue in the dataset. The augmentation procedure was applied by randomly rotating some training images by 30°C, zooming by 20%, shifting horizontally 10% and shifting vertically 10% to make the model more robust to slight variations.

3.3 Model Architecture

1) InceptionV3. A sequence of convolutional and pooling operations are performed on the input data by a succession of modules, organized into blocks, that make up the InceptionV3 model. Since our dataset only allowed for binary classification, we modified the InceptionV3 architecture by removing its top layers and adding two dense layers. There are 256 neurons present in the dense layer that comes before the output layer. To avoid overfitting, we've used the ReLu activation function 1, with a dropout of 0.5.

$$f(x) = max(0, x) \tag{1}$$

The dense layer employs the 'he_uniform' kernel initializer. The output layer classifies the images into two groups, 'ASD' and 'Normal' using Sigmoid activation function 2. The model has been trained utilizing Adam optimizer with the given specifications: learning rate = 0.001, beta_1 = 0.9, beta_2 = 0.999 and epsilon = 0.1. In addition, 'binary crossentropy' was chosen as the loss function.

$$S(x) = \frac{1}{1 + e^{-x}} \tag{2}$$

2) VGG19. The foundation of the VGG19 model is a convolutional layer, which is followed by ReLU activation function as discussed previously in 1 and a max pooling layer.

We slightly changed the architecture by deleting the top layers and adding a dense layer followed by a flatten layer. Using Sigmoid activation function, the output layer categorizes the images into two groups: 'ASD' and 'Normal'. Adam optimizer was used to train the model with the following parameters: learning rate = 0.001, beta_1 = 0.9, beta_2 = 0.999 and epsilon = 0.1. 'Binary crossentropy' was selected as the loss function that is calculated using the equation given in 3.

$$Loss = abs(Y\_pred - Y\_actual) \tag{3}$$

3) Xception. Xception has been designed to be more efficient than standard CNNs, with fewer parameters and computational resources, while still producing satisfactory results.

The input layer passes the image data through a stack of depthwise seperable convolutional blocks and skip connections. The blocks consist of a pointwise convolution and rectified linear unit (ReLU) activation function that is presented in 1. The skip connections skip additional processing and directly pass the data to the output. Following that, the output layer produces a prediction.

We fine-tuned the architecture by not including the top layers and adding one dense layer with a dropout of 0.5 followed by on flatten layer. Using the Adam optimizer, the model has been trained with the following parameters: learning rate = 0.001, beta_1 = 0.9, beta_2 = 0.999 and epsilon = 0.1. 'Binary crossentropy' was selected to be used as the loss function.

4 Experimental Results and Discussion

Precision, recall, specificity, F1-score, accuracy, cohen kappa score and roc-auc score were some of the performance metrics used to evaluate the described models. Table 1 contains a comparison of the models' performances for the mentioned parameters.

Table 1. A comparison among the models on performance evaluation metrics

InceptionV3			VGG19			Xception		
Accuracy		0.62	Accuracy		0.95	Accuracy		0.98
F1 score	ASD	0.44	F1 score	ASD	0.97	F1 score	ASD	0.98
	Normal	0.71		Normal	0.97		Normal	0.98
ROC AUC score		0.80	ROC AUC score		0.96	ROC AUC score		0.98
Cohen Kappa score		0.25	Cohen Kappa score		0.93	Cohen Kappa score		0.97

In short, Table 1 illustrates that the Xception architecture outperforms other two architectures by achieving 36% and 2% higher accuracy than InceptionV3 and VGG19 respectively. The cohen's kappa value of InceptionV3 is 0.25, which interprets the test as fair. However, the model obtained an average ROC AUC score, that is 0.80. On the other hand, ROC AUC scores of both VGG19 and Xception are between 0.95 to 1.00, which suggest that both of the models are capable of identifying ASD from handwriting images perfectly. Additionally, Xception obtained the highest kappa score out of the three models that is close to 1, indicating great concordance with the assigned labels.

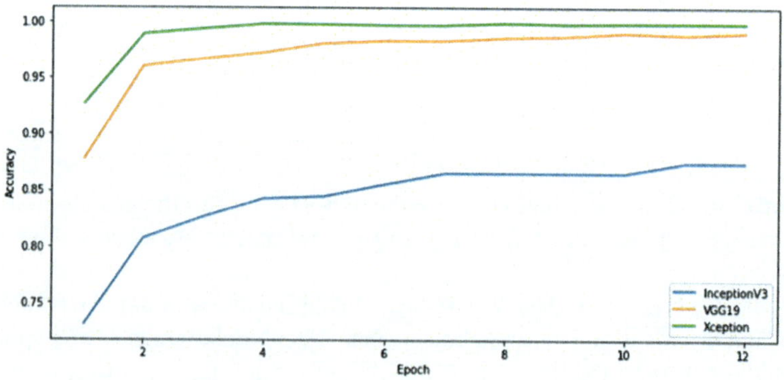

Fig. 2. Training Accuracy graph of three models.

Besides, Fig. 2 exhibits a graph comparing training accuracy of the three models. The graph demonstrates that the training accuracy of Xception is superior to that of the other two models at each epoch. Training accuracy of InceptionV3 is comparatively lower at each epoch. On the other hand, Fig. 3 displays a graph representing the training losses of the models per epoch. The graph illustrates that the training loss of Xception becomes close to zero after four epochs. Although VGG19's training loss is initially higher than that of the other two models, it improves significantly after the first six iterations.

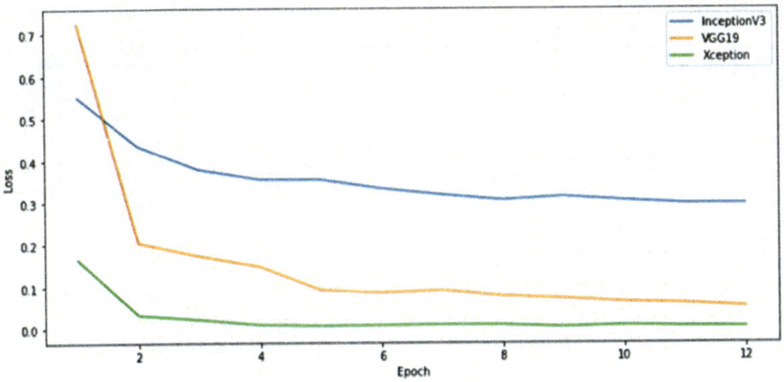

Fig. 3. Training Loss graph of three models.

Furthermore, Fig. 4 presents a diagram of validation accuracy of three models. It depicts that the accuracy of both VGG19 and Xception become 100% after four epochs. However, similar to the training accuracy, the validation accuracy of InceptionV3 is lower. Figure 5 exhibits the validation losses of the three models per epoch. The graph signifies that validation loss of InceptionV3, in comparison to the other models, is higher at every epoch.

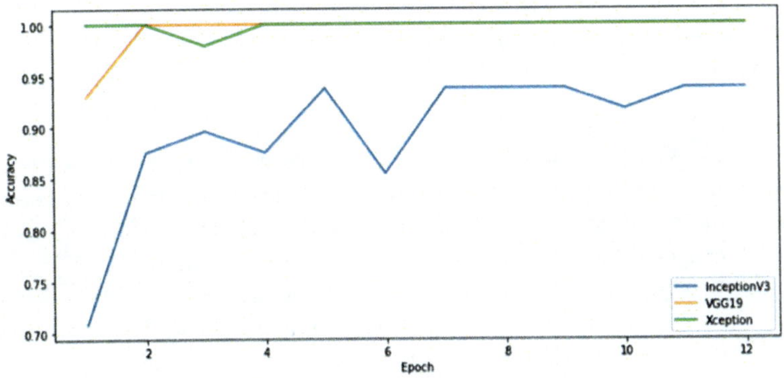

Fig. 4. Validation Accuracy graph of three models.

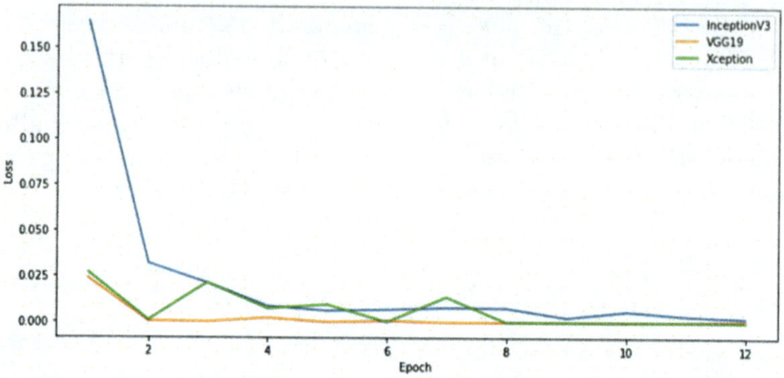

Fig. 5. Validation Loss graph of three models.

From the confusion matrices of the three models demonstrated in Fig. 6, it is visible that InceptionV3 showed overall poor outcome as evidenced by its 190 failed prediction on the test set. Conversely, Xception has accurately predicted 11 more images labeled as 'ASD' than VGG19. However, both VGG19 and Xception predicted all handwritings of normal children accurately.

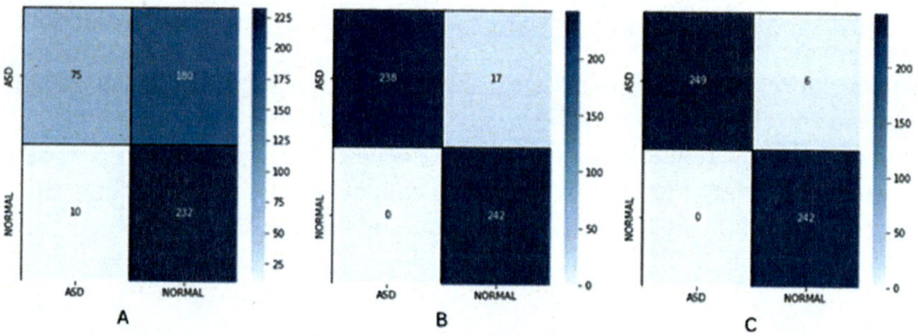

Fig. 6. Confusion matrix of the three models on test set. (A) InceptionV3 (B) VGG19 (C) Xception

One potential reason why VGG19 has outperformed InceptionV3 is because it has a deeper and more narrow architecture, with a larger number of convolutional layers and smaller filters. This allows it to capture more detailed features in the input data which makes the model more computationally expensive to train and deploy. In that case, Xception in much efficient since it utilizes depthwise separable convolutions that decompose the standard convolution operation into a depthwise convolution and a pointwise convolution, which allows the model to achieve a similar level of performance with fewer parameters and computational resources. Additionally, the architecture of Xception uses skip connections that allow it to incorporate information from multiple layers of the network and improve the flow of gradients during training.

5 Conclusion

In this research, we set out to automate the difficulty of distinguishing children with autism spectrum disorder from healthy subjects by utilizing a novel approach. Studies convey that children diagnosed with ASD often struggle with both fine and gross motor skills, that include hand-wrist movements. Therefore, handwriting impairments are generally present in children diagnosed with autism. As a result, handwriting traits can be a new bio-marker for identifying ASD.

To provide evidence in support of the assertion, we gathered handwriting images of children aged between 7 to 10 years. Following that, we incorporated three architectures in order to successfully predict ASD from handwritten text images. Among the three architectures, VGG19 and Xception have shown promising outcomes for diagnosing ASD from handwriting with an accuracy rate of 95% and 98% respectively. The proposed handwriting features based automated, non-invasive, and rapid detection protocol will help screening children with autism spectrum disorder.

When doing research on forecasting ASD, we ran into certain challenges that are intended to overcome in the future. Lack of sufficiently large data with more variation to train the prediction model is the study's primary weakness. Again, the dataset only contain images of handwriting in Bangla language. Our future work will emphasize on collecting more handwriting in different languages from reliable sources so that the prediction becomes more robust.

References

1. El-Yacoubi, M.A., Garcia-Salicetti, S., Kahindo, C., Rigaud, A.S., Cristancho-Lacroix, V.: From aging to early-stage Alzheimer's: uncovering handwriting multimodal behaviors by semi-supervised learning and sequential representation learning. Pattern Recogn. **86**, 112–133 (2019)
2. Moetesum, M., Siddiqi, I., Vincent, N., Cloppet, F.: Assessing visual attributes of handwriting for prediction of neurological disorders-A case study on Parkinson's disease. Pattern Recogn. Lett. **121**, 19–27 (2019)
3. Gornale, S., Kumar, S., Siddalingappa, R., Hiremath, P.S.: Survey on handwritten signature biometric data analysis for assessment of neurological disorder using machine learning techniques. Trans. Mach. Learn. Artif. Intell. **10**, 27–60 (2022)
4. Faundez-Zanuy, M., Fierrez, J., Ferrer, M.A., Diaz, M., Tolosana, R., Plamondon, R.: Handwriting biometrics: applications and future trends in e-security and e-health. Cogn. Comput. **12**, 940–953 (2020)
5. Rosenblum, S., Ben-Simhon, H.A., Meyer, S., Gal, E.: Predictors of handwriting performance among children with autism spectrum disorder. Res. Autism Spectrum Disorders **60**, 16–24 (2019)
6. Islam, S., Akter, T., Zakir, S., Sabreen, S., Hossain, M.I.: Autism spectrum disorder detection in toddlers for early diagnosis using machine learning. In: Proceedings of 2020 IEEE Asia-Pacific Conference on Computer Science and Data Engineering, Gold Coast, Australia, pp. 1–6 (2020)
7. Alwidian, J., Elhassan, A., Ghnemat, R.: Predicting autism spectrum disorder using machine learning technique. Int. J. Recent Technol. Eng. **8**, 4139–4143 (2020)

8. Shinde, A.V., Patil, D.D.: Content-centric prediction model for early autism spectrum disorder (ASD) Screening in Children. In: Proceedings the ICT Infrastructure and Computing, Singapore, pp. 369–378 (2022)
9. Hossain, M.D., Kabir, M.A., Anwar, A., Islam, M.Z.: Detecting autism spectrum disorder using machine learning techniques: an experimental analysis on toddler, child, adolescent and adult datasets. Health Inf. Sci. Syst. **9**, 1–13 (2021)
10. del Mar Guillén, M., Amador, S., Peral, J., Gil, D., Elouali, A.: Overcoming the lack of data to improve prediction and treatment of individuals with autistic spectrum disorder and attention deficit hyperactivity disorder. In: Proceedings the International Conference on Ubiquitous Computing and Ambient Intelligence, Córdoba, Spain, pp. 760–771 (2023)
11. Karri, V.S., Remya, S., Vybhav, A.R., Ganesh, G.S., Eswar, J.: Detecting autism spectrum disorder using DenseNet. In: Proceedings of the ICT Infrastructure and Computing, Singapore, pp. 461–467 (2022)
12. Karunakaran, P., Hamdan, Y.B.: Early prediction of autism spectrum disorder by computational approaches to fMRI analysis with early learning technique. J. Artif. Intell. **02**, 207–216 (2020)
13. Li, C., Zhang, T., Li, J.: Identifying autism spectrum disorder in resting-state fNIRS signals based on multiscale entropy and a two-branch deep learning network. J. Neurosci. Methods **383**, 109732 (2023)
14. Aulia, M.R., Djamal, E.C., Bon, A.T.: Personality identification based on handwritten signature using convolutional neural networks. In: Proceedings the 5th NA International Conference on Industrial Engineering and Operations Management Detroit, Michigan, USA, pp. 1761–1772 (2020)
15. Diaz, M., Moetesum, M., Siddiqi, I., Vessio, G.: Sequence-based dynamic handwriting analysis for Parkinson's disease detection with one-dimensional convolutions and BiGRUs. Expert Syst. Appl. **168**, 114405 (2021)
16. Nolazco-Flores, J.A., Faundez-Zanuy, M., Velázquez-Flores, O.A., Del-Valle-Soto, C., Cordasco, G., Esposito, A.: Mood State Detection in Handwritten Tasks Using PCA-mFCBF and Automated Machine Learning. Sensors **22**, 1686 (2022)
17. Rahman, A.U., Halim, Z.: Identifying dominant emotional state using handwriting and drawing samples by fusing features. Appl. Intell. **53**, 2798–2814 (2022)
18. Chai, J., Wu, R., Li, A., Xue, C., Qiang, Y., Zhao, J., Zhao, Q., Yang, Q.: Classification of mild cognitive impairment based on handwriting dynamics and qEEG. Comput. Biol. Med. **152**, 106418 (2023)

A Brief Summary of Selected Link Prediction Surveys

Ahmed Rawashdeh(✉)

Applied Science Private University (ASU), Amman, Jordan
ah_rawashdeh@asu.edu.jo

Abstract. This paper summarizes several surveys of Link Prediction methods. It starts with a background introduction and problem definition, then provides information about several Link Prediction methods found in many surveys. It has been written with the aim of providing an assistive summary of Link Prediction methods for researchers in this field. Link Prediction is important since it has many applications including recommending friends in social networking and recommending products for customers to buy in e-commerce. It works by predicting which links are more likely to form in the future based on the local (neighborhood) or the global structure of the graph. This paper is a surveys' summary. It is beneficial because surveys are important in providing a very good review, reference, and comprehensive coverage of the topic. By having a good survey, researchers and readers can save a great amount of time by only looking at fewer papers. Several methods found in survey papers have been summarized in this work including Common Neighbors, Preferential Attachment, Jaccard, Adamic/Adar, SimRank, PageRank, Probabilistic, Node-based, Topology, Path-based, Random Walk, Learning, Quasi, and others. It has been found out that the survey paper with the highest citation has 2827 citations, followed by the second highest which is 643. This paper is a summary of survey papers, and should be distinguished from traditional surveys, that summarize Link Prediction methods discussed in one or more non-survey papers. This paper is the first paper of its kind in this field.

Keywords: Survey · Link Prediction · Social Network · Dynamic Networks · Surveys Summary

1 Introduction

The Link Prediction problem was first introduced by [1] and later by [2], and since then it has gained popularity. The reader needs to be introduced to this problem first. The next section provides a formal definition of Link Prediction. However, prior to that, it is helpful to know the importance of this area. Research in this field is important since Link Prediction has a variety of applications including, to name a few, friends' recommendation in social networking, authors recommendation in co-authorship networks, videos recommendation in media streaming websites (the people also watched this video feature), item recommendation in retail websites (the people who bought this item also bought the following items feature). This paper represents a survey of surveys, but first what is a survey of surveys?

K. Daimi and A. Al Sadoon (Eds.): ICR 2023, LNNS 721, pp. 175–184, 2023.
https://doi.org/10.1007/978-3-031-35308-6_15

There is a variety of survey papers, that cover "survey papers". Several of these have provided information about surveys, but in a different area than this paper. A survey on one topic reviews all papers in that topic, and a survey of surveys reviews survey papers. For example, the reader may refer to [3, 4, 5] for surveys of surveys. They are all characterized by the vast number of surveys they have reviewed, and the variety of comparative tables, visuals and figures they have included. However, this paper differs in being more compact and briefer, but at the same time to the point and useful for researchers.

Why this paper? there is still a demand for a review and a detailed survey of Link Prediction methods. Therefore, comes this research paper with the aim to help researchers of Link Prediction to know the required background information about this field and to stay updated on the latest in this field. Moreover, this research paper summarizes and reviews several surveys, and it could be considered as a summary of surveys. This paper is the first of its kind since it is the first survey of Link Prediction methods' surveys. However, what is Link Prediction? The problem needs to be formally defined first. The following section provides an introductory definition of the problem.

1.1 Link Prediction Problem

The problem of Link Prediction can be briefly and formally summarized as follows:

Given a graph (G) which consists of two sets: the set of vertices (V) and the set of edges (E), which links are going to be formed in the future, and what are the missing links which have been dropped/erased. The former version of this problem is concerned about predicting new links, the latter is concerned about predicting missing links. So, there are two types of links to be predicted: either new links or missing links. For more details the reader may refer to [6, 7], and [8] which also list several Link Prediction applications. Also, the reader may refer to [9].

Since the motive of research is as important as the research itself, and to be clearer about the importance of Link Prediction, the reader is encouraged to continue and read the next section.

1.2 Why Link Prediction

Why is there a need to predict future or missing links? The answer is as the networks' sizes continue to grow, and as the structure, of the different types of networks, dynamically changes, it has been proved to be beneficial to be able to infer which links are about to form between any two nodes in the future or to restore the lost links of the graph. This helps in improving the services provided by the website which implements/provides the Link Prediction services (such as recommender systems described in Sect. 1). Application of which, allows for predicting links in social networks, generally known as friends' recommendations, and also helps in the case of Facebook, which uses common friends between the users in recommending friends, it is known as the "people you may know" feature [10]. Another application is recommending items which customers are more likely to buy in online retail websites [11, 12].

The next question, which may rise, is what methods of Link Prediction were surveyed in survey papers? And how do these survey papers differ in terms of their coverage of Link Prediction methods? and what are the characteristic of each paper (citation and references for example)? The next section provides answers to all these questions and includes tables summarizing that.

2 Link Prediction Surveys

This section provides information about Link Prediction surveys. The following tables: Table 1, Table 2, Table 3, Table 4, and Table 5 summarize the list of Link Prediction methods discussed and surveyed in several survey papers [8, 9, 13–15].

Several Link Prediction methods were surveyed in multiple papers. For instance, Common Neighbors, Jaccard, and Adamic/Adar Index were discussed in all survey papers (the five papers). Salton was mentioned in all except for [9, 14]. Kats is in all survey papers. Random walk has been explained in all except for [14]. Probabilistic methods are in [5, 8, 14, 16]. Supervised Machine Learning methods were surveyed in [9, 13, 15] and not in [8, 14].

Link Prediction methods are either: Node based, Path based, Topological based, Local, Global, Learning, Random Walk, Probabilistic, or Quasi. Also, they have been classified based on the type of network they can be used in as either Homogeneous, Heterogeneous, or Aligned network-based Link Prediction methods [9]. The following paragraphs explain each type.

2.1 Node Based

Node based are Link Prediction methods which uses the nodes part of the graph. Graphs, as explained in Sect. 1.1, consists of two sets, the nodes set (vertices) and the edges set (connections). Nodes represent the profile content in social networks. Example of such methods are: Common Neighbors, Jaccard, Preferential Attachment, and Adamic Adar. Information about each methods follow.

Common Neighbors: Considers the number of common adjacent neighbors of the two nodes of the graph. The more the number of Common Neighbors, the more likely that a link (connection) will be formed and thus the link should be recommended.

Jaccard: Considers the ratio of the number of shared direct neighbors between the two nodes of the graph to overall number of neighbors of the two nodes.

Preferential Attachment: Is the probability of forming a link calculated as the product of the number of neighbors of the first node multiplied by the number of direct neighbors of the second node. The more the nodes are connected the more likely to predict the link.

Adamic/Adar: The more the number of shared links between the pair of the nodes the more likely to predict the link.

For the math formula of each of the method above, the reader may refer to [7, 6].

2.2 Path-Based (Global)

Path-based are methods that look at ensembles of all paths between the pair of nodes. Example is Katz and FriendLink [17].

2.3 Probabilistic

This method uses probability in predicting the link. The probability is defined as plausibility which has reference to reasonableness of belief or expectation. The other meaning of probability, which is attributed to it by statisticians, has reference to random ~~and~~ chance phenomena [16].

2.4 Learning

Learnings are methods that use Machine Learning algorithms to classify pairs of nodes, after training on a labeled training-data (i.e., examples where the output is known), in order to predict the formation of a link or not between the nodes in the pair. The trained models are evaluated using a testing-dataset, to select a good model for predicting the formation of the link.

2.5 Random-Walk

Random-Walks are methods that predict the links using Random Walk. This method, in its simplest form, executes a Random Walk from the first node recursively vising its next adjacent neighbor node at each step. Then perform another Random Walk from the second node. If the two walks meet, then a link will be predicted. Another version is to start the walk from the first node and predict a link if the walk reaches the second node.

2.6 Homogeneous

Homogeneous methods are node-based methods or path-based methods.

2.7 Heterogenous

Heterogenous methods are machine learning methods.

Table 1. Link Prediction methods in [8]

Lü L, Tao Z. [8]				
Local	Global	Quasi-Local Indices	Maximum Likelihood Methods	Probabilistic Models
1. Common Neighbors 2. Salton index 3. Jaccard index 4. Sorensen index 5. Hub promoted index 6. Hub depressed index 7. Leicht-Holme_newman index 8. Adamic-Adar Index 9. ResourceAllocation index	1. Katz 2. Leicht-Holme_newman Index 3. Average Commute time (ACT) 4. Cosine based on L + 5. Random walk 6. SimRank 7. Marix Forest Index (MFI) 8. Quasi-Local Indices	1. Local Path Index (LP) 2. Local Random Walk (LRW) 3. Superposed Random Walk (SRW)	1. Hierarchical Structure Model . Stochastic Block Model	1. Probabilistic Relational Models 2. Probabilistic Entity Relationship Models 3. Stochastic Relational Models

Table 2. Link Prediction methods in [13]

Wang, P, et al.[13]			
Topology-based	Path based	Random Walk	Learning Based
1. Common Neighbors (CN) 2. Jaccard Coefficient (JC) 3. Sorensen Index 4. Salton Cosine Similairty 5. Hub Promoted (HP) 6. Leicht_holme_Nerman 7. Parameter-Dependent (PD) 8. Adamic-Adar Coefficient 9. Preferential Attachment (PA) 10. Resource Allocation (RA)	1. Local Path 2. Katz 3. Relation Strength Similarity (RSS) 4. FriendLink (FL)	1. Hitting Time (HT) 2. Commute Time (CT) 3. Cosine Similarity Time (CST) 4. SimRank 5. Rooted PageRank (RPR)	1. Feature-based Classification 2. Probabilistic Graph Model 3. Matrix Factorization

2.8 Topological

Topological methods are either node-based or global based. They are methods which are based on the structure of the graph. According to [15] they are classified as either Local or Global. Local methods rely on the structures of the graph such as neighborhood nodes, while Global methods rely on the overall structural information, and they are not restricted to two node distance as Local methods. However, their complexity increases by network size.

Table 3. Link Prediction methods in [9]

Zhang J, S Yu P. [9]			
Homogeneous Network	Heterogeneous Network	Aligned Network	
Unsupervised (local): 1. Preferential Attachment Index (PA) 2. Common Neighbors 3. Jaccard Coefficient 4. Adamic/Adar Index 5. ResourceAllocation Index Unsupervised (Global): 6. Shortest path (SP) 7. Katz Random 8. Random Walk ProximityMeasures based on random Walk: 9. Hitting time (HT) 10. Commute time (CT) 11. Cosine Similarity 12. RandomWalkwith Restart	Supervised: 1. Feature Extraction 2. Social Meta Path Classification Algorithms Collective Link Prediction	Anchor Link Prediction 1. Heterogeneous Feature Extraction across Networks 2. Extended Jaccard Coefficient 3. Extended Adamic/Adar Link Transfer Across Aligned Networks: 1. Supervised Link Prediction	
Local Neighbor Based Predicators	**Global Path based Predicator**	**Random Walk based Link Prediction**	**Proximity Measures based Random Walk**
1. Preferential Attachment Index (PA) 2. Common Neighbors 3. Jaccard Coefficient 4. Adamic/Adar Index 5. ResourceAllocation Index	1. Shortest Path (SP) 2. Katz	Random Walk	1. Hitting Time 2. Commute Time 3. Cosine Similarity 4. Random Walk with Restart

Table 4. Link Prediction methods in [14]

Hasan MA, Mohammed J [14]		
Node-wise similarity	Topological pattern based	Probabilistic model based
1. Similarity measure in binary classifier 2. Pairwise kernel matrices 3. Statisticalrelational learning	1. Node based patterns • Common Neighbors • Jaccard • Adamic/Adar • Preferential Attachment 2. Graph based patterns 3. Path based patterns • Katz • Page rank • SimRank	1. Probabilistic relational models (dependency/Markov Networks) 2. Bayesian relational models (parametric/non-parametric) 3. Stochastic relational models

Table 5. Link Prediction methods in [15]

Samad A, et al. [15]			
Topological based (local)	Topological based (global and path based)	Random Walk	Quasi
1. Common neighbor 2. Jaccard coefficient 3. SAM 4. Adamic/Adar 5. Resource Allocation 6. Preferential Attachment 7. Sorensen Index 8. Salton Cosine 9. Hub Promoted 10. Hub Depressed 11. Leicht-Holme-Nerman 12. Parameter-Dependent 13. Individual Attraction 14. Local Naïve Bayes 15. CAR-based 16. Functional Similarity Weight	1. Local path 2. Katz 3. Relation Strength 4. Shortest Path 5. FriendLink	1. Random Walk 2. RandomWalkwith Restart 3. Hittime time 4. Commute Time 5. Cosine Similarity 6. SimRank 7. Rooted pageRank 8. PropFlow 9. SepctralLink	1. Local Random Walk 2. Supervised Random Walk
Hybrid	**Learning Based**	**Probabilistic model**	**Preprocessing**
1. Evidential Measurement 2. Methods in Weighted Networks	1. Classification 2. Matrix Factorization 3. Meta-Heuristics 4. Kernel-based	1. Hierarchical Structure Model 2. Stochastic Block Model 3. Cycle Formation Model 4. LocalCo-Occurrence Model	1. LowRank Approximation 2. Unseen Biagrams 3. Filtering

3 Discussion

The formulas for the different Link Prediction methods can be found in [15, 18, 19]. Also, the paper [18] provides an experimental survey of Link Predictions which the reader may find useful as well. On the other hand, the author in [19] provided details about the progress of Link Prediction research including local similarity indices, link predictability, networking embedding, and more. A recent survey paper [20] categorized temporal Link Prediction methods into six different main types: Matrix Factorization, Probabilistic, Spectral Clustering, Time Series, Deep Learning, and others. It also included a comparison between several Link Prediction techniques. Moreover, it listed the pros and cons of the different Link Prediction techniques and their categories. Another recent survey paper [21] presented a comprehensive review of the usage of matrix factorization in biomedical link prediction. In which, the authors conducted a systematic empirical comparison on a dataset to evaluate the performance of the methods. Martinez, et al. [22] grouped Link Prediction methods into four main categories: Similarity-based methods, Probabilistic and Statistical methods, Algorithmic methods, and Preprocessing methods. Similarity based methods are either Local, Global or Quasi-local. Algorithmic methods are further classified as either Classifier-based, Metaheuristic-based, or Factorization-based. The authors also included, in their paper, a comparison between the complexity of different types of Link Prediction techniques. Also, Zhou [19] covered the complexity of different Link Prediction methods too.

Table 6 provides a comparison between the studied survey papers in terms of which methods they have surveyed. The comparison considers the following Link Prediction methods: common Neighbors, Jaccard coefficient, Adamic/Adar, Preferential Attachment, Salton, Katz, and random walk, SimRank, PageRank, Probabilistic and cosine. These methods were found in almost all these survey papers. All of the methods were included in all papers except Preferential Attachment is not in [8], Salton cosine, SimRank, PageRank and Probabilistic are not in [9]. Cosine is not in [14], and all remaining methods are in all papers.

Table 6. Link Prediction methods in survey papers

Link Prediction method	Paper				
	[8]	[13]	[9]	[14]	[15]
Common Neighbors	yes	yes	yes	yes	yes
Jaccard coefficient	yes	yes	yes	yes	yes
Adamic/Adar	yes	yes	yes	yes	yes
Preferential Attachment	No	yes	yes	yes	yes
Salton Cosine	yes	yes	No	Yes	yes
Katz	yes	yes	yes	yes	yes
Random Walk	yes	yes	yes	No	yes
SimRank	yes	yes	No	yes	yes
PageRank	No	yes	No	yes	yes
Probabilistic	yes	yes	No	yes	yes
Cosine	yes	yes	yes	No	yes

Table 7 is a comparison between the survey papers in terms of the publication year, the number of references. The number of citations of the paper, and if it is a journal or not. The papers from the most recent to the oldest are as follows: [15] which was published in 2020, then [13] which was published in 2015, after that comes [9] which was published in 2014, finally comes the oldest among them [14] and [8] which were published in 2011. The paper with the highest citation count is [8] with a total number of citations equals to 2877, and the one with the lowest number of citations is [15].

The survey paper with the largest number of references is [8]. All the survey papers are journal papers.

Table 7. Comparison between the survey papers.

Paper	Year	Number of references	Number of Citations (scholar.google.com)	Journal
[8]	2011	166	2827	yes
[13]	2015	131	643	yes
[9]	2014	62	22	yes
[14]	2011	29	716	yes
[15]	2020	108	8	yes

4 Conclusion

This paper summarized several Link Predictions surveys. Survey papers include variety of Link Prediction methods such as Common Neighbors, Jaccard, Preferential Attachment, Adamic-Adar, Katz, Probabilistic, Random-Walk, and Classification methods (Learning based). Some methods are common to all survey papers while the others can only be found in few papers. Moreover, different survey papers use different classification of Link Prediction methods. For example, in some papers, the Link Prediction methods are classified as either Local or Global, while in other papers, the same methods are classified as Topological or as Node-based and Path-based. Finally, in this paper, the survey papers were classified based on the number of citation and references. The paper with the highest number of citations has 2827 and the one with the lowest number of citations has 8.

5 Future Work

Future work is to extend this survey to a comprehensive survey that will cover additional survey papers. Additionally, an experimental survey of Link Prediction methods can be conducted too.

References s

1. Liben-Nowell, D., Kleinberg, J.: The link prediction problem for social networks. In: Proceedings of the twelfth international conference on Information and knowledge management. New York, pp. 556–559 (2003)
2. David, L.N., Kleinberg, J.: The link-prediction problem for social networks. J. Am. Soc. Inf. Sci. Technol., 1019–1031 (2007)

3. Giraldo, J., et al.: Security and privacy in cyber-physical systems: a survey of surveys. IEEE Design Test, 7–17 (2017)
4. Chatzimparmpas, A., et al.: A survey of surveys on the use of visualization for interpreting machine learning models. Information Visualization, 207–233 (2020)
5. McNabb, L., Robert, S.L.: Survey of surveys (SoS)-Mapping the landscape of survey papers in information visualization. Comput. Graph. Forum, 589–617 (2017)
6. Rawashdeh, A.: An Experiment with Link Prediction in Social Network: Two New Link Prediction Methods, San Francisco CA, USA, pp. 563–581 (2019)
7. Rawashdeh, A.: Performance based Comparison between Several Link Prediction Methods on Various Social Networking Datasets (Including Two New Methods). Int. J. Adv. Comput. Sci. Appl. (IJACSA), pp. 1–8 (2020)
8. Lü, L., Tao, Z.: Link Prediction in complex networks: a survey. Physica A: Stat. Mech. Appl., 1150–1170 (2011)
9. Zhang, J., S Yu P. Link Prediction across heterogeneous social networks: A survey. [Internet]. 2014 March 20[cited2022Nov10].http://bdsc.lab.uic.edu/docs/2014_survey_paper.pdf
10. CenterH.PeopleYouMayKnow.[Internet] (2022). https://www.facebook.com/help/336320879782850
11. Krysik, A.: Amazon's Product Recommendation System In 2021: How Does The Algorithm Of The eCommerce Giant Work? [Internet] (2021). https://recostream.com/blog/amazon-recommendation-system
12. Recommendations.[Internet] (2022).https://www.amazon.com/gp/help/customer/display.html?nodeId=GE4KRSZ4KAZZB4BV
13. Wang, P., et al.: Link Prediction in social networks: the state-of-the-art. Science China Information Sciences, 1–38 (2015)
14. Hasan, M.A., Mohammed, J.: A survey of Link Prediction in social networks. Social network data analytics, pp. 243–275 (2011)
15. Samad, A., et al.: A comprehensive survey of Link Prediction techniques for social network. EAI Endorsed Trans. Ind. Networks Intell. Syst. **7**(23), e3–e3 (2020)
16. Anscombe, F.J., Aumann, R.J.: A definition of subjective probability. Ann. Math. Stat., 199–205 (1963)
17. Papadimitriou, A., Panagiotis, S., Yannis, M.: Friendlink: Link prediction in social networks via bounded local path traversal. In: International Conference on Computational Aspects of Social Networks (CASoN), Salamanca, Spain, pp. 66–71 (2011)
18. Wu, H., Song, C., Ge, Y., et al.: Link prediction on complex networks: an experimental survey. Data Sci. Eng. **7**, 253–278 (2022)
19. Zhou, T.: Progresses and challenges in link prediction. Iscience **24**(11), 103217 (2021)
20. Divakaran, A., Mohan, A.: Temporal link prediction: a survey. N. Gener. Comput. **38**, 213–258 (2020)
21. Ou-Yang, L., et al.: Matrix factorization for biomedical link prediction and scRNA-seq data imputation: an empirical survey. Briefings Bioinform. **23**(1) 2022
22. Martínez, V., Berzal, F., Cubero, J.-C.: A survey of link prediction in complex networks. ACM Comput. Surv. (CSUR) **49**(4), 1–33 (2016)

A Taxonomy for Efficient Electronic Medical Record Systems Using Ubiquitous Computing

Y. Yasmi[1], Nawzat Sadiq Ahmed[2], Razwan Mohmed Salah[3](✉), Qurat Ul Ain Nizamani[4], and Shaymaa Ismail Ali[5]

[1] Study Group Australia, Darlinghurst, Australia
[2] Duhok Polytechnic University, Duhok, KRI, Iraq
nawzat.ahmed@dpu.edu.krd
[3] The University of Duhok, Duhok, KRI, Iraq
razwan.mayi@uod.ac
[4] Kent Institute Australia, Sydney, Australia
qurat.nizamani@kent.edu.au
[5] Cihan University, Duhok, KRI, Iraq
shayma.ali@duhokcihan.edu.krd

Abstract. Electronic medical records (EMR) when accessed over cloud from many sources can have issues of incomplete and inaccurate information. This research aims at providing a taxonomy for EMR by identifying components that can constitute EMR systems by integrating medical entities. The system should be able to provide relevant information to the patients, medical practitioners and relevant authorities without any loss of data. Integrated medical records accessed using the cloud computing provides availability of data at any time and place.

Keywords: Electronic Medical Records (EMR) · Particle Swarm Optimization (PSO) · Transfer Data Mart (TDM) · Ubiquitous Computing · Name Entity Recognition (NER)

1 Introduction

The records related to the medical health of the patients stored electronically over the cloud, is known is *EMR*. Ubiquitous computing is used for retrieval of EMR of patients with ease from the cloud. However, it may result into incomplete and inaccurate data of the patient's medical records. This paper proposes a taxonomy for EMR of patients and comprise of components such as data, extraction and validation. The data component allows to identify the type of data available for extraction of medical records. For the timely detection and error management for the documentation of data, various frameworks have been considered. The proposed system uses data extraction to retrieve important and relevant data and is validated on the grounds of its reliability, accuracy and consistency. This was not available in the previous state-of-art solutions. This further helps in easy interoperability of patient data for easy transfer without any quality degradation. Through literature, it has been identified that for ubiquitous computing Transport

K. Daimi and A. Al Sadoon (Eds.): ICR 2023, LNNS 721, pp. 185–195, 2023.
https://doi.org/10.1007/978-3-031-35308-6_16

Data Mart (TDM) integrated with Parallel Particle Swarm Optimization (PPSO) [11] is the state-of-the-art solution that can be used for making the data accurate and complete. The main contribution of the paper is identification of key components for an EMR system that will provide complete information. The evaluation and validation of the components is also reported in this paper together with the efficiency achieved in the proposed system.

The rest of the paper is organized as follows: The literature survey of the prominent works in EMR systems is reported in Sect. 2. Section 3 defines our own proposed taxonomy with system's major components and their relationships. Discussion regarding the proposed components and limitations of systems is carried out in Sect. 4. The paper is concluded in Sect. 5.

2 Literature Review

Jimenez-Molina et al. suggested ProFUSO for the efficiency of a healthcare application system [1]. Since there are huge volumes of data to be stored, data retrieval for the process consumes more time. Parallel index building method was introduced for the same purpose which provided real-time data access but was not successful for large-scale data [2]. Peckham suggested Leeds Cystic Fibrosis EPR (LCFEPR) to prevent exploitation of medical records [3]. The proposed system could not overcome the issue of data leakage but provided enhanced accuracy of medical data. Ubiquitous Healthcare Management System with Health Diet Control (UHMS-HDC) was proposed by Kan et al. for better integration of data [4]. The proposed system enabled accessibility of health records on mobile phones. A Name Entity Recognization (NER) model was proposed for natural language processing (NLP) of the patient's data collected electronically [5]. The paper also worked on transferability of data and achieved performance of $FI = 0.762$. Computer aided Diagnosis [CAD) that is CT based nodule detection for providing accurate and clear image in lungs nodule detection was proposed in [6]. Pre-Anaesthesia-Testing (PAT) clinic was proposed for prevention of Obtrusive Sleep Apnea in undiagnosed patients [7]. This system proved helpful in improvising the prevention of risk factors but still faced time delay in the provided information. Lee et al. proposed Prediction module for the purpose of electronic critical care flow sheet data that provided appropriate graph frequencies but could not overcome time consumption limitation [8]. Lee et al. suggested that heart blood flow reduction or sudden blockage cannot be predicted and to overcome this and Risk prediction with HER system was proposed [9]. Fleddermann et al. proposed Best Practice Alert (BPA) which provided alerts on the initial stages for risk prevention in the cardiac treatment [10]. Elhoseny et al. state that management of data on the cloud IoT should be precise and introduced Parallel Particle Swarm Optimization (PPSO) for the same purpose. This reduced execution time but the time taken for data retrieval is still considered high [11]. EMR for post-operative-care unit (PACU) for acceptance of data format directly was proposed by Lingren et al. [12]. This system is more reliable than the traditional manual search but lack of documentation has been observed. E-critical system (E-Critical Tracer, E-Critical Meta-Vision) was suggested by Brundin-Mather et al. which maintained data quality but transactional errors were still found [13]. The process of readmission in the hospital is costly for which Clustering and Logistic regression was proposed in [14]. Smoking cessation technique was proposed by Bae et al. for curing the patients of smoking in E-clinics by sending reminders to the patient [15], but lack of information still remained a limitation. The results of the patients relied on accuracy of medical codes for which Prediction Task Guided Health Record Aggregation (PTGHRA) was proposed by Cui & Shen that provided more accurate results according to availability of previous data but the inaccurate presentation still served as a limitation [16].

The management of the clinical database in the clinics is important and it led to the introduction of Research Electronic Data Capture (REDC) which provided data retrieval with ease but could not achieve a lower loading time [17]. Since data accounting heterogeneity is difficult for hospitals, Composite Mixture Model (CMM) was proposed by Mayhew et al. which provided analysis on a high scale but was still required experts for the same using Bayesian information criterion, Akaike information criterion (AIC), Partitioning Around Medoids (PAM), and Multivariate Imputation using Chained Equations (MICE) [19].

Durable Power of Attorney for Health Care (DPOAHC) was introduced to make advanced planning for care. This helped in development of different caring methodologies but could also possibly provide false information which could prove to be life-threatening [20].

3 Proposed System and Evaluation

Based on the works studied and reported in Sect. 2, we have identified the components that can be considered while devising an efficient and synchronized EMR system. Our proposed taxonomy for EMR systems comprises of three factors, i.e., Data, Extraction and Validation. The proposed factors with subclasses are reflected Fig. 1. The arrows with solid lines depict the subclass inter relationships. The dashed lines show the relationship between the sub classes of different factors and the process followed by them for validation. Data component has 4 sub components i.e., Mining, Clustering, Construction and Collaboration. The techniques used for extraction of only relevant data can be Real time Indexing, NLP, Clinical Decision Support Systems (CDSS) and Prediction. The data extracted must be validated on the grounds of consistency, accuracy and reliability before it can be sent to the applications. The Mining data can be extracted using NLP techniques. The evaluation criteria for this purpose can be consistency. Clustering is used for predication and must be evaluated for reliability.

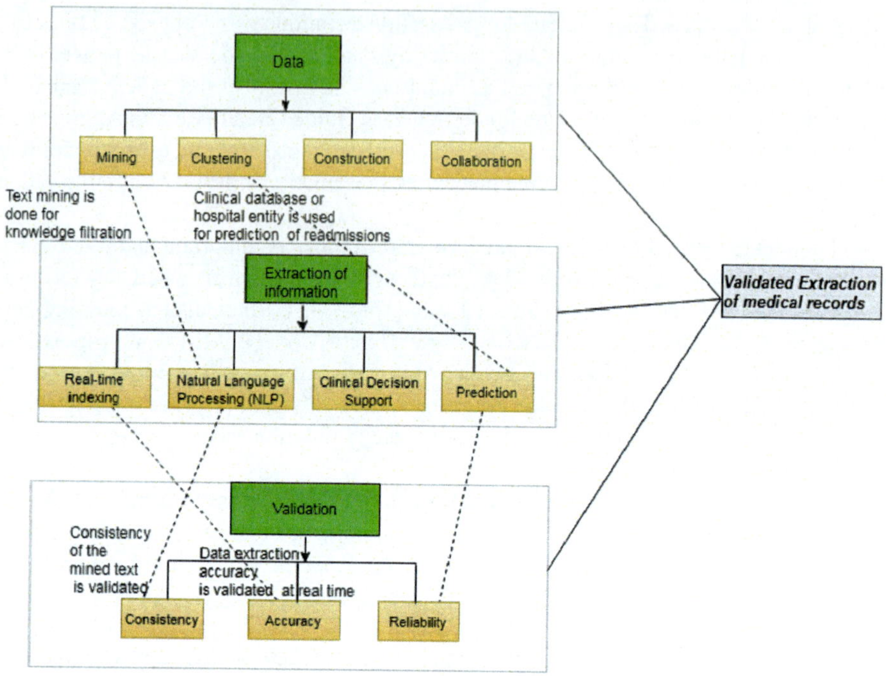

Fig. 1. Proposed System Components

3.1 Classification of Data

The data related to patient reports can be classified as mined data, clustered data, constructed data or collaborated data, as shown in Fig. 2. This classification allows to identify the type of data available for extraction of medical records. The works considered in Sect. 2, suggested the sources that can provide data for the application implementing EMR systems.

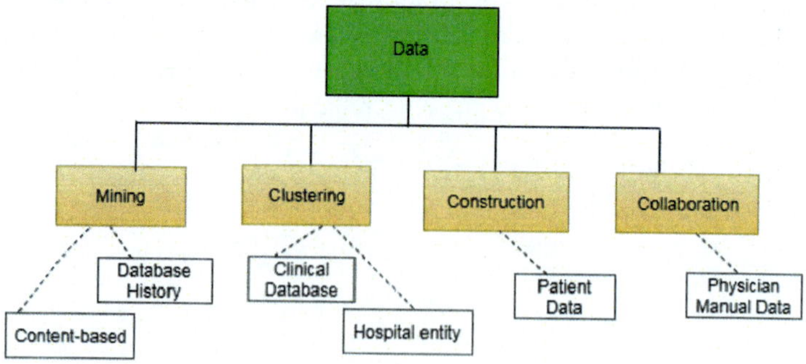

Fig. 2. Sub-factors of Data

Table 1. Proposed Taxonomy components and Evaluation

Ref	Data			Extraction of Information	Evaluation		
	Technique	In	DT		Data evaluated	Method	Results
[1]	BPMN	PD	Con	Using bio-signal or medical information	Enhancing patient data gathering system	Four-layer process for data of patient & hospital	Efficiency up to 58%
[3]	LCFEPR	DH	Con	Primary care platform, EMIS	Modifying the EMIS web	Ease of access for clinician/ patients	58% increased efficiency
[4]	MySQL, JAVA	HE	Cl	Dietary plan/ health condition data are provided to UHMS-HDC	Services for metabolic syndrome to reduce heart disease/ diabetes	Improves information update with mobile device/web portal of hospital	Improvised updates increased by 1-2mm
[5]	NER	DH	M	Data trained to recognize text for 7 classes	Data from MIMIC-III Corpora	NER model for NLP	Performance of FI = 0.957
[6]	CAD	PD	Con	Radio frequencies emitted by CT scanning machine to detect nodules	CT machine providing accurate imaging	Improving sensitivity and reduction of false imaging using CAD	False imaging is reduced by 43%
[7]	PAT	DH	M	Disorder in surgical histories, assessments using manual EMR	PAT procedure to help reduce the risks factors of sleep apnea	Evaluating sleep apnea for different patients for integrated EMR	Better integration with EMR
[8]	Care flow sheet data	DH	M	Patient's related frequencies projected to ICU's digital screens	Data to predict the risks of the extubation among the patient	Provides information for patients for lowering risks related to extubation	Risk lowered by 3 times
[9]	Thrombolysis, GRACE	DH	M	Patient's acute coronary syndrome analyzed by data recorded at the admission stage	Provides patient's medical history, risk level, physical tests	Help hospitals in lowering risks of coronary syndrome	Death rates reduction, by 5 out of 7 patients
[10]	Chi-Square, E-Alert	HE	Cl	Chronic patient's data for go into BPA alert	Analysis for heart diseases of patients readmitted to hospitals	(TTE) is obtained with images of modality providing easy treatment	Easy retrieval of clinical data using GUI

(continued)

Table 1. (*continued*)

Ref	Data			Extraction of Information	Evaluation		
	Technique	In	DT		Data evaluated	Method	Results
[11]	MATLAB, PSO	DH	M	Comparison of algorithm for retrieval time over the cloud	Improved storage, scalability and execution time	Optimizing the VM, choosing suitable application for data retrieval	Optimization of data with 3 times faster result
[12]	EMR	PD	Con	The manual records replaced by the EMR	Healthcare date	Less computation time using EMR	Improved computation time
[13]	Cohen's kappa	HE	Cl	Patient information gathered from EMR to evaluate further research	Obtaining Secondary data from clinical information portal	Completeness/ accuracy of data in retrieval, migration, uploading, etc	Completeness/accuracy of data achieved
[14]	Big data analytics	DH	M	Patient's information during the admission process checked in EMR	Evaluates patient's condition for making improved decisions	Prediction for readmission of same patient /similar case	Accuracy increased by 48%
[15]	Meditech	PD	Con	Analysis of the patient for smoking status	Recording status for counselling	Ethnicity impact on cessation	2 times increased validity
[16]	NLP	DH	M	Demographic information about the patient's hospitalization criteria	Enhances reliability of observations done by medical staff	PTGHRA improves prediction with the decrement in training set size	Prediction accuracy up to 50%
[17]	ASP, REDCap	HE	Cl	Patient reports which are on REDCap	Evaluating effect of assessment reports	Audit tool for expert evaluation	Enhanced evaluation
[18]	Prognosis Prediction	PD	Con	POPCORN provides multi-centre collaboration gateway	Prediction for research by collaborative learning process	Discriminating similar values of a multi-center collaborative network	Improved Prognosis Prediction in cancer

In Input**PD** Patient Data**DH** Database History**HE** Hospital Entity **DT** Data type **M** Mining **Cl Clustering H** Hospital.

Mining of the data can be done using database history or utilizing content-based data. The former utilizes big data analysis and the latter relies on tools like mapping of the medical report, logistic regression mining and text mining. The **clustering** of the medical records is done in two forms, viz., clinical database and hospital entities. Clinical database records are obtained through meta-analysis and hospital entity records are clustered using techniques like REDCap [17] and BPMN [1]. **Construction** of data involves collection, categorization and then recording it for further processing. The data recording is done using the Audit tool or the Antimicrobial Stewardship Program (ASP) [17]. The ASP tool used for construction of data decreases the infection spread that is caused by organisms of multidrug resistance. The data can have a form of collaborated source that is usually the manual data of the patients prepared by the physicians in the clinics. These data are firstly collaborated and fed into the EMR after collaboration through the use of Bayesian framework or the technique of POPCORN.

3.2 Extraction of Data

Extraction of the data leads to retrieval of only important and relevant information. It allows the retrieval of data of a specific pattern from the database that can include structured as well as unstructured data. The activity can be performed using Real-time indexing, NLP, CDSS and the prediction. The tools used for this purpose can be TDM, Name Entity Recognition (NER), CDA engine, Care-flow data, etc. The sub factors of extraction are reported in Fig. 3.

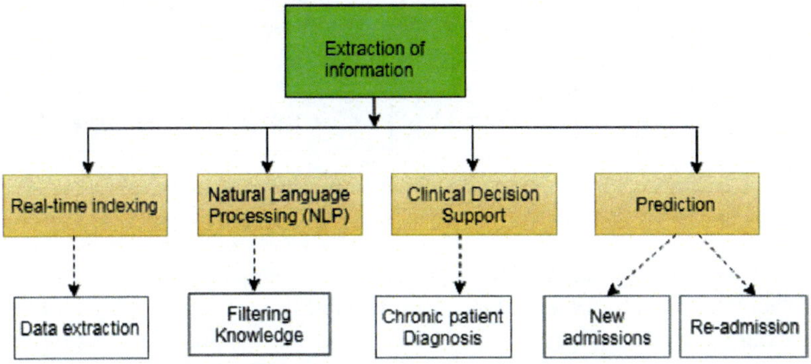

Fig. 3. Subfactors of Extraction of Information

Real-time indexing process enables extraction of the valuable and hidden information from the databases that are large enough to be accessed without extraction processing. The tools used for this purpose are Parallel index building, Web Access to DICOM Objects (WADO service) and logistic regression. **NLP** is a process wherein the computers analyses, understand and derive the sense from language of the humans. The NLP in this work is used with different techniques like Text mining and NER. The NER is one of the sub-tasks that is used for extraction of information based on the name of the value such as a person, time expression, percentage etc. **CDSS** is sometimes conducted with data mining for examination of the medical history of a patient. This is helpful in prediction of potential events relating to interaction of the patient with drug or symptoms of flag diseases. The different techniques used for diagnosis of chronic patient are Chi-square set and TDM. **Prediction** of the admission of a new patient or the readmission of a previously admitted patient is done with the help of data extraction. The technique used for this purpose are Thrombolysis & Global Registry of Acute Coronary Events

(GRACE) [9]. The readmission is predicted with the help of Care-flow data and Logistic Regression.

3.3 Validation of Data

Validation of data means that the data that is collected for sending to an application is accurate, consistent and reliable. This is done by use of validation's check of the data and the routinely validity check of data. Data validation can also be called as input validation. The different attributes of subclasses (consistency, accuracy and reliability) are storage optimization, data retrieval, computerized and manual data. The subclasses of the validation factor are discussed below (Fig. 4):

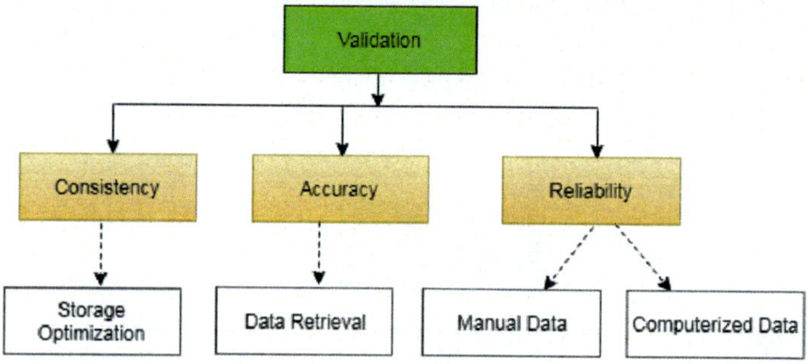

Fig. 4. Validation classification components

Consistency of the data ensures that there are no unexpected or unusual values. During tabulation or cross tabulation of the variables the data checking is done. The main attribute of consistency is storage optimization. The techniques used for achieving consistency are MATLAB, PSO, Cloud Sim package, and PPSO. **Accuracy** ensures that extracted data is correct in results and produces no vague values. The main attribute of accuracy is retrieval of data. The techniques used for achieving accuracy of the data are Cohen's kappa, E-critical system (E-Critical Tracer, E-Critical Meta Vision), and Intraclass correlation coefficient. The extracted data can be validated through **reliability** while having categorized into two types, i.e., manual data or computerized data. Most of the works have considered computerized data for the purpose of reliability.

The components of proposed system together with the evaluation and validation is reported in Table 1. This table includes the different criteria used for data extraction and validation and the method of evaluation used in the research works has been specified. The last column of the table reports results with achieved efficiencies.

4 Discussion

The discussion is focused on three components of the taxonomy to explore the strengths and weaknesses of various systems and how the gap can be filled.

Data is classified as Mining, clustering, Construction and Collaboration. The sub-factors of these sub-components are content based, database history, clinical database, hospital entity, patient data and physician manual data. Only some of the publications have considered physician's manual data [18] and clinical database [4, 10, 13, 17] as the sub-factors of their findings. The reliability of the manual data was not considered as a sub-factor by most of the publications. The manual data generated by Physicians after diagnosis of a patient require lengthier and longer processes to make it equivalent to electronic records. [12] used the health record of patients, where they replaced the manual records of patients with the Electronic medical Records using Electronic Computer system. In addition, clinical databases, are usually the records from remote locations and smaller health facilities, which could not provide proper diagnosis mechanisms. Hence, they need extensive filtration to obtain the accurate records of patient health. In **Extraction of data,** re-admission is a sub-factor, which cannot be considered for all of the cases as patients may have been cured with some treatment or might have expired after the treatment of a particular disease. A few works have considered inclusion of chronic patients' diagnosis & readmissions [14] for the part of their research. [1] worked on the domain of Chronic Patients where they used BPMN as their tool for identification of four-layer process in which the patient's data was captured using bio-signal **Validation** is the last factor of the taxonomy table, which have consistency, accuracy and reliability as its components. The sub-factors of these components are Storage optimization, data retrieval, manual data and computerized data. Manual data is not considered by many authors as it needs time and effort to convert it to into an equivalent electronic form for the purpose of reliability. of When transferring data from one location to another, the issues such as loss of data, inaccurate and incomplete data can be avoided using state of the art works that uses PPSO and TDM.

5 Conclusion

EMR is beneficial for health care as it has rich database of clinical data. The data causes problem of integration between the healthcare system and applications. The device source, which is used, is very costly and has low sensitivity [11]. The advantage of ubiquitous computing can be used to overcome problems and limitations and also for detection of error in proper documentation of data. The data can be maintained by frameworks from remote locations using mobile devices and different data formats. With the increased use of cloud technologies, synchronization of the data is essential before it can be inputted in the application working on Electronic Medical Records. The state-of-art solutions use TDM and PPSO for data transfer, which improves the completeness and accuracy of the patient's medical records. We have proposed a system that provides classification based on the essential components viz., data, extraction, validation required for EMR applications. An EMR system based on these components will be beneficial for both doctors and patients. The taxonomy will allow the system designers to choose efficient sub-factors. The retrieval time hence can be reduced and the data will also be complete and accurate.

References

1. Jimenez-Molina, A., Gaete-Villegas, J., Fuentes, J.: ProFUSO: business process and ontology-based framework to develop ubiquitous computing support systems for chronic patients' management. J. Biomed. Inf. **82**, 106–127 (2018). Doi:https://doi.org/10.1016/J.JBI.2018.04.001
2. Liu, L., Liu, L., Fu, X., Huang, Q., Zhang, X., Zhang, Y.: A cloud-based framework for large-scale traditional Chinese medical record retrieval. J. Biomed. Inform. **77**, 21–33 (2018). https://doi.org/10.1016/J.JBI.2017.11.013
3. Peckham, D.: Electronic patient records, past, present and future. Paediatr. Respir. Rev. **20**, 8–11 (2016). https://doi.org/10.1016/J.PRRV.2016.06.005
4. Kan, Y.C., Chen, K.H., Lin, H.C.: Developing a ubiquitous health management system with healthy diet control for metabolic syndrome healthcare in Taiwan. Comput. Methods Programs Biomed. **144**, 37–48 (2017). https://doi.org/10.1016/J.CMPB.2017.02.027
5. Kormilitzin, A., Vaci, N., Liu, Q., Nevado-Holgado, A.: Med7: A transferable clinical natural language processing model for electronic health records. Artif. Intell. Med. **118**, 102086 (2021)
6. urRehman, M. Z., Javaid, M., Shah, S.I.A., Gilani, S.O., Jamil, M., Butt, S. I.: An appraisal of nodules detection techniques for lung cancer in CT images. Biomedical Signal Processing Control **41**, 140–151 (2018). https://doi.org/10.1016/J.BSPC.2017.11.017
7. Stubberud, A.B., Moon, R.E., Morgan, B.T., Goode, V.M.: Using the electronic medical record to improve preoperative identification of patients at risk for obstructive sleep apnea. J. Perianesth. Nurs. **54**, 62–68 (2018). https://doi.org/10.1016/J.JOPAN.2018.04.002
8. Lee, J.Y., Park, H.A., Chung, E.: Use of electronic critical care flow sheet data to predict unplanned extubation in ICUs. Int. J. Med. Informatics **117**, 6–12 (2018). https://doi.org/10.1016/J.IJMEDINF.2018.05.011
9. Huang, Z., Ge, Z., Dong, W., He, K., Duan, H., Bath, P.: Relational regularized risk prediction of acute coronary syndrome using electronic health records. Inf. Sci. **465**, 118–129 (2018). https://doi.org/10.1016/J.INS.2018.07.007
10. Fleddermann, A., Jones, S., James, S., Kennedy, K.F., Main, M.L., Austin, B.A.: Implementation of best practice alert in an electronic medical record to limit lower-value inpatient echocardiograms. Am. J. Cardiol. **53**. 98–103. https://doi.org/10.1016/J.AMJCARD.2018.07.017
11. Elhoseny, M., Abdelaziz, A., Salama, A.S., Riad, A.M., Muhammad, K., Sangaiah, A.K.: A hybrid model of internet of things and cloud computing to manage big data in health services applications. Future Generation Comput. Syst. **86**, 1383–1394 (2018). https://doi.org/10.1016/J.FUTURE.2018.03.005
12. Lingren, T., Sadhasivam, S., Zhang, X., Marsolo, K.: Electronic medical records as a replacement for prospective research data collection in postoperative pain and opioid response studies. Int. J. Med. Inf. **111**, 45–50 (2018). https://doi.org/10.1016/J.IJMEDINF.2017.12.014
13. Brundin-Mather, R., et al.: Secondary EMR data for quality improvement and research: a comparison of manual and electronic data collection from an integrated critical care electronic medical record system. J. Critical Care **47**, 295–301 (2018). doi.https://doi.org/10.1016/J.JCRC.2018.07.021
14. Zolbanin, H.M., Delen, D.: Processing electronic medical records to improve predictive analytics outcomes for hospital readmissions. Decis. Support Syst. **112**, 98–110 (2018). https://doi.org/10.1016/J.DSS.2018.06.010
15. Bae, J., Ford, E.W., Kharrazi, H.H., Huerta, T.R.: Electronic medical record reminders and smoking cessation activities in primary care. Addict. Behav. **77**, 203–209 (2018). https://doi.org/10.1016/J.ADDBEH.2017.10.009

16. Cui, L., Xie, X., Shen, Z.: Prediction task guided representation learning of medical codes in EHR. J. Biomed. Inform. **61**, 112–119 (2018). https://doi.org/10.1016/J.NEDT.2017.11.018
17. Kragelund, S.H., Kjærsgaard, M., Jensen-Fangel, S., Leth, R.A., Ank, N.: Research Electronic Data Capture (REDCap®) used as an audit tool with a built-in database. J. Biomed. Inf. **81**, 112–118 (2018). https://doi.org/10.1016/J.JBI.2018.04.005
18. Tian, Y., et al.: POPCORN: a web service for individual PrognOsis Prediction based on multi-center clinical data CollabORatioN without patient-level data sharing. J. Biomed. Inform. **86**, 1–14 (2018). https://doi.org/10.1016/J.JBI.2018.08.008
19. Mayhew, M.B., Petersen, B.K., Sales, A.P., Greene, J.D., Liu, V.X., Wasson, T.S.: Flexible, cluster-based analysis of the electronic medical record of sepsis with composite mixture models. J. Biomed. Inform. **78**, 33–42 (2018). https://doi.org/10.1016/J.JBI.2017.11.015
20. Walker, E., McMahan, R., Barnes, D., Katen, M., Lamas, D., Sudore, R.: Advance care planning documentation practices and accessibility in the electronic health record: implications for patient safety. J. Pain Symptom Manage. **55**(2), 256–264 (2018). https://doi.org/10.1016/J.JPAINSYMMAN.2017.09.018

Machine Learning-Based Trading Robot for Foreign Exchange (FOREX)

Fatima Mohamad Dakalbab[1], Manar Abu Talib[1](✉), and Qassim Nasir[2]

[1] Department of Computer Science, University of Sharjah, Sharjah, United Arab Emirates
{falbab,mtalib}@sharjah.com

[2] Department of Computer Engineering, University of Sharjah, Sharjah, United Arab Emirates
nasir@sharjah.com

Abstract. Financial markets are extremely complex due to their non-linear, non-stationary, and time-variant nature. Researchers are increasingly investigating the automation of financial trading as AI capabilities advance particularly in complicated markets such as Foreign Exchange. (FOREX). Traders typically use three types of trading analysis: technical analysis, which uses historical price data to perform mathematical computations; fundamental analysis, which investigates economic factors influencing price movement; and sentiment analysis, which investigates the emotional movement due to market news. There have been a variety of integration techniques utilized in prior attempts to combine AI prediction models with these approaches. Federated learning, which might integrate the learning capacity of dispersed models, has not yet been used by anyone. This study proposes a FOREX trading robot that uses federated learning to aggregate trading analysis methodologies, specifically analyzing market news sentiment and technical calculations based on historical prices for a specific currency pair to determine when to buy or sell for maximum profit. The implementation of federated learning is a future work that we intend to test in the near future. This is the first research work to study the deployment of federated learning in the financial trading field.

Keywords: Automated Trading · Algorithmic Trading · Artificial Intelligence · Machine Learning · FOREX Trading

1 Introduction

Financial markets are one of the most complex systems in the world, due to their non-linear, non-stationary, and time-variant nature. They are sensitive and vulnerable to a variety of variables, such as economic news, political events, and international influence [1]. Artificial Intelligence (AI) advancements have enabled the application of AI techniques in financial markets, which has been termed Financial Technology. (FinTech). FinTech has automated a wide range of financial activities, including investing, insurance, trading, financial services, and risk management. Investments, insurance, trade, financial services, and risk management have all been automated using this technology. AI has numerous applications in trading markets, including forecasting future prices or trends of financial assets, analyzing social media and news sentiment, optimizing financial portfolios, and assessing and avoiding risks for financial assets [2].

K. Daimi and A. Al Sadoon (Eds.): ICR 2023, LNNS 721, pp. 196–210, 2023.
https://doi.org/10.1007/978-3-031-35308-6_17

The Foreign Exchange (FOREX) market is one of the largest financial markets globally, with a daily average volume of $6.6 trillion [3]. The market operates on a decentralized system, which allows traders to buy or sell currencies from their devices, anywhere and at any time. Unlike other markets, FOREX is open 24/5, with trading sessions spanning four different time zones. Each of these zones has its own set of opening and closing times. Due to the market's high volatility and risk, it is challenging for human traders to monitor and engage in trading activities 24/7. To address this challenge, expert advisors or trading robots have been developed to automate the trading process. These robots use predetermined formulas based on trading techniques to make decisions. They eliminate the psychological component of trading, such as the sense of tension and ambiguity, resulting from the trader's uncertainty caused by the significant danger of losing investment funds. Furthermore, they help to eliminate human emotions such as greed, fear, and other biases that may affect trading decisions. Algorithmic trading robots that incorporate machine learning models have become popular in predicting the future price direction and increasing the speed of buying and selling profitable positions. These models implement technical analysis indicators such as moving averages, trendlines, and other mathematical calculations to predict the market's movement [4]. The machine learning models used in algorithmic trading have the advantage of adapting to changing market conditions, unlike traditional trading strategies, which may not be flexible enough to adjust to the market's high volatility [5]. In summary, the FOREX market is a highly volatile market that operates 24/5, making it challenging for human traders to monitor and engage in trading activities 24/7. To address this challenge, expert advisors or trading robots have been developed to automate the trading process. Algorithmic trading robots that incorporate machine learning models have become popular in predicting the future price direction and increasing the speed of buying and selling profitable positions. These models implement technical analysis indicators to make decisions, and they are not influenced by human emotions such as fear, greed, and other biases that may affect trading decisions.

Since forecasting is a difficult process due to market properties such as excessive volatility, noise, and economic shocks, we plan to investigate the construction of a FOREX trading robot in this study. Motivated by federated learning's capability to integrate the learning potential of heterogeneous and distributed models, we propose a federated learning approach in integrating trading analysis methods. To the best of our knowledge, no research work has used the federated learning mechanism in the FOREX market. As a result, this study purposes a FOREX trading robot that uses the federated learning mechanism in aggregating trading analysis methodologies. The proposed FOREX trading robot aims to analyze the sentiment of the news that may affect the price market. In addition, it computes the technical calculations that are based on the historical prices for a specific currency pair. Considering these analysis types, the trading robot will determine whether to buy or sell a currency pair at a specified time, resulting in the maximum profit.

The paper is structured as follows: Sect. 2 provides an introduction to the fundamental principles of trading. Section 3 reviews research articles that utilize machine learning for FOREX prediction. Section 4 outlines the proposed research methodology. Section 5 presents preliminary results. Finally, Sect. 6 concludes with insights and suggestions for future research.

2 Background

2.1 Trading Analysis Types

Traders employ many sorts of trading analyses to forecast market moves and evaluate patterns. Traders typically employ one or a mix of these analysis techniques to suit their trading style. These categories are broadly classified as technical analysis and fundamental analysis as shown in Fig. 1 [1]:

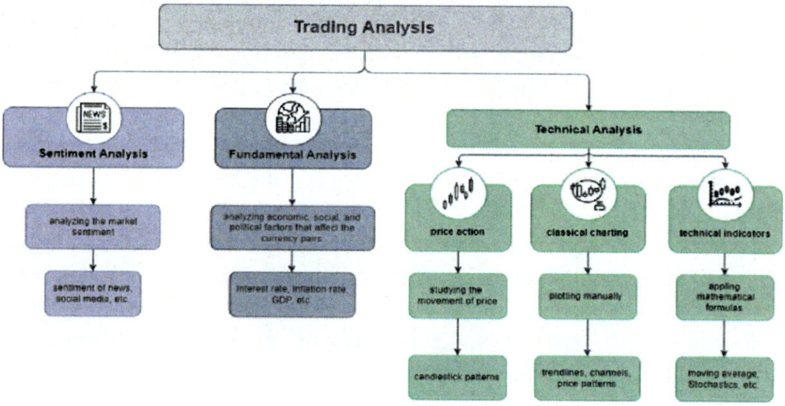

Fig. 1. Trading Analysis Types.

Investor sentiment toward a specific market or financial instrument is referred to as market sentiment. If traders start acting negatively, the sentiment of the market also decreases. As a result, traders utilize sentiment analysis to categorize markets as bullish or bearish, with a bull market being characterized by rising prices and a bear market by decreasing asset values. Market sentiment can be assessed by traders using a variety of methods, such as sentiment indicators, as well as by simply observing the movement of the markets and using the ensuing data to guide their actions [6].

Sentiment indicators are numerical or graphical depictions of traders' levels of positivity or negativity regarding the state of the market. This could be the proportion of trades in each currency pair that has taken a specific position. For instance, if 20% of traders go short and 80% of traders go long, it simply means that 80% of traders are long the currency pair. On the other hand, the fundamental analysis approach consists of analyzing the impact of economic factors that affect the market. Fundamental factors are used to determine an estimation of the intrinsic values of financial instruments that are used to trade in a specific market. Fundamental factors could include information about central bank statements, and economic data indicators that determine the growth of the economy such as inflation rate, gross domestic product, politics, seasonality, and natural disasters. Two essential indices of the condition of an economy are interest and inflation rates. People frequently purchase investment products that boost the economy when interest rates are low. The economy weakens in the opposite scenario. When supply and demand are not balanced, inflation takes place and interest rates rise [19]. The technical analysis is based on statistical methods and charts that depict the price movement of a market over one year, with each point on the graph representing the closing price for each trading day. In the financial markets, technical analysts look for price patterns and market trends that they might exploit. The overall goal of this analysis is to discover (non-linear) patterns which will be utilized to produce trading strategies from the price series of financial assets, capturing meaningful market movements while disregarding random variations.

2.2 Federated Learning

The concept of federated learning started with the aim of providing more security for sensitive data. However, it is gradually becoming one of the most effective approaches for aggregating outputs and identifying similar patterns across multiple models. Federated learning aims to facilitate decentralized learning. It trains machine learning models locally without explicitly sharing the local instance's data. Instead, the trained model's weights and parameters will be exchanged with the main server, which will aggregate the various weights obtained from different instances. The workflow of federated learning begins when the server distributes the global model to the various nodes. Moving forward, the nodes will train that shared model using their local data. Instead of exposing their data, the models complete their training and share the trained model's parameters. The server will then aggregate the local models, and this procedure may be repeated until the global model converges. The security of data is not the only advantage federated learning achieves. The usage of different types of data allows it to provide data diversity which enhances the prediction of the model [7]. In addition, the decentralized and collaborative environment allows it to be more scalable compared to centralized learning. Furthermore, it minimizes latency since it accelerates the training learning process which saves time.

3 Related Work

This section summarizes 41 research papers from 2016–2022 on using machine learning models for FOREX trading. It discusses analysis types, indicators, factors, sentiment sources, asset pairs, datasets, and machine learning models used in each study.

3.1 FOREX Prediction Based on Time-Series Price Data

Researchers have conducted several studies using machine learning to predict Opening, Highest, Lowest, and Closing price (OHLC) price time series data. Authors Ye and Duo [8], along with several others, utilized ARIMA and trading strategies in their studies on statistical machine learning models. Whereas Sidehabi, Indrabayu, and Tandungan [9] applied adaptive spline threshold autoregressive and other classical machine learning models. Conversely, the Long Short Term Memory (LSTM) model has shown great popularity in FOREX prediction as presented in several studies [10–14]. Results of this study's use of OHLC price data for FOREX prediction are presented in Table 1.

Table 1. FOREX Prediction using OHLC Price Data.

Ref	Analysis	Asset Pairs	Method
[9]	✗	not mentioned	Adaptive Spline Threshold, Auto regression, SVM, GANN
[15]	✗	USD/CHF	Modified Fuzzy Relational Model
[16]	✗	USD/EUR, JPN/USD, USD/GBP	Neural Network
[17]	✗	EUR, USD, DKK, NZD, CAD, JPY, GBP, CHF, AUD, SEK, NOK	SVM, Random Forest, Bayesian Autoregressive Trees Dense-layer Neural Network, Naïve Bayes
[18]	✗	EUR/USD	Gaussian Process Kernel
[19]	✗	EUR/USD	Q-network
[2]	✗	up to 21 currencies	ENMX (elastic network model)
[21]	✗	EUR/USD, GBP/USD, AUD/USD,	Gaussian Mixture Model Initialized Neuro-Fuzzy autonomous learning multi-model
[14]	✗	EUR/USD, GBP/USD, USD/JPY, USD/CHF, AUD/USD, USD/CAD	RNNN, GRU, LSTM, MLP, Random Forest, XGBoost, AdaBoost, SVM
[8]	✗	GBP/USD, USD/CHF, USD/JPY, EUR/USD,	ARIMA, trading strategies: GARCH, Kalman filter, Akaike Information Criterion, Bayesian Information Criterion
[10]	✗	EUR/USD	LSTM loss function
[11]	✗	USD/CHF, EUR/USD, USD/CAD, GBP/USD	GRU, LSTM
[22]	✗	EUR/USD	Reinforcement Learning: Fitted Q Iteration, Extra-trees (feature selection)
[12]	✗	EUR/USD, GBP/USD, USD/JPY, USD/CHF	Deep recurrent neural network compared with LSTM, FNN, GRU
[13]	✗	22 currencies against USD	Bidirectional LSTM
[23]	✗	INR/USD	ANN + GA, ANN, GA
[24]	✗	EUR/USD, EUR/CHF, CHF/JPY, USD/JPY	Elliott wave, Fast Fourier Transform, Artificial Neural Networks (ANN)

3.2 FOREX Prediction Based on Fundamental or Sentiment Analysis

A few research have been carried out using sentiment analysis or fundamental analysis. To improve the ability to forecast the FOREX market, Korczak, Hernes, and Bac [25] presented research on a multi-agent trading system that incorporates fundamental analysis. With correlations of the various time series indicators and algorithms of fundamental factors, the authors construct a neural network model. It is important to keep in mind that building models only based on fundamental analysis does not produce satisfactory results, which explains why there are few numbers of studies conducted in this direction. On the other hand, Ranjit et al. [26] used an ANN and the naive Bayes model to study the sentiment analysis of tweets relating to USD against the Nepalese Rupee currency. The authors assert that using fundamental and sentiment analysis alone is insufficient to get accurate FOREX predictions as technical analysis outperforms sentiment analysis in terms of results.

3.3 FOREX Prediction Based on Fundamental or Sentiment Analysis

In comparison to fundamental and sentiment analysis, technical analysis is widely more adapted in FOREX prediction due to its successful returns. Numerous studies incorporated technical indicators with the OHLC charting prices data in building their machine learning models. The widest machine learning algorithm utilized with technical indicators is the Genetic Algorithm (GA) [27–31]. Özorhan et al. [29] and Almeida et al. [31] both considered Support Vector Machine (SVM) with GA which reflects the strong potential of developing hybrid models. One of the interesting techniques utilized with machine learning algorithms is wavelet denoising as presented by these studies [32, 33]. The most widely technical indicators that are almost applied in all the studies are the MA and its derivates such as Simple Moving Average (SMA), Exponential Moving Average (EMA), Weighted Moving Average (WMA), and Moving Average Convergence/Divergence (MACD). In addition to the RSI, Williams Percent Range (WillR), Commodity Channel Index (CCI), Stochastic Oscillator (STOC), Average True Range (ATR), and some other specialized indicators. Table 2 provides a summary of the research findings obtained from the thorough investigation of the studies that consider technical analysis with the OHLC chart pricing.

Table 2. FOREX Prediction using OHLC Price Data.

Ref	Technical Analysis	Asset Pairs	Method
[27]	Not mentioned	(EUR, GBP) /USD	Genetic algorithm with greedy heuristic search
[34]	Not mentioned	(EUR, GBP) /USD, USD/JPY	CART algorithm, C4.5 algorithm
[28]	Not mentioned	EUR/(GBP, JPY, USD) GBP/(CHF,USD)	genetic programming
[29]	MACD, RSI, SMA, WMA, WMA/SMA, crossover CCI, SK%	EUR/(CHF, GBP,USD) GBP/(CHF,USD) USD/CHF	SVM Genetic Algorithm
[35]	EMA, WillR, RSI	EUR/USD	ARIMA, deep recurrent neural network

(continued)

Table 2. (*continued*)

Ref	Technical Analysis	Asset Pairs	Method
[31]	RSI, ROC, MACD, MA, EMA	EUR/USD	Genetic Algorithm, SVM
[36]	MA, RSI, CCI, WillR	EUR/USD	ANN
[32]	RSI, MACD, K, WillR, ROC, CCI, ATR, NATR	USD/JPY	Wavelet Denoised-ResNet with LightGBM
[33]	28 TI derived from MACD, SMA, ADX, WillR	EUR/GBP, AUD/USD, CAD/CHF	(RNN) baseline model, LSTM, bidirectional (BiLSTM), GRU
[30]	16 TI: MA, EMA, DEMA, TEMA, VI, Momentum: RSI, STOC Volatility: Bollinger bands, Ichimoku indicators	(EUR,GBP,AUD)/USD, USD/(JPY,CAD, CHF)	Genetic Algorithm Maximizing Sharpe and Sterling Ratio mode
[33]	ADX, absolute price oscillator, Aroon oscillator, BOP, CCI, momentum oscillator, PPO, MACD, WillR, RSI, STOC, TRIX, ATR normalized ATR	USD/JPY	Wavelet denoising, Attention-based Recurrent Neural Network (ARNN), (ARIMA)
[38]	RSI	EUR/USD, USD/JPY, USD/CHF, GBP/USD USD/CAD, AUD/USD	Fuzzy Inference System, compared against RNN, LSTM, GRU, MLP, RF, AdaBoost, XGBoost, SVM
[39]	MA (EMA, AMA, MACD…) Don-chain Channel, ATR, WillR, RSI	(GBP, EUR)/USD, (USD,GBP)/JPY, USD/CHF, EUR/GBP,	Convolutional network for image classification, ResNet50 Attention-based network, vision transformer
[40]	STOC, WillR, RSI, MA, MACD	EUR/USD	Ensemble machine learning, fuzzy logic, and multi-objective evolutionary computation, Ensemble multi-class SVM
[41]	MA, WillR, RSI, price oscillator, CCI	EUR/USD	Artificial neural network
[42]	MA, SMA, EMA	(EUR,AUD, GBP)/USD	Conventional

3.4 FOREX Prediction Based on Multiple Trading Analysis Types

The combination of trading analysis types is considered to be a new direction in the FOREX prediction market. Two studies presented by Semiromi et al. [43] and Anbaee et al. [6] combined sentiment analysis with technical analysis. Whereas three studies combined fundamental analysis with technical analysis [4, 32, 44]. Almost all the papers used LSTM, except for [43] used XG-boost, random forest, and SVM. Whereas the authors in [3] built their model using Multilayer Perceptron (MLP) and linear regressing. The common fundamental factors that are utilized in this direction are inflation and interest rate, federal funds rate, and gross domestic product. Table 3 summarizes the findings of the extensive investigation in this study. It presents research studies that considered two trading analysis types.

Table 3. FOREX Prediction using OHLC Price Data.

Ref.	TA	FA	SA	Aggregation	Asset Pairs	Method
[43]	✓	✗	✓	-	USD/JPY, EUR/USD, GBP/USD, USD/CHF	XGB, Random Forest, SVM
[6]	✓	✗	✓	Concatenation fusion strategy	BTC/USD, EUR/USD, USD/JPY, GBP/USD	Fin BERT-based Sentiment and Informative Market Feature, LSTM
[45]	✓	✓	✗	Rule-based mechanism	EUR/USD	LSTM
[46]	✓	✓	✗	Automatically	USD/EUR	LSTM, ANN
[3]	✓	✓	✗	Combined as one dataset	EUR/USD	MLP, Linear Regression
Our Work	✓	✗	✓	Federated learning	EUR/USD	LSTM

As shown in Table 3, there have been attempts to build a FOREX prediction system utilizing more than one trading analysis approach. However, to the best of our knowledge, none of the existing work implemented a FOREX prediction utilizing a federated learning mechanism. This study aims to contribute to the field of research by developing a FOREX trading model based on a federated learning mechanism. The proposed model integrates two types of trading analysis commonly used by traders in their daily actions. The primary objectives of this study include investigating the potential of developing a FOREX trading robot based on the two types of trading analysis and assessing the market sentiment and the impact of news on a currency pair. Furthermore, the study will analyze historical price data and employ mathematical technical indicators to predict trends. The sentiment-based and technical-based trading models will then be aggregated using a federated learning mechanism, and the performance of the aggregated FOREX trading model will be evaluated. Finally, the study aims to demonstrate the findings of this research work and provide insights into the potential benefits of utilizing federated learning in FOREX trading.

4 Proposed Technique

We propose a comprehensive FOREX trading robot that integrates technical, fundamental, and sentiment analysis. The robot analyzes news events and historical price data through sentiment and technical analysis, using federated learning to aggregate trading analysis models and make buy, sell, or hold decisions based on statistical analysis. The framework of the proposed approach is shown in Fig. 2, and the methodology consists of three phases: sentiment analysis, technical analysis, and federated learning, each explained in detail in Fig. 3. The next sections go through the specifics of each phase.

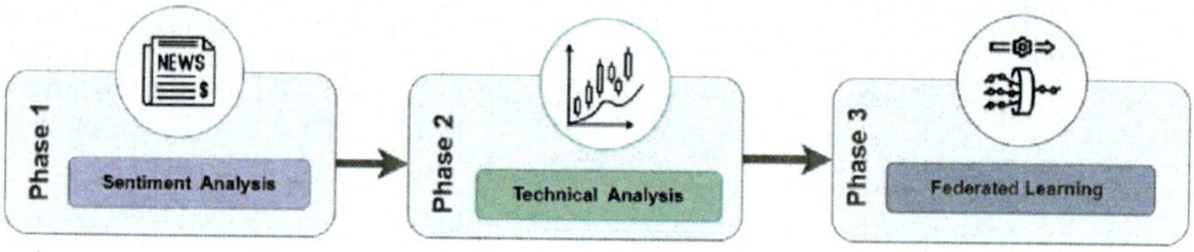

Fig. 2. Federated Learning Workflow.

For the first phase, market sentiment can be assessed by traders using a variety of methods, such as sentiment indicators, as well as by simply observing the movement of news to guide their actions. In this phase, we will explore two types of data: economic calendar, and news reports. Scraping news articles from FOREX sources such as Yahoo Finance would be the first step. Understanding the chosen data is one of the most crucial aspects in data analysis and machine learning applications to guarantee that the model is constructed on valid data that does not mislead the machine learning model. Therefore, we will preprocess the scraped data by cleaning and formatting it. Moving forward, we will use a text summarization tool by Hugging Face Transformers models to build and calculate the sentiment of the summarized articles. According to the sentiment prediction, we can have an overview prediction about the coming trend of the currency pair we are tackling.

The technical analysis is based on statistical methods and charts that depict the price movement of a market over one year, with each point on the graph representing the closing price for each trading day. In the financial markets, technical analysts are the most widely applied analysis type with historical currency pair data. As the initial step in this phase, we will gather the historical pricing data. Moving forward we will utilize libraries for calculating technical indicators on these historical data. TA-Lib is a wellknown python library for calculating technical indicators. There are many different forms of technical indicators in TA-Lib. Technical indicators include three distinct varieties. Trend technical indicators emphasize processing the trend direction. Another type is processing the volume of market actions. The last type is known as oscillator technical indicators. Meanwhile, for this phase, the opening, high, low, and closing prices will be obtained to calculate several technical indicators. Consequently, feature engineering will be used to concentrate on the inputs that the model will benefit from the most. We intend to investigate two machine learning methods. Starting with reinforcement learning's potential because research suggests that it has significant financial implications. Moving on to deep learning techniques and approaches. We will inspect their performance in terms of financial performance evaluation metrics such as profit and loss.

The final phase will mainly explore aggregating the predictions from the trading analysis modules. We will investigate the approach of federated learning. To the best of our knowledge, federated learning has not been investigated with financial markets, as a result, we will explore its feasibility. In this phase, after training each module based on their local data, the shared model's parameter will be shared with the global server which will integrate these weights. Then the updated shared model will be shared again back to the modules to train and share their results until the convergence of the global model. Moving forward, we will test the global FOREX trading model by performing back-testing on historical data that has not been exposed to the model. Finally, performance analysis will be conducted to evaluate the forex trading model.

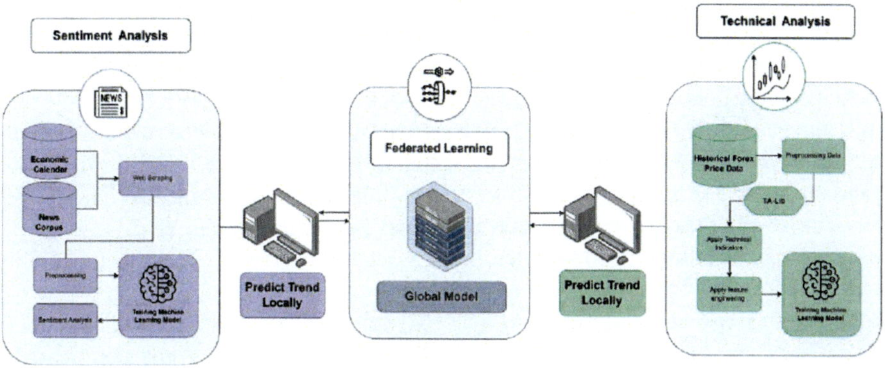

Fig. 3. Federated Learning Workflow.

5 Preliminary Results

The feasibility of the technical and sentiment analyses came early among the three phases. We used the financial summarization Pegasus model from the hugging face transformer in the sentiment analysis section to summarize each news article. Using beautiful soup, news articles from Yahoo Finance were obtained and the latest news article related to the USD/EUR currency pair were scraped. The data was scraped then cleaned and processed. Next, we used the news article summary as input for the summarization model to estimate the sentiment of the article. The model is capable of determining confidence value in its calculation of the sentiment of the news. A sample of the initial sentiment analysis phase implementation is shown in Table 4.

Table 4. FOREX Prediction using OHLC Price Data.

Currency	Article Summary	Sentiment Label	Confidence	Article URL
EUR	Management Board narrows sales expectations for 2022 to EUR 290 to 310 million	NEGATIVE	0.9756190776 8249	Link
USD	The demand for building and construction plastics will grow at an incredible rate in the years to come	POSITIVE	0.9997821450 2334	Link

As for the technical analysis phase, we obtained historical USD/EUR price data from the MarketWatch website. The data spans between the years 2007 through 2023 and it includes features for opening, high, low, close, and volume. We added the following technical indicators to the dataset: on balance volume, Bollinger bands, Stochastic RSI, and 200 Smooth moving average. Figure 4 presents the dataset along with the added technical indicators. To build the predictive model, the dataset is preprocessed and then split into three sets: a training set, a testing set, and a validation set. The sequence length, defined as the number of time steps in the input sequence, is set to 13. The training set, consisting of 1583 samples, is utilized to train the model's parameters. The testing set, with 26 samples, is used to assess the model's accuracy on unseen data, while the validation set, containing 370 samples, helps monitor the model's generalization ability and prevent overfitting. The model architecture is based on a recurrent neural network (RNN) with Long Short-Ter Memory (LSTM) cells. The input shape of the model is set to (None, 1), where the first dimension represents the number of time steps, and the second dimension represents the number of features, which is one in this case. The RNN model consists of two LSTM layers, each with an output dimension of 40. The activation function used in the model is Rectified Linear Unit (ReLU). The recommended optimizer for RNN, RMSprop, is chosen with a learning rate of 0.001. The model is trained using a mean squared error (MSE) loss function for 200 epochs with a batch size of 512. Overall, the model has a total of 101,321 trainable parameters. Figure 5 presents the results of the trained model. Whereas Table 5 presents a sample of the actual price prediction of the test dataset.

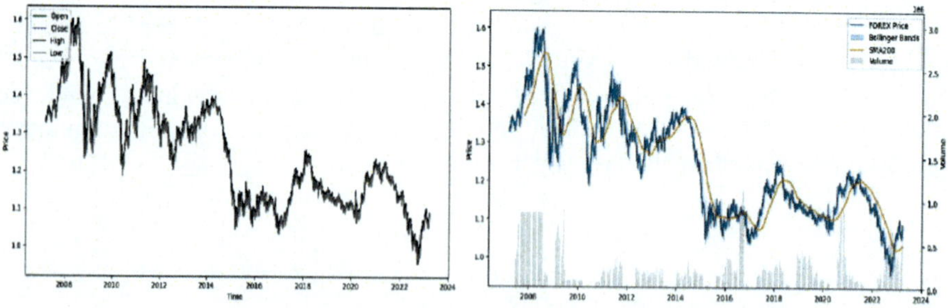

Fig. 4. EUR/USD Price with Technical Indicators.

Table 5. The Predicted and the Actual EUR/USD Prices.

Date	Prediction	Actual Price
2023–03-09	1.060016	1.05967
2023–03-10	1.054500	1.06387
2023–03-12	1.054400	1.07168
2023–03-13	1.059230	1.07025
2023–03-14	1.059304	1.07508
2023–03-15	1.064728	1.05985

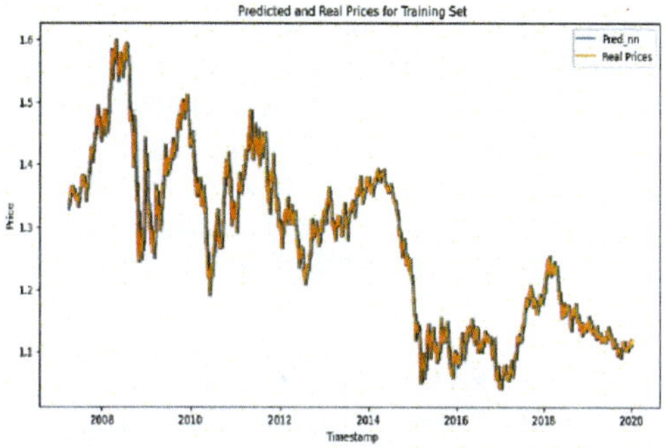

Fig. 5. Training Set Prediction with Real Prices

6 Future Work

Our current work focuses on refining the model and experimenting with different technic indicators and parameter values to improve its accuracy. We also plan to enhance the sentiment analysis component by incorporating real-time web scraping modules for the latest news updates. Once both phases are complete, we aim to leverage federated learning techniques to aggregate the model's performance across multiple currency pairs. This approach is scalable and efficient as it enables learning without sharing the underlying data. Additionally, we plan to include more historical price data with 1-, 3-, and 5-min candlestick charts to enhance the model's predictive power.

7 Conclusion

As a result of its capacity to manage the complexity of financial markets, notably the FOREX, AI has become widely used in financial trading. Traders generate forecasts using three types of trade analysis: technical, fundamental, and sentiment analysis. Various methodologies have been used in previous studies to integrate AI prediction models with these approaches. However, the use of federated learning in this context has not been investigated. This paper proposes a FOREX trading robot that aims to utilize federated learning to integrate market news sentiment analysis and technical calculations based on past prices to make profitable trading decisions. The application of federated learning is a promising area for future research, and this is the first study to look into its use in financial trading. Overall, this study emphasizes the potential benefits of adding federated learning into financial trading.

References

1. Leles, M.C.R., Sbruzzi, E.F., De Oliveira, J.M.P., Nascimento, C.L.: Trading switching setup based on reinforcement learning applied to a multiagent system simulation of financial markets. In: SysCon 2019 - 13th Annual IEEE International Systems Conference, Proceedings. Institute of Electrical and Electronics Engineers Inc. (2019)

2. Dang, Q.-V.: Reinforcement learning in stock trading. In: Le Thi, H.A., Le, H.M., Pham Dinh, T., Nguyen, N.T. (eds.) ICCSAMA 2019. AISC, vol. 1121, pp. 311–322. Springer, Cham (2020). https://doi.org/10.1007/978-3-030-38364-0_28
3. Chantarakasemchit, O., Nuchitprasitchai, S., Nilsiam, Y.: Forex rates prediction on EUR/USD with simple moving average technique and financial factors. In: 17th International Conference on Electrical Engineering/Electronics, Computer, Telecommunications and Information Technology, ECTI-CON 2020. Institute of Electrical and Electronics Engineers Inc., pp. 771–774 (2020)
4. Baek, S., Glambosky, M., Oh, S.H., Lee, J.: machine learning and algorithmic pairs trading in futures markets. Sustain 12 (2020)https://doi.org/10.3390/SU12176791
5. Neely, C.J., Weller, P.A.: Lessons from the evolution of foreign exchange trading strategies. J. Bank Financ. **37**, 3783–3798 (2013). https://doi.org/10.1016/j.jbankfin.2013.05.029
6. Anbaee Farimani, S., Vafaei Jahan, M., Milani Fard, A., Tabbakh, S.R.K.: Investigating the informativeness of technical indicators and news sentiment in financial market price prediction. Knowledge-Based Syst. **247**, 108742 (2022). https://doi.org/10.1016/j.knosys.2022.108742
7. Zhang, T., Gao, L., He, C., et al.: Federated learning for the internet of things: applications, challenges, and opportunities. IEEE Internet Things Mag. **5**, 24–29 (2022). https://doi.org/10.1109/iotm.004.2100182
8. Ye, W., Duo, W.: Autonomous FOREX trading agents. In: Proceedings of the 2019 3rd International Conference on Advances in Image Processing. ACM, New York, NY, USA, pp. 205–210 (2019)
9. Sidehabi, S.W., Indrabayu, Tandungan, S.: Statistical and Machine Learning approach in forex prediction based on empirical data. In: Proceedings CYBERNETICSCOM 2016: International Conference on Computational Intelligence and Cybernetics. Institute of Electrical and Electronics Engineers Inc., pp. 63–68 (2017)
10. Ahmed, S., Hassan, S.U., Aljohani, N.R., Nawaz, R.: FLF-LSTM: A novel prediction system using Forex Loss Function. Appl. Soft Comput. J. **97**, 106780 (2020). https://doi.org/10.1016/j.asoc.2020.106780
11. Islam, M.S., Hossain, E.: Foreign exchange currency rate prediction using a GRU-LSTM hybrid network. Soft Comput. Lett. **3**, 100009 (2021). https://doi.org/10.1016/j.socl.2020.100009
12. Dautel, A.J., Härdle, W.K., Lessmann, S., Seow, H.-V.: Forex exchange rate forecasting using deep recurrent neural networks. Digit. Financ. **2**, 69–96 (2020). https://doi.org/10.1007/s42521-020-00019-x
13. Datta, R.K., Sajid, S.W., Moon, M.H., Abedin, M.Z.: Foreign currency exchange rate prediction using bidirectional long short term memory. In: Studies in Computational Intelligence. Springer Science and Business Media Deutschland GmbH, pp. 213–227 (2021)
14. Munkhdalai, L., Munkhdalai, T., Park, K.H., et al.: Mixture of activation functions with extended min-max normalization for forex market prediction. IEEE Access **7**, 183680–183691 (2019). https://doi.org/10.1109/ACCESS.2019.2959789
15. AmirAskari, M., Menhaj, M.B.: A modified fuzzy relational model approach to prediction of foreign exchange rates. In: 2016 4th International Conference on Control, Instrumentation, and Automation, ICCIA 2016. Institute of Electrical and Electronics Engineers Inc., pp. 457–461 (2016)
16. Galeshchuk, S.: Neural Networks performance in exchange rate prediction. Neurocomputing **172**, 446–452 (2016). https://doi.org/10.1016/j.neucom.2015.03.100
17. Petropoulos, A., Chatzis, S.P., Siakoulis, V., Vlachogiannakis, N.: A Stacked Generalization System for Automated FOREX Portfolio Trading. Expert Syst. Appl. **90**, 290–302 (2017). https://doi.org/10.1016/j.eswa.2017.08.011

18. Ploysuwan, T., Chaisricharoen, R.: Gaussian process kernel crossover for automated forex trading system. In: ECTI-CON 2017–2017 14th International Conference on Electrical Engineering/Electronics, pp. 802–805. Telecommunications and Information Technology. Institute of Electrical and Electronics Engineers Inc., Computer (2017)
19. Carapuço, J., Neves, R., Horta, N.: Reinforcement learning applied to forex trading. Appl. Soft Comput. J. **73**, 783–794 (2018). https://doi.org/10.1016/j.asoc.2018.09.017
20. Contreras, A.V., Llanes, A., Pérez-Bernabeu, A., et al.: ENMX: an elastic network model to predict the FOREX market evolution. Simul. Model Pract. Theory **86**, 1 (2018). https://doi.org/10.1016/j.simpat.2018.04.008
21. Yong, Y.L., Lee, Y., Gu, X., et al.: Foreign currency exchange rate prediction using neuro-fuzzy systems. In: Procedia Computer Science. Elsevier, pp. 232–238 (2018)
22. Bisi, L., Liotet, P., Sabbioni, L., et al.: Foreign exchange trading: a risk-averse batch reinforcement learning approach, 20. https://doi.org/10.1145/3383455
23. Sarangi, P.K., Chawla, M., Ghosh, P., et al.: FOREX trend analysis using machine learning techniques: INR vs USD currency exchange rate using ANN-GA hybrid approach. In: Materials Today: Proceedings. Elsevier, pp. 3170–3176 (2020)
24. Jarusek, R., Volna, E., Kotyrba, M.: FOREX rate prediction improved by elliott waves patterns based on neural networks. Neural Netw. **145**, 342–355 (2022). https://doi.org/10.1016/j.neunet.2021.10.024
25. Korczak, J., Hernes, M., Bac, M.: Fundamental analysis in the multi-agent trading system. In: Proceedings of the 2016 Federated Conference on Computer Science and Information Systems, FedCSIS 2016, pp. 1169–1174 (2016)
26. Ranjit, S., Shrestha, S., Subedi, S., Shakya, S.: Foreign rate exchange prediction using neural network and sentiment analysis. In: Proceedings IEEE 2018 International Conference on Advances in Computing, Communication Control and Networking, ICACCCN 2018. Institute of Electrical and Electronics Engineers Inc., pp. 1173–1177 (2018)
27. Ozturk, M., Toroslu, I.H., Fidan, G.: Heuristic based trading system on forex data using technical indicator rules. Appl. Soft Comput. J. **43**, 170–186 (2016). https://doi.org/10.1016/j.asoc.2016.01.048
28. Adegboye, A., Kampouridis, M., Johnson, C.G.: Regression genetic programming for estimating trend end in foreign exchange market. In: 2017 IEEE Symposium Series on Computational Intelligence, SSCI 2017 Proceedings. Institute of Electrical and Electronics Engineers Inc., pp. 1–8 (2018)
29. Özorhan, M.O., Toroslu, İH., Şehitoğlu, O.T.: A strength-biased prediction model for forecasting exchange rates using support vector machines and genetic algorithms. Soft. Comput. **21**(22), 6653–6671 (2016). https://doi.org/10.1007/s00500-016-2216-9
30. Zhang, Z., Khushi, M.: GA-MSSR: genetic algorithm maximizing sharpe and sterling ratio method for robotrading. In: Proceedings of the International Joint Conference on Neural Networks. Institute of Electrical and Electronics Engineers Inc. (2020)
31. Jubert de Almeida, B., Ferreira Neves, R., Horta, N.: Combining Support Vector Machine with Genetic Algorithms to optimize investments in Forex markets with high leverage. Appl. Soft Comput. J. **64**, 596–613 (2018). https://doi.org/10.1016/j.asoc.2017.12.047
32. Zhao, Y., Khushi, M.: Wavelet Denoised-ResNet CNN and LightGBM method to predict forex rate of change. In: IEEE International Conference on Data Mining Workshops, ICDMW. IEEE Computer Society, pp. 385–391 (2020)
33. Zeng Z, Khushi M (2020) Wavelet Denoising and Attention-based RNNARIMA Model to Predict Forex Price. In: Proceedings of the International Joint Conference on Neural Networks. Institute of Electrical and Electronics Engineers Inc.
34. Przemyslaw, J., Jan, K., Katarzyna, T.: Decision trees on the foreign exchange market. In: Smart Innovation, Systems and Technologies. Springer Science and Business Media Deutschland GmbH, pp. 127–138 (2016)

35. Weerathunga, H.P.S., Silva, A.T.P.: DRNN-ARIMA approach to short-term trend forecasting in forex market. Institute Electr. Electron. Engineers (IEEE), pp. 287–293 (2019)
36. Zafeiriou, T., Kalles, D.: Intraday ultra-short-term forecasting of foreign exchange rates using an ensemble of neural networks based on conventional technical indicators. In: ACM International Conference Proceeding Series. Association for Computing Machinery, pp. 224–231 (2020)
37. Qi, L., Khushi, M., Poon, J.: Event-Driven LSTM for forex price prediction. In: 2020 IEEE Asia-Pacific Conference on Computer Science and Data Engineering, CSDE 2020. Institute of Electrical and Electronics Engineers Inc. (2020)
38. Hernandez-Aguila, A., Garcia-Valdez, M., Merelo-Guervos, J.J., et al.: Using Fuzzy inference systems for the creation of forex market predictive models. IEEE Access **9**, 69391–69404 (2021). https://doi.org/10.1109/ACCESS.2021.3077910
39. Fisichella, M., Garolla, F.: Can deep learning improve technical analysis of forex data to predict future price movements? IEEE Access **9**, 153083–153101 (2021). https://doi.org/10.1109/ACCESS.2021.3127570
40. Sadeghi, A., Daneshvar, A., Madanchi Zaj, M.: Combined ensemble Multi-class SVM and Fuzzy NSGA-II for trend forecasting and trading in forex markets. Expert Syst. Appl. **185**, 115566 (2021). https://doi.org/10.1016/j.eswa.2021.115566
41. Zafeiriou, T., Kalles, D.: Ultra-short-term trading system using a neural network-based ensemble of financial technical indicators. Neural Comput. Appl. **35**, 1–26 (2021). https://doi.org/10.1007/s00521-021-05945-4
42. Hansun, S., Kristanda, M.B.: Performance analysis of conventional moving average methods in forex forecasting. In: Proceeding of 2017 International Conference on Smart Cities, Automation and Intelligent Computing Systems, ICON-SONICS 2017. Institute of Electrical and Electronics Engineers Inc., pp. 11–17 (2017)
43. Naderi Semiromi, H., Lessmann, S., Peters, W.: News will tell: forecasting foreign exchange rates based on news story events in the economy calendar. North Am. J. Econ. Financ. **52**, 101181 (2020). https://doi.org/10.1016/j.najef.2020.101181
44. Das, S.R., Mishra, D., Rout, M.: A hybridized ELM-Jaya forecasting model for currency exchange prediction. J King Saud Univ Comput Inf Sci **32**, 345–366 (2020). https://doi.org/10.1016/j.jksuci.2017.09.006
45. Yıldırım, D.C., Toroslu, I.H., Fiore, U.: Forecasting directional movement of Forex data using LSTM with technical and macroeconomic indicators. Financial Innovation **7**(1), 1–36 (2021). https://doi.org/10.1186/s40854-020-00220-2
46. Pornwattanavichai, A., Maneeroj, S., Boonsiri, S.: BERTFOREX: Cascading Model for Forex Market Forecasting Using Fundamental and Technical Indicator Data Based on BERT. IEEE Access **10**, 23425–23437 (2022). https://doi.org/10.1109/ACCESS.2022.3152152

Computer and Network Security

A Decentralized Solution for Secure Management of IoT Access Rights

Yi-Chun Yang(✉) and Ren-Song Tsay

Logos Lab, Department of Computer Science, National Tsing Hua University, Hsinchu, Taiwan
k16272002@gmail.com

Abstract. As the Internet of Things (IoT) grows, there is a pressing need for secure and efficient management of device access rights. This paper presents Ureka, an open system that uses blockchain technology to manage IoT access rights in a transparent and bidirectional way. Ureka consists of a personal private system, a blockchain smart contract system, and a ticket processing system on an IoT device. Each user and IoT device are identified and authenticated through a unique asymmetric key pair, and access to devices is mediated through smart contracts and tickets. Ureka also implements regulation mechanisms to govern user behavior and prevent rule violations. Our evaluation shows that Ureka effectively manages IoT access rights and prevents unauthorized access. The contributions of this paper include the Ureka open standard, the implementation of a transparent and bidirectional smart contract and ticket system, and the regulation mechanisms for governing user behavior.

Keywords: Access Control · Blockchain · Decentralization · General Data Protection Regulation (GDPR) · Internet of Things (IoT) · Privacy · Security

1 Introduction

The Internet of Things (IoT) has become a ubiquitous and crucial technology affecting daily life due to its embedded digital intelligence for precise and accurate identification of objects or people, sensing, actuation, and communication [1]. The IoT technology connects not just things but also people into a network, promising to revolutionize current service models such as e-Health, smart homes, smart stores, smart vehicles, and smart cities. However, when all people can connect to all things [2], ensuring information security y and privacy becomes a significant challenge [3].

Like the Internet industry, the IoT ecosystem is dominated by prominent players and far from the expected many-small-player case. A few enterprises have established their proprietary IoT framework and become the primary device manufacturers and service providers. These big players have created centralized cloud-based access centers for managing users' data and access rights. While users are supposed to own their personal data, they have no direct control rights as the enterprise providers' proprietary systems control the data. Users have no choice but to trust the centralized enterprise providers.

K. Daimi and A. Al Sadoon (Eds.): ICR 2023, LNNS 721, pp. 213–224, 2023.
https://doi.org/10.1007/978-3-031-35308-6_18

The centralization of the management scheme presents a significant problem. These few enterprise providers who dictate the entire IoT system's operations become the weakest point susceptible to security attacks. Most dominant enterprise providers offer nontransparent unidirectional contracts, leaving users with no choices. This system has frequently raised concerns about user privacy and human rights violations. Furthermore, the high risk of privacy leakage due to the centralization of these valuable data-containing systems makes them attractive targets for malicious attackers.

This paper proposes an efficient user-self-managed IoT access method that utilizes blockchain smart contracts and P2P personal networks to address the issues. Our solution, Ureka, adopts a user-centric approach and an access authorization ticket protocol to design a P2P-based open system for decentralized access management. Ureka employs a blockchain-based smart contract for access accounting management for each IoT device. Users can directly request access to an IoT device from the device owner and record the transactions on the tamper-proof blockchain through the smart contract.

Ureka employs a ticket-based protocol to execute access authorization. These transportable and unforgeable tokens, signed by the device owner, represent the permissions of all device access requesters for specific IoT devices. Target IoT devices verify the tickets and grant access to authorized requesters upon validation.

Ureka offers a standardized, privacy-preserving framework with user-centric tickets, allowing users to manage and preserve their personal data. The P2P-based contract and ticket system provides users with a transparent and bidirectional transaction platform, eliminating potential privacy violations. With Ureka, users no longer rely on enterprise providers to safeguard their personal data and privacy, as they now have practical means to do so themselves.

The paper is structured as follows: Section 2 overviews the current IoT ecosystem and existing IoT access systems. Section 3 uses Google's IoT access system as a case study to illustrate potential privacy and security issues. Section 4 references literature to elucidate the fundamental design principles of Ureka. Section 5 details the proposed Ureka concept. Section 6 introduces the Ureka standard. Section 7 presents the Ureka system design. Section 8 discusses regulations for governing user behavior. Finally, in Sect. 9, we conclude the work.

2 Existing IoT Access Solutions

The Internet of Things (IoT) market is still in its early stages, but many companies are already racing to sell products to consumers, with the smart home segment being the first target market. Around 2016, major corporations such as Google, Apple, Amazon, and Xiaomi launched their IoT product lines to capture commercial opportunities in the smart home market. These products include Google Home, Apple HomeKit, Amazon Echo, and Xiaomi MIJIA [4–7].

The current IoT business model involves selling devices and associated property rights to individual consumers, who become the device owners and have the right to access them or share access with family members or tenants. These family members or tenants become device users with limited access rights but not property rights. When using the devices, the users generate personal data they should own and manage.

Although device owners hold property rights, service agreements typically allow the enterprise providers to access the sold devices for product responsibility and to offer product updates through Internet connections. This situation also allows these companies to access the users' private information, despite their claims of big data analysis and value-added services for the ecosystem.

In conclusion, multiple parties besides the owner or authorized users can access an IoT device. It raises the issue of avoiding unauthorized access by illegal users and malicious attackers. Thus, a secure and reliable IoT access system is crucial.

Although initial projections for the IoT market predicted fragmentation with numerous small players, the current landscape indicates an oligopoly dominated by a few large companies. These companies have launched proprietary IoT products and development frameworks to attract partners and developers to their ecosystem. While each company's framework differs, nearly all cloud-based IoT systems employ a centralized control approach for distributed devices.

However, as depicted in Fig. 1, this centralized system approach presents a significant security threat. In this scenario, device owners have limited control over their devices, while the enterprise providers effectively hold the reins and pose substantial risks to user privacy.

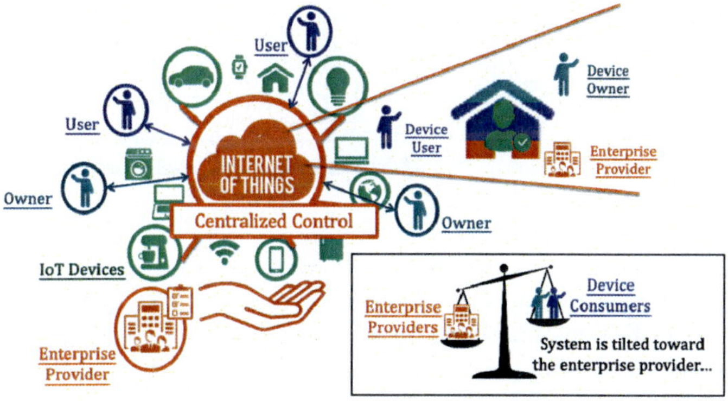

Fig. 1. Existing centralized IoT access systems may intrude on user privacy.

In the following section, we will use the well-known Google IoT solution as a case study for reference.

3 Google's IoT Access System

Google has entered the smart home market with its Google Home product line [4]. Like other IoT players, Google acts as the device manufacturer and service provider, selling devices to individual consumers and collecting user-generated data to enhance its services. Google's proprietary IoT development framework offers a solution for managing device access rights.

All Google IoT devices are connected and regulated by Google's proprietary cloud system. Google utilizes its Google Cloud Identity and Access Management (IAM) System [8] in the Google Cloud Platform to centrally manage both its cloud and IoT resources. As illustrated in Fig. 2, the IAM system enables Google consumers to manage resources and authorize access to specific resources centrally. While initially designed for cloud resource management, Google has adapted it for similarly handling IoT devices. A Google consumer can become an IAM system administrator, granting users permission. The IAM system will automatically transfer device configurations from the cloud to the target IoT devices, updating their permission configurations accordingly.

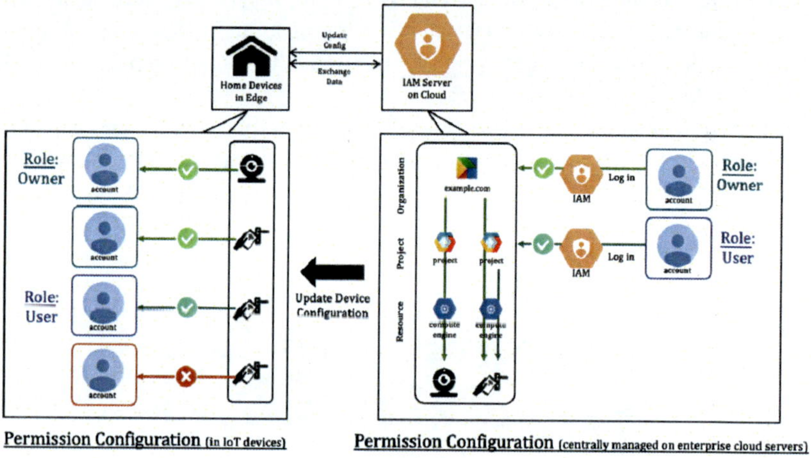

Fig. 2. Cloud IAM system regulates all Google IoT devices.

Suppose a Google consumer wishes to share or rent out their Google devices to other users. In this case, the transaction must be regulated by Google's proprietary system and cannot be completed solely by the original device owner and potential users. For instance, if a company wishes to implement a smart door or lock system using Google's IoT system for access control, the company can define an access policy on the IAM system and assign an administrator. The administrator can then establish access management roles based on the company's access policy in the IAM system. The cloud-connected IoT devices will receive device configuration commands for permission management from the IAM system. After verifying these commands are from Google's cloud server, the IoT devices will comply with the commands and accept the new authorized requesters. The IoT devices will update their permission configurations, partition their internal data or resources based on the access policy, and ensure that different requesters have appropriate permissions to utilize their allocated resources.

Google only offers the Cloud IAM service to enterprise partners or developers, but it also provides an alternative service, called Multi-user service [9], for individual consumers of smart home products. For example, after a homeowner purchases Google Home devices, they can link the devices to their Google account and invite other users, such as family members, to join. Although this Multi-user service is currently limited in its capabilities, Google plans to support the same access control functions as the IAM system in the future.

The central management of Google's Cloud IAM system allows easy control over users' data and personal access rights. However, as previously discussed, this centralized access control system presents several security concerns. In this article, we will focus on the two most critical issues.

The first issue is about the nontransparent and unfair transaction model. Google's Cloud IAM system controls the transactions between Google and its consumers, as well as between consumers themselves. However, the amount of information shared during these transactions is limited. Consumers may not be aware of the data being exchanged between their IoT devices and the Google cloud server. While the terms of service are meant to clarify the services offered, they often contain ambiguous language that can be difficult to understand. In practice, Google is the only entity with access to and control over the collected data, which raises concerns about privacy and data protection. Although Google does provide options for data sharing and the ability to opt out of data collection, these controls are limited, and the management system is opaque, meaning the enterprise provider controls it. This situation can result in potential issues, such as the sale of user data to advertisers or government surveillance.

The second issue is about vulnerable privacy management. The centralized management model used by Google's IoT access system poses a potential risk of privacy breaches. Users have limited options to safeguard their personal data and must rely on the trustworthiness of the host Google cloud server. It makes the centralized server an attractive target for attackers who can access sensitive information from all users. Unfortunately, large-scale security breaches at major enterprise providers are frequently reported, harming many end users. It's worth noting that while Google's IoT access system serves as an example, similar issues exist in most other IoT systems that adopt a similar system architecture.

4 Smart Contracts for Access Management

The concept of smart contracts provides an opportunity to manage IoT devices in a decentralized manner. Nick Szabo first introduced the idea of smart contracts in his works [10, 11]. A contract is a set of promises between parties that regulate their relationships in traditional markets. However, with the advent of digital technology, contracts have evolved into "smart" contracts. The development of blockchain technology [12], a decentralized, secure, and transparent transaction technology, made the implementation and execution of smart contracts possible.

A smart contract is a digital representation of rules defined by specific terms and conditions. Many researchers in the blockchain field are exploring new ways to use this technology beyond supporting decentralized digital currencies. The processing of traditional contracts relies on specific legal or financial entities, making them susceptible to monopolies. In contrast, smart contracts rely on openly registered and executable code, serving as the rules for transactions, payment, accounting, and regulation. The blockchain-based smart contract approach provides a more open, transparent, and bidirectional tool for future transactions, making it more suitable for individual consumers and device owners. Unlike traditional IoT systems, which require centralized regulation, smart contracts are a universal standard that can be easily prepared, registered, and executed without intermediaries. With the blockchain smart contract protocol, even personal device owners can easily expand their business at a low cost to serve a wider audience.

The potential for the blockchain-based smart contract approach extends beyond the virtual digital world and into the physical world, where tangible goods and services can be controlled and monitored through these contracts. By embedding standard contractual clauses, such as property rights, collateral, and bonding, into hardware devices or software applications, smart contracts make it difficult and expensive for parties to breach the agreement.

Szabo theorized that any valuable asset that could be digitally managed could be integrated with a smart contract. This concept is becoming a reality with the advancement of IoT technologies, and Szabo utilized the example of a vending machine to demonstrate the fundamental principles of smart properties.

A smart property or manageable IoT device has three critical components: a medium of exchange, software automata, and hardware automata. For example, the Ethereum blockchain platform [13] allows anyone to create and register executable smart contracts on the blockchain. Ethereum addresses these components by utilizing Ether as a medium of exchange, smart contracts, and the Ethereum Virtual Machine (EVM) as software and hardware automata.

However, there is a challenge in applying smart contracts to IoT devices that blockchain cannot directly regulate. A ticket system has been proposed in our solution to address this challenge. These transportable and unforgeable tokens, digitally signed based on the smart contract, represent the access rights of device users and serve as a bridge between the online blockchain and offline physical objects. By implementing the concept of a "contract with bearer" from Szabo's smart property theory, the Ureka ticket system aims to bring practical and secure smart property systems into daily life.

5 The Proposed Approach

Ureka proposes an alternative approach to managing access to IoT devices by utilizing an open, peer-to-peer (P2P) system instead of relying on centralized, proprietary cloud systems. This approach aims to reduce the risk of attacks targeted at centralized service centers.

The Ureka P2P system proposes an approach where all participants, including enterprise providers and consumers, are considered equal. Under this model, the device owner has complete control over how their device is used and who has access to it. Any individual can negotiate access to a device with the owner. The proposed framework allows multiple users to access an IoT device simultaneously. This fair transaction model eliminates the need for centralized service models, as device owners can self-manage access rights.

We have implemented Ureka using P2P technology and a blockchain-based smart contract framework to manage access to IoT devices. Our approach ensures device owners completely control who can access their devices. Smart contracts record access on a decentralized ledger system for transparency and security.

Smart contracts are publicly accessible and immutable, enabling transparent tracking of IoT device access. We authorize access using digitally signed, tamper-proof, portable tokens called tickets. Once a ticket is validated, the target device can establish secure communication sessions for authorized requesters.

By leveraging tickets and secure communication sessions, Ureka provides a privacy-preserving mechanism that allows device owners and users to manage access rights independently and protect their personal data. Furthermore, our decentralized solution distributes system risk, reducing vulnerability by avoiding a single point of failure.

6 The Proposed Ureka Open Standard

This section introduces the Ureka open standard, which includes contract and ticket specifications, verification, and communication protocols. Ureka ensures secure and efficient management of IoT access rights by implementing a transparent and bidirectional smart contract and ticket system and a dedicated contract and ticket management protocol. As illustrated in Fig. 3, all users can negotiate access rights for IoT devices, sign agreements based on the Ureka open protocol, and receive authorization tickets automatically generated from the contract details. Ureka employs specific verification and communication protocols to ensure a trustworthy communication process.

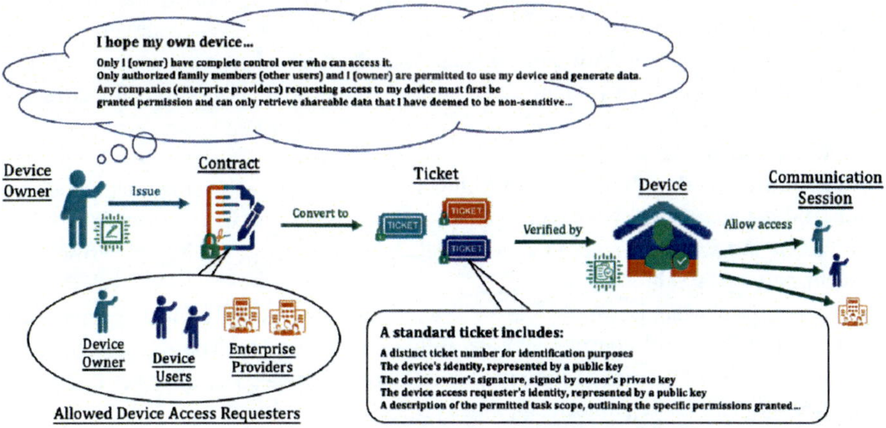

Fig. 3. Illustrations of the Ureka approach.

6.1 Contract and Ticket Content

For a device access requester, the most crucial aspect of a ticket is the authorization to access the targeted IoT device upon successful transaction completion. A sample smart contract can entail the device owner (a homeowner), the device users (homeowner's family members or tenants), and the enterprise providers (companies providing update services and data analysis services on the cloud). The contract lets the family members or tenants access the smart home and its household devices for a specified leasing period. The contract also allows the homeowner to regularly deduct the agreed rental fee from the tenant's account. Additionally, the contract grants the companies the right to update the software and collect agreed data from the smart home devices.

The ticket protocol closely mirrors the contract protocol, resulting in similar content. The critical element in the ticket, the access permission, should align with the corresponding entry in the contract. The only distinction between the contract and the ticket is the format; the contract is written in a human-readable format, while the ticket content is in a machine-readable format, such as the JSON format [14]. To ensure compatibility with various IoT devices, the ticket data must be in a commonly used data interchange format, like JSON, for easy readability.

6.2 Verification Protocols

To change its access privileges, a device must successfully complete three verification procedures. These procedures are contract, ticket, and communication session verification, as depicted in Fig. 3. The following sections provide further detail on each of these procedures.

1) **Contract Verification**
   Blockchain frameworks have established effective verification methods for smart contracts through decentralized validation. Block validators, who are deemed to be trustworthy jointly, verify the records of the smart contract. These validators follow a consensus protocol and validate the records collectively. This ensures that once the records are recorded, they cannot be modified, and access permissions for different devices can be confirmed and validated through notarization.
2) **Ticket Verification**
   To ensure a ticket's validity, it must follow the agreed contract and is not altered. As the contract has already been confirmed on the blockchain network, once the ticket is signed by the device owner and validated, there is no need for additional verification by the network's validators.

   The device owner is responsible for issuing tickets that comply with the conditions specified in the smart contract and are authorized for access. The IoT devices will only accept the ticket signed with the device owner's private key after verifying that the ticket holder is the authorized requester per the authentication process.
3) **Communication Session Verification**
   Upon successfully verifying the ticket and the authorized requester, the target IoT device adjusts its permission configurations to ensure that each ticket holder is granted the necessary permissions to execute the commands specified in the ticket. Sometimes, the IoT device may need to initiate a separate secure communication session with the requester. This is achieved by generating unique session key pairs to encrypt all messages between them. The session key pairs establish a verifiable channel between the IoT device and the requester, and their secure storage is essential to ensure the communication's confidentiality and integrity.

6.3 Communication Protocols

Implementing IoT applications requires various communication protocols depending on the specific use case. For example, a webcam or surveillance camera requires a well-established Wi-Fi environment to record and transmit video over the Internet instantaneously. In contrast, a wearable device continuously exchanging body information with a user's smartphone requires a Bluetooth module. The Ureka open standard is not restricted to any particular communication protocol and may be adapted to support different protocols. References to existing systems are primarily to prototype and test our proposed concept.

7 The Proposed Ureka Open System

This section presents the Ureka open system, comprising three key components: a personal private system that users manage, a blockchain-based smart contract system, and a ticket processing system on an IoT device, as depicted in Fig. 4.

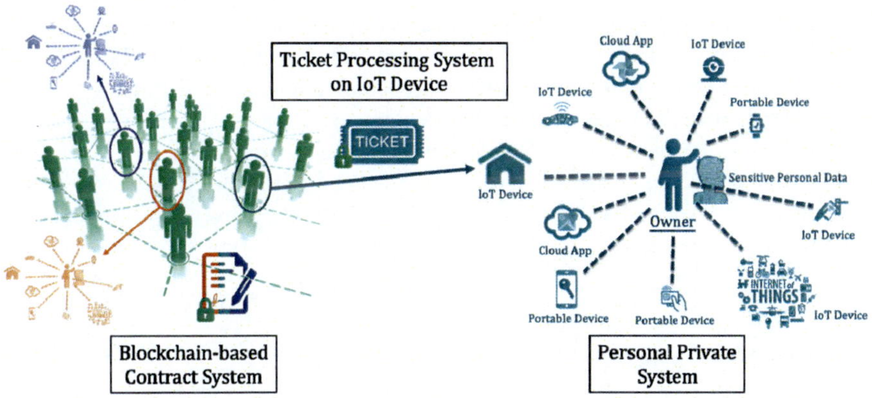

Fig. 4. The ticket system serves as a bridge, connecting the IoT device to the external world.

7.1 Personal Private System

A personal private system is a system that is exclusively accessible to its owner. With such a system, individuals can securely manage their personal key files, passwords, tickets, health information, and personal data with peace of mind.

We assume that Trusted Platform Module (TPM) [15] or Trusted Execution Environment (TEE) [16] based devices, most likely smartphones, can be the means of communication and interface for managing personal systems, while more secure personal devices may become available in the future. Presently, secure smartphones are used to demonstrate the fundamental concepts of the proposed Ureka system.

Individuals can also back up their data in a personal cloud system or offline storage for added security. A secure and convenient recovery system should be implemented in addition to the backup system to make the system more robust.

People can also set up a personal hosting system on the cloud. This hosting system can store their identity, allowing them to sign contracts or process transactions based on their identities automatically. A device owner or an enterprise provider can use this hosting system to offer their device for business services.

A private personal system must be designed with security in mind to protect users' privacy. To increase its credibility, it is recommended to be based on an open-source project that anyone can verify and has an active development community to ensure the absence of hidden backdoors or security vulnerabilities.

7.2 Blockchain-Based Contract System

The contract system operates as a global and publicly accessible cloud system on the Internet, allowing anyone to process smart contracts or transactions based on the blockchain.

A user must generate a unique asymmetric key pair to establish a unique identity for accessing devices and the blockchain network. The private key of this key pair serves as the user's identity and should be kept secure and protected. Similarly, IoT devices require an asymmetric key pair for identification and authentication, which various standardization organizations can standardize during manufacturing.

Each access to an IoT device is treated as a transaction on the blockchain network. Before accessing the device, a requester must send a request to the device's smart contract, which will mediate the ticket-issuing process and prevent any fraudulent or non-repudiable actions. The ticket-issuing process and procedure will be explained in the following section.

7.3 Ticket Processing System on IoT Device

Each IoT device has its dedicated ticket processing system, serving as the sole connection between the device and the external environment. This system provides security protection for the IoT device, safeguarding it from unauthorized access.

The ticket system is different from the contract system. A contract system is a global and publicly accessible cloud system. In contrast, the ticket system is a local system specific to each IoT device and can only be accessed by authorized device requesters approved by the device owner.

The ticket system validates the U-ticket (Use ticket) issued by the owner and authenticates the ticket holder to safeguard the device's security. Once the U-ticket task is completed, the ticket system signs an R-ticket (Receipt ticket) using the device's unique private key for the user to return to audit the smart contract to close the access transaction.

In general, four types of U-tickets cover all possible device usage scenarios: initialization, ownership transfer, access authorization, and revocation. The first step in the proposed scheme is to establish ownership of the device. Typically, the manufacturer is set as the first owner and assigns an initialization U-ticket to store the manufacturer's public key in the device. This process can only be executed once and is irreversible. Therefore, as the first device owner, the manufacturer is fully accountable for ensuring the device's integrity before selling it to a buyer.

Furthermore, the device ownership can be transferred to a new owner using an ownership transfer U-ticket. Upon successful validation, the device updates the stored owner's public key from the old to the new device owner.

The ticket system verifies and authenticates the authorized user for the access authorization U-ticket. The device will perform the instructed operation if the ticket is for a one-time operation. For ongoing access, the device and user will establish a secure session to execute commands within the specified permission scope and under valid operating conditions.

8 User Behavior Regulations

Blockchain smart contracts are capable of automating execution by embedding codes that define usage rules and associated penalties for rule violations. However, managing human behavior is more challenging than controlling hardware devices. Despite well-defined rules, people may still violate them intentionally or unintentionally. Therefore, regulation mechanisms are needed to govern the behavior of device requesters.

Commercial and legal methods have provided acceptable regulation outcomes. For example, penalties can be linked with each violation, and smart contracts can enforce fines or confiscate deposits for rule violations. While this approach does not guarantee total prevention, it can reduce criminal activities. Additionally, automated execution and integration with the financial system make smart contracts a more efficient means of handling deposit confiscation. Traditional legal enforcement systems still apply for rules that cannot be automated.

The legal status of smart contracts is not yet accepted in most countries. Still, Ureka has implemented a basic regulation flow based on economic incentives, a common practice in free markets. However, endorsement from legislatures is required to enforce legal fines or penalties. The recently implemented General Data Protection Regulation (GDPR) [17], which sets international data privacy and human rights standards, provides a reference for designing smart contracts. Practical design experiences in implementing GDPR are still evolving, and much can be learned from its implementation.

9 Conclusion

In conclusion, this paper presented the Ureka open system, which addresses the security and privacy challenges associated with IoT device access control. The Ureka system provides a secure and efficient way to manage IoT device access rights using smart contracts and tickets. The system ensures that only authorized requesters can access IoT devices, and any access is recorded as a transaction on the blockchain.

One of the main contributions of this paper is the design of a transparent and bidirectional smart contract and ticket system that ensures the secure and efficient management of IoT device access rights. This system enables device owners to issue tickets that comply with the conditions specified in the smart contract. IoT devices will only accept the ticket signed with the owner's private key.

Another contribution of this paper is the implementation of specific verification and communication protocols to guarantee a trustworthy communication process. This includes generating unique session key pairs for encrypting all messages and protecting their storage in both the IoT device and the requester's system.

Overall, the Ureka open system provides a comprehensive solution for managing IoT device access rights that address security and privacy challenges. The contributions of this paper have the potential to advance the field of IoT device access control and facilitate the development of more secure and efficient IoT systems.

Acknowledgment. The authors would like to thank Taiwan National Science and Technology Council (NSTC) for sponsoring grant 111–2221-E-007–077.

References

1. Atzori, L., Iera, A., Morabito, G.: The internet of things: a survey. Comput. Netw. **54**(15), 2787–2805 (2010)
2. Satyanarayanan, M.: Pervasive computing: vision and challenges. IEEE Pers. Commun. **8**(4), 10–17 (2001)
3. Miorandi, D., Sicari, S., De Pellegrini, F., Chlamtac, I.: Internet of things: vision, applications and research challenges. Ad Hoc Netw. **10**(7), 1497–1516 (2012)
4. Google Home. https://store.google.com/us/category/connected_home?hl=en-US. [Retrieved: March 2023]
5. Apple HomeKit. https://www.apple.com/tv-home/. [Retrieved: March 2023]
6. Amazon Echo. https://www.amazon.com/smart-home-devices/b?node=9818047011. [Retrieved: March 2023]
7. Xiao-mi MIJIA. https://home.mi.com/. [Retrieved: March 2023]
8. Google cloud identity and access management (IAM) system. https://cloud.google.com/iam/docs. [Retrieved: March 2023]
9. Google Home: Multi-user service. https://www.youtube.com/watch?v=15_DCzw_vHU. [Retrieved: March 2023]
10. Szabo, N.: The Idea of Smart Contracts. https://www.fon.hum.uva.nl/rob/Courses/InformationInSpeech/CDROM/Literature/LOTwinterschool2006/szabo.best.vwh.net/idea.html. [Retrieved: March 2023]
11. Szabo, N.: Formalizing and securing relationships on public networks, First Monday, (1997)
12. Bashir, I.: Mastering blockchain. Packt Publishing Ltd, (2017)
13. Buterin, V.: A next-generation smart contract and decentralized application platform, white paper, vol. 3, no. 37, pp. 2–1 (2014)
14. Bray, T.: The javascript object notation (JSON) data interchange format, 2070–1721, (2014)
15. Tomlinson, A.: Introduction to the TPM, pp. 173–191. Smart Cards, Tokens, Security and Applications (2017)
16. Sabt, M., Achemlal, M., Bouabdallah, A.: Trusted execution environment: what it is, and what it is not. In: 2015 IEEE Trustcom/BigDataSE/Ispa, vol. 1, pp. 57–64. IEEE (2015)
17. General Data Protection Regulation (GDPR) Compliance. https://gdpr.eu/. [Retrieved: March 2023]

Multi Factor Authentication as a Service (MFAaaS) for Federated Cloud Environments

Sara Ahmed AlAnsary, Rabia Latif(✉), and Tanzila Saba

Artificial Intelligence and Data Analytics Laboratory, College of Computer and Information Sciences (CCIS), Prince Sultan University, Riyadh, Saudi Arabia
{221421242,rlatif,tsaba}@psu.edu.sa

Abstract. Growing needs of organizations have left them looking for innovative solutions in cloud computing. One of the methods currently being used to meet those demands is federated cloud computing. Described as the linking of many service providers' cloud environments to load balance traffic and respond to spikes in server demand, this environment provides great solutions for those in need of them. However, cloud computing generally uses single factor authentication which has proven to be less effective. This paper proposes a multi factor authentication framework for federated cloud environments to address the security issues surrounding federated cloud computing. The proposed method will be implemented on a simulated cloud environment to evaluate its strength and ability of protection against various simulated attacks and all results will be recorded.

Keywords: Cloud Computing · Federated Cloud Computing · Service Provider · Security Framework · Authentication · Multifactor Authentication

1 Introduction

Srivastava and Khan (2018) describe cloud computing as the "most powerful computation architecture" which is based on Internet [1] The concept of cloud computing is executed where there is a mediator providing the service to users which pay exclusively for the services used. Cloud computing has improved their services from the traditional platforms and with that improvement came the development of the federated cloud computing environment. Federated cloud computing is the interconnection of cloud environments of two or more service providers to load balance traffic and manage sudden surges in server demand [5]. Federated cloud computing also allows several forms of cloud scenarios, hybrid-cloud, multi-cloud, and aggregated cloud, to merge in an integrated environment.

With the ever-growing popularity of cloud computing in general and federated cloud computing specifically, the question of security mechanisms is raised. A security measure that is highly effective is multi factor authentication. Described as "a widely recommended authentication mechanism for the protection of valuable online assets" [6]. Multi factor authentication provides three forms of authentication factors (1) knowledge, (2) ownership, and (3) inherence. However, individually, each authentication factor poses

K. Daimi and A. Al Sadoon (Eds.): ICR 2023, LNNS 721, pp. 225–236, 2023.
https://doi.org/10.1007/978-3-031-35308-6_19

no value. Whereas, when two of the factors are combined, this creates the spectrum of multi factor authentication. This combination lessens the impact of the various vulnerabilities that can be encountered, which include all of phishing, shoulder sniffing, and man-in-the-middle attacks.

User authentication, authorization, and the assignment of specific privileges are all necessary for user identity management in the digital sphere. This paper proposes a framework using multi factor authentication to combat the security issues that may be faced in a federated cloud environment. The contribution of this paper is to provide a clear and straightforward method to implementing multifactor authentication in federated cloud computing.

The lay out of this paper is as follows. Section 2 presents the related work which provides insights on existing work. Section 3 presents the proposed framework alongside the cases that discuss the framework. Section 4 addresses possible privacy and security issues that may be faced with the framework and its implementation. Section 5 discusses the implemented questionnaire on a select number of companies alongside the results presented and then discusses the evaluation of those results. Section 6 covers the conclusion and possible future work.

2 Related Work

Hassan et al. [7] centered their research on a secure multi-factor user authentication method for electronic payment systems. The authors analyzed the challenges regarding secure authentication measures for protection measures for protection of private user information from threats. The system that was proposed was composed of three phases that was found to improve security effectiveness for multiple types of attacks tiers of authentication that were vulnerable to passcode-based attacks.

Olanrewaju et al. [8] focused their study on frictionless and secure user authentication technique in web-based premium application. They analyzed how many other methods either provide security at increasing resource resilience or have low intensity full implications. Additionally, they investigated unknown assault environments. The research proposed that based on user behavior login occurrences, an automated verification method was created. Their solution, in comparison to existing techniques, determined to give roughly ten percent decrease in latency, seven percent quicker reaction time, and eleven percent lower memory consumption.

Zhang et al. [9] proposed a secure and usable 2FA with magnetic wrist wearables to improve the security and usability of password-based authentication for mobile touch-screen devices with magnetic bands were given. The basis of the research was done in consideration to advanced hacking methods that posed serious challenges to the conventional passcode-based authentication mechanisms. The average true-positive rate for MagAuth was 96.3% and the average false-positive rate was 8.4%. Additionally, it showed that MagAuth was quite resilient to numerous attacks.

Moepi et al. [10] suggested a multi-factor authentication method regarding online banking services in South Africa alongside traditional pin-code identification. They based their method on implementing a second security layer of authentication where they combined user biometrics alongside "bank-registered devices" to achieve their goal which included an attempt to lessen the security concerns associated with virtual banking.

Halim et al. [11] with the aid of OpenCV, presented a facial identification-based door security system. They used human facial identification alongside Twillio service to deliver a One-Time Password (OTP) as the foundation of their project's design. Results revealed that the Local Binary Pattern Histogram (LBPH), which was incorporated into their system, identified features quickly. A "failure" file and an accompanying CSV sheet was also created in the case of an unidentified face being detected. The testing revealed a flaw in its inability to identify faces with greater.

Khalid et al. [12] proposed an approach for creating a safe system founded on an asymmetric cryptographic technique which was better suited than other relevant techniques at the time through safeguarding real-time data. This was done to address the, at the time, remote uses of authentication and key distribution regarding Internet of Drones (IoD), which were discovered to lead to possible loss of access due to corruption regarding the key management system. Their proposed approach showed both the complications of communication and the computing costs were reduced. Their approach also displayed resistance. Table 1 summarizes the strength and weaknesses of the approaches that were discussed.

Table 1. Literature Review

Ref	Strengths	Weaknesses
[7]	Proposed method improved security effectiveness for multiple types of attacks and tiers of authentication	Did not speak of which attacks and the mention of attacks was very minimal and general
[8]	Technique presented increase in reaction time and reduction in latency and memory consumption	There was no discussion of attacks or mention of how the technique held up against attacks
[9]	The results displayed a high true-positive rate and a low false-positive rate. It was also stated that the 2FA method was quite resilient to numerous attacks	Mention of attacks was extremely broad
[10]	The method attempted to lessen security concerns associated with virtual banking	There was no mention of attacks, even though the topic speaks of an extremely sensitive topic which is banking
[11]	Features were identified quickly	Inability to identify faces with greater accuracy and no speak of attacks at all
[12]	Proposed approach showed decrease in complication of communication and computing costs as well as resistance towards many threats	Threats were not listed and spoken of very vaguely

Based on the weaknesses in the existing approaches, we proposed the framework in Sect. 3 to address the issues related to multifactor authentication in federated cloud environment.

3 Proposed Framework and Scenarios

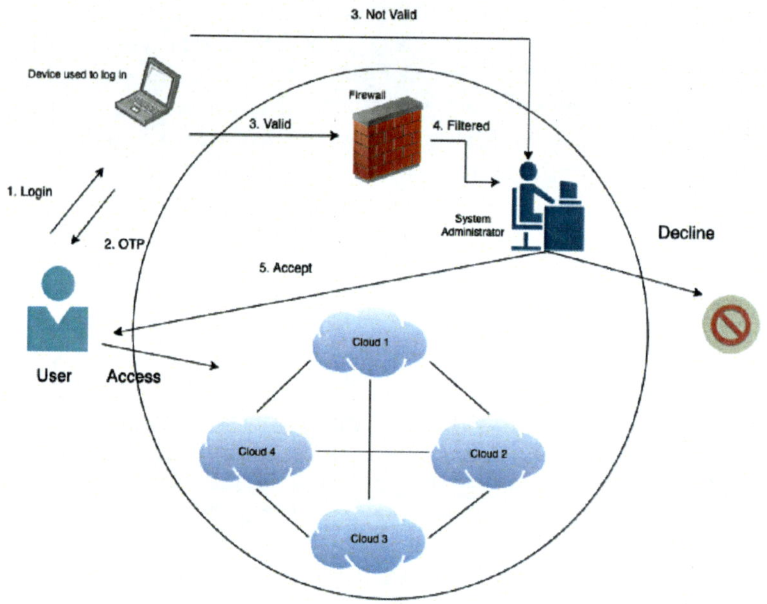

Fig. 1. Proposed Framework

The proposed framework illustrated in Fig. 1 is presented as a multi factor authentication method for accessing federated cloud environments. The process begins where a user will attempt to access the cloud environment by presenting the appropriate user credentials to the front end of the cloud infrastructure. This may be presented in the form of a username and password, biometric recognition, pin, etc.

Once the user submits this information, the credentials are checked within the database for approval of their accuracy and authenticity. If the credentials are corrected the user will be presented with the second factor of authorization. In the form of a one-time password, authentication email, token, phone call, etc.

If the information presented is not approved, the request will be sent to the system supervisor for reviewing. The request must be checked within a five-minute time frame, or it will be timed out and automatically canceled. If the system supervisor accepts the request, the user will be presented with the second factor of authorization.

If the system supervisor declines the request, the request will be aborted, and the user will not be granted access to the federated cloud infrastructure. Similarly, if the second form of authorization is not passed, the request will be aborted, and the user will be denied access.

If the second form of authorization is passed appropriately, the user may access the appropriate cloud service within the federated cloud environment as per their permissions.

A. *Authentication cloud*

The initial framework discusses how the federated cloud environment interacts with external users. The following framework will address how the interaction works between the clouds within the federated cloud environment.

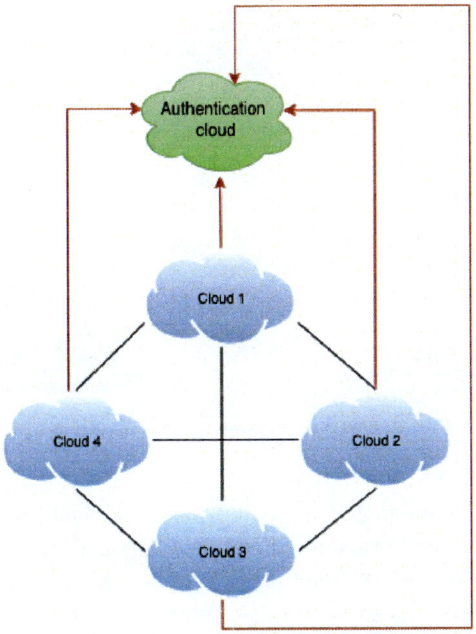

Fig. 2. Intercloud Communication

Figure 2 presents the concept of an authentication cloud alongside digital certificates for the interaction between clouds within the federated cloud environment. The process begins when a cloud wants to interact with another cloud. Cloud 2 and Cloud 3 will be used as an example (Fig. 3).

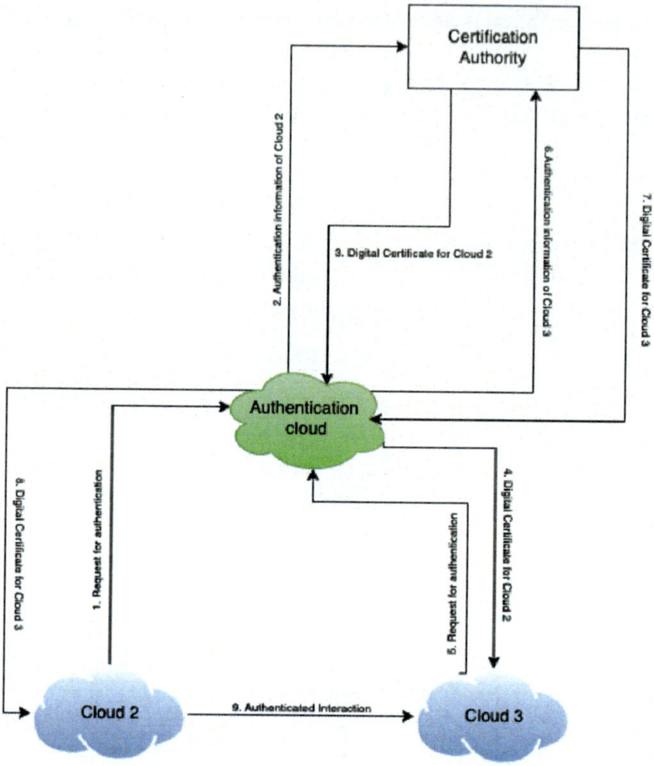

Fig. 3. Proposed Intercloud Communication

Cloud 2 will initiate the interaction with Cloud 3. To interact with Cloud 3, Cloud 2 will interact with the authentication cloud first. The authentication cloud will send Cloud 2's authentication information to the Certification Authority, which will in turn send the digital certificate for Cloud 2.

Once Cloud 2 is authenticated it may present its digital certificate to Cloud 3, or whichever cloud it chooses to interact with, and start interaction.

As for Cloud 3, Cloud 2 may only interact with it if it has its own digital certificate to ensure safety and integrity. Cloud 3 will go through the same process of authentication where it will communicate with the authentication cloud to receive the digital certificate and will present it to Cloud 2 at the initiation of interaction.

This authentication procedure ensures that interactions between clouds within the federated cloud are accurate and unaffected by malicious or unintentional external sources. It also ensures that the necessary security controls are put in place. This also presents the concept of "trusted federation" [13].

B. *Trusted federation*

A requirement for inter-cloud communication is the management of trust. Therefore, to acquire consumers' trust in a federation, it is essential to address the issues raised by the cloud-to-cloud trust model. Several trust models for both traditional and multi-cloud computing scenarios were previously presented, however, their concern was mainly on consumer requirements rather than giving federated cloud computing a standpoint.

The concept of "trusted federation" is presented when two or more clouds are interacting from different CSPs (Cloud Service Providers), where there is a provision of digital certificates presented by the CA, Certification Authority.

4 Handling Privacy and Security Issues Using Proposed MFAaaS Framework

With federated cloud environments there are always issues that may be encountered. They will be listed and discussed in this section.

4.1 Handling Privacy and Security Issues

Although the quick development of cloud computing has increased product flexibility, cost efficiency, and scalability, it also presents a huge number of privacy and security problems. As an emerging concept that is constantly changing, there are security vulnerabilities that have not yet been identified that must be resolved.

One of the main issues presented are the privacy issues associated with cloud computing, especially in a federated environment. There are a variety of different privacy issues that will be discussed.

a. Data Confidentiality Issue

When externalizing and outsourcing exceedingly delicate and sensitive data to the cloud service provider, confidentiality of the user's data is a crucial problem to consider. Users who do not have the required authorization to access private data should not be able to access it, and using strict access control policies and regulations is one way to ensure that secrecy. This issue is one of the main issues facing federated cloud computing. The proposed method of authentication discussed earlier is a method of addressing this problem.

b. Data Loss Issues

One of the biggest security concerns that cloud companies confront is data loss or data theft. More than 60% of consumers would refuse to use the cloud services offered by a provider if they had previously reported data loss or theft of crucial or sensitive information. Ensuring that all data shared is protected from loss to a cloud service provider and between different clouds withing the federated environment is crucial to obtain the trust of the cloud users and ensuring the trust in the use of the cloud services. Especially amongst the different clouds.

c. Hypervisor Relatied Issues

Virtualization is the logical separation of computing resources from real restrictions and limitations. However, there are still some issues with individual authentication, accountability, and authorization. The hypervisor is a target for attackers because it manages multiple virtual machines. Instead of physical machines that are independent, virtual machines in the cloud usually reside on a single physical machine that is managed by the same hypervisor. Several virtual machines will therefore be in danger if the hypervisor is compromised.

Additionally, because the hypervisor technology is new and incorporates features like isolation, security hardening, access control, etc., attackers have additional opportunities to exploit the system.

4.2 Handling Transparency Issues

Transparency in cloud computing security refers to a cloud service provider's willingness to disclose various facts and features regarding its level of security readiness. Some of these specifics violate security, privacy, and service level guidelines. When measuring transparency, it's crucial to consider the actual accessibility of the security readiness data and information in addition to the willingness and disposition.

No matter how readily available security information is, if it is not organized and presented in a way that cloud service customers and auditors can easily understand it, the organization's transparency can also be assessed as low.

4.3 Possible Exploitation of the Authentication Mechanism

Many federated authentication environments are being abused by malicious cyber criminals to gain access to secured data. After the actors have secured initial access to a victim's on-premises network, the exploitation takes place. The actors employ privileged access in the on-premises environment to compromise administrator credentials with the capacity to control cloud resources or to undermine the processes the business uses to grant access to cloud and on-premises resources. When using authentication-based solutions, it is crucial that the server and any dependent services are properly configured for secure operations.

4.4 Different Authentication Technologies May Present Challenges to Customers

With the placement of different authentication technologies on the cloud environment, although they are placed to ensure security, authenticity, integrity, and availability, their presence may cause some issues for users in terms of inconvenience or difficulty. Users may have issues with multi factor authentication seeing that it requires additional steps at log in to ensure the authenticity of the user attempting to access the system. However, some users may find this process tedious.

For these users it should be made clear how important the use of multi factor authentication is in an environment such as the federated cloud environment and the importance of confidentially, authenticity, and integrity should also be highlighted.

5 Questionnaire and Evaluation

This paper implemented a questionnaire over one main company and its partner companies for a variety of reasons. First, to validate if the purpose of this paper is being achieved. Second, to asses the use, levels, and value of multi-factor authentication within the companies. Lastly, to assess the use, levels, and value of authentication for cloud services wiithin the companies. The following section will break down how and where the data was collected, the results of the questionnaire, and the response rates of each question.

5.1 Target Companies

The questionnaire was launched on one main company and three partner companies in Saudi Arabia. The main compaany is a security consultancy company, when asked to submit the questionnaire to the partner companies, the answer was yes. However, the partner companies and their respected sectors were not disclosed. The only information received was that the questionnaire would be sent to the information security department or that equivalent to it in the partner company. The reason four companies were chosen was to gain insight, perform comparative analysis, and evaluate the suggested variables in a variety of work settings.

5.2 Questionnaire Design

The objective of this research is to evaluate the effectiveness of multi factor authentication in cloud computing environment and to present it as a service for federated cloud environments. The questionnaire design is based on the evaluation of authentication measures generally in a company's network and more specifically for their cloud computing uses.

The questionnaire evaluates multi factor authentication within the companies on two scales. An internal scale which views how multi factor authentication is used on the internal system/s of the company, and on an external scale, which evaluates how the company uses multi factor authentication on cloud services. The questionnaire consists of eight (8) yes/no questions and two (2) rating questions. The ratings are both from one to five (1–5), where one question is weighed as least effective to most effective and the second question asks the level of importance from "not important" to "extremely important". The questionnaire will be presented in more detail in the results section.

5.3 Questionnaire Results

The questionnaire resulted in a total of fourteen (14) answers from the information security departments, or that equivalent to it, in four companies. The results are displayed in the table below.

Table 2 displays the results of the yes/no multiple-choice questions whereas Table 3 displays the results of the rating questions. Question 3 presented the rating from one to five (1–5) where one is "non-effective" and five is "extremely effective". Question 8 presented the rating from one to five (1–5) where 1 is "not important" and five is "extremely important".

Table 2. Questionnaire Multiple Choice

No	Question	Yes	No
1	Do you use any special authentication measures for accessing the system within your organization?	71.4%	28.6%
2	Does your organization use any forms of multi factor authentication? (OTP, token, biometrics)	64.3%	35.7%
4	Do you have any kind of preventative methods for unauthorized access currently in place?	64.3%	35.7%
5	Would you consider multi factor authentication a necessity to your organization?	78.6%	21.4%
6	Does your organization use any form of cloud computing?	92.9%	7.1%
7	Does your organization use specified/pre-authorized devices to access the cloud services?	64.3%	35.7%
9	Would you consider the implementation of a multi factor authentication framework for your organization?	85.7%	14.3%
10	Would the implementation of a multi factor authentication framework be well received by the employees of your organization?	64.3%	35.7%

Table 3. Questionnaire Ratings

No	Question	1	2	3	4	5
3	How would you rate the current authorization methods in place for your organization?	7.1%	14.3%	42.9%	28.6%	7.1%
8	How important in the authentication process to accessing cloud services in your organization?	0%	0%	28.6%	21.4%	50%

5.4 Evaluation and Comparison

The survey results show that, for the most part, the companies have some form of authorization set in place, some have multi factor authentication while others just have regular authorization, i.e., regular username and password without extra measures. They also show how much the companies value multi factor authentication and how they would like to implement it within their processes. However, there was a clear majority that thought their employees would not be to open to the implementation. This was discussed as one of the difficulties or issues that are presented with implementing multi factor authentication. Users tend to get annoyed with it or find it as a nuisance to have to go through the various steps of authorization. However, the added security outweighs the disturbance which was already discussed.

As for the cloud computing, the results showed that almost all the companies use cloud computing services and that a majority don't have specified devices that access these services. The results also show that the companies value the authentication to these services greatly. The results were very promising in terms of the companies wanting to implement added security like multi factor authentication and viewing it as an essential feature for the security of both their internal and external processes.

This research presented a conceptual framework that addressed many of the issues that were not addressed by the techniques discussed in the related work. It covers many factors of attacks that were discussed in Sect. 4 and presented the associated solutions and how the framework tackles said issues.

6 Conclusion and Future Work

This paper presented a multi factor authentication framework for both federated cloud environments interaction with external users as well as a framework for internal communication between the clouds within the federated environment.

It addressed the security issues brought up with the authentication process of federated clouds. This will be done to ensure the confidentiality, integrity, and availability of information as well as the value of information that is to be protected. The appropriate security of the federated cloud environments will provide greater sustainability to the entire infrastructure of the cloud. For the future there are aspirations to implement the framework and evaluate the durability through various simulated attacks.

References

1. Dollarhide, M.: Social Media. Investopedia.Com (2021, December 7). https://www.investopedia.com/terms/s/social-media.asp
2. Surmelioglu, Y., Seferoglu, S.S.: An examination of digital footprint awareness and digital experiences of higher education students. World J. Educ. Technol.: Curr. Issues **11**, 48–64 (2019). https://doi.org/10.18844/jet.v11i1.4009
3. Huang, S.-Y., Ban, T.: Monitoring social media for vulnerability-threat prediction and topic analysis. In: 2020 IEEE 19th International Conference on Trust, Security and Privacy in Computing and Communications (TrustCom) (2020)
4. Gurunath, R., Klaib, M.F.J., Samanta, D., Khan, M.Z.: Social media and steganography: use, risks and current status. IEEE Access **9**, 153656–153665 (2021)
5. Alotaibi, S., Alharbi, K., Alwabli, H. Aljoaey, H., Abaalkhail, B., Khediri, S.E.: Threats, crimes and issues of privacy of users' information shared on online social networks. In: 2021 International Symposium on Networks, Computers and Communications (ISNCC), pp. 1-8 (2021). https://doi.org/10.1109/ISNCC52172.2021.9615815

6. (N.d.-b). Researchgate.Net. Retrieved December 10, 2021. https://www.researchgate.net/profile/Subhi-Zeebaree/publication/348930053_Social_Media_Networks_Security_Threats_Risks_and_Recommendation_A_Case_Study_in_the_Kurdistan_Region/links/6017c23545851517ef2eb05b/Social-Media-Networks-Security-Threats-Risks-and-Recommendation-A-Case-Study-in-the-Kurdistan-Region.pdf
7. Ghazinour, K., Ponchak, J.: Hidden privacy risks in sharing pictures on social media. Procedia Comput. Sci. **113**, 267–272 (2017)
8. Ali, S., Islam, N., Rauf, A., Din, I., Guizani, M., Rodrigues, J.: Privacy and security issues in online social networks. Future Internet **10**(12), 114 (2018)
9. Social media as a tool for malware propagation, cybercrime, and data loss, Techgenix.com, 24-Jul-2020. https://techgenix.com/social-media-malware/. Accessed: 09 Dec 2021
10. Vinayakumar, M., Alazab, A., Jolfaei, S., Poornachandran, P.: Ransomware triage using deep learning: twitter as a case study. In: 2019 Cybersecurity and Cyberforensics Conference (CCC) (2019)
11. Chaudhary, P., Gupta, B.B., Gupta, S.: Cross-site scripting (XSS) worms in Online Social Network (OSN): taxonomy and defensive mechanisms. In: 2016 3rd International Conference on Computing for Sustainable Global Development (INDIACom), pp. 2131–2136 (2016)
12. Khan, Z.R., Rakhman, S., Bangera, A.: Who stole me? Identity theft on social media in the UAE. GATR J. Manage. Market. Rev. **2**(1), 79–86 (2017). https://doi.org/10.35609/jmmr.2017.2.1(11)
13. Kaubiyal, J., Jain, A.K.: A feature based approach to detect fake profiles in twitter. In: Proceedings of the 3rd International Conference on Big Data and Internet of Things - BDIOT 2019 (2019)
14. Why social media awareness training in the workplace is a good idea, Associationofmbas.com, 02-Jul-2019. https://www.associationofmbas.com/why-social-media-awareness-training-in-the-workplace-is-a-good-idea/. Accessed 09 Dec 2021
15. Greenman, C.: Top seven reasons why you should not share your passwords - SolarWinds, Logicalread.com, 12-Jul-2017. https://logicalread.com/top-seven-reasons-why-you-should-not-share-your-passwords/. Accessed 09 Dec 2021
16. 5 reasons why general software updates and patches are important, Norton.com. https://us.norton.com/internetsecurity-how-to-the-importance-of-general-software-updates-and-patches.html. Accessed 09 Dec 2021

Exploring User Attitude Towards Personal Data Privacy and Data Privacy Economy

Maria Zambas, Alisa Illarionova, Nikoletta Christou, and Ioanna Dionysiou(✉)

Department of Computer Science, School of Sciences and Engineering, University of Nicosia, Nicosia, Cyprus
{zampa.m,illarionova.a,christou.n5}@live.unic.ac.cy,
dionysiou.i@unic.ac.cy

Abstract. This paper explores digital privacy and its related concept of personal data economy as perceived by consumers. Online personal data sharing, data protection, and ethics are investigated, and a survey was designed and conducted to gather opinions, primarily from university students, on the aforementioned topics. Research findings re-reinforce the significance of the General Data Protection Regulation (GDPR) towards data protection but also urge that further regulation and transparency are required. Digital privacy education should become part of security awareness initiatives, aiming to cultivate an ecosystem among all involved parties (consumers\users, businesses, governments, third parties, etc.) to share, manage, and store personal data in a responsible, lawful, and ethical manner.

Keywords: Digital Privacy · Data Privacy Economy · Price Discrimination · Data Protection · Ethics

1 Introduction

As data-driven products and services become more widespread and integrated into our lives, digital privacy and personal data protection have become more important than ever. Digital privacy concerns how one chooses to share personal data online and how it is being protected. Personal data is any identifying information about an individual, which is often disclosed to companies or websites, following some terms and conditions, sold, or kept private by alternative means.

While many consumers choose to share their data in exchange for accurate personalized recommendations/ads, concerns exist about the lack of control over personal data. The importance is emphasized by the recent launch of the General Data Protection Regulation (GDPR), operating within EU jurisdiction, and other national and international data privacy laws. Users mistakenly believe that government regulation will protect them from the worst of harm and fail to understand the cumulative nature of sharing their data. In reality, *"There is no federal regulation specifically targeted at geolocation tracking, including Bluetooth and Wi-Fi, in retail stores"* [1]. Additionally, consumers are prepared to trade privacy for convenience and discounts and can make decisions about the

K. Daimi and A. Al Sadoon (Eds.): ICR 2023, LNNS 721, pp. 237–244, 2023.
https://doi.org/10.1007/978-3-031-35308-6_20

issues associated with such plans, despite the lack of transparency and full understanding of the consequences of sharing their private data in the long term.

This paper examines and assesses digital privacy as perceived by the consumer, with focus on university students attending technical-oriented programs of study, and its main contributions are:

- Examining the attitude of university students towards personal data privacy, five years after the GDPR adoption [17]
- Exploring the practice of price discrimination from the consumer perspective.

The rest of the paper is organized as follows: Section 2 provides an overview of current practices in the area of data privacy, with emphasis on data collection as well as on the newly emerged market of personal data exchanges. Section 3 briefly discusses the survey research methodology that was followed for collecting feedback from participants regarding digital privacy concepts. Section 4 presents and assesses the survey findings, whereas Section 5 concludes with recommendations and future research directions.

2 Digital Privacy Concepts Overview

A. Data Collection

User personal data is collected both in the physical and digital worlds. Starting with the former, an example is related to a common practice that businesses and commercial stores deploy; by offering Bluetooth and free in-store Wi-Fi, they track individuals and collect their data, mostly for advertising purposes [1]. Even though the customer does give consent prior the use of the services, still there are doubts that he\she is always fully aware of the consequences. As far as the latter is concerned, apps usually request consent, when downloaded, to collect, store and process data (location, access to folders, messages, geolocation, etc.) to use the app. Companies often choose to sell that data to businesses, which in turn utilize the information to match app users to online profiles in order to customize users' future online experience with the enterprise, thus yielding increased profits [1, 2].

Another approach to gathering data is through cookies. A cookie that is combined with an individual identifier qualifies as personal data [3]. Cookies and other information collected such as IP addresses further contribute to online profiling, as discussed in subsequent sections. It is noteworthy to mention that information can be involuntarily and unknowingly obtained from a customer or website visitor. Customers are often unable to make fully informed and rational decisions about their privacy because of imperfect or asymmetric information [4].

B. Third Parties

The vast amount of data that consumers produce by using everyday items that are now connected to the Internet (Internet of Things IoT) and Bluetooth have increased the amount of data and information accessible for collection, analytics, and transfer to third parties. Third parties use that data to precisely determine consumer preferences and identify potential customers for online profiling [3].

Based on how the third-party policy is currently applied, a person who has voluntarily or otherwise disclosed information to a third party, cannot claim to have a reasonable expectation of privacy in the information. The data collected by third parties may be monitored and accessed by the government or other agencies without the owner's consent or knowledge [5]. From the legal side, companies are not allowed to process any data that falls into any special categories such as racial or ethnic origin, political opinions, religious beliefs, or sexual orientation. However, other types of personal data have very limited legal protection. A fair balance between the company's interests and the consumer's interests must be considered when discussing third parties' legal access to personal data [3].

C. Price Discrimination

Price discrimination is the practice of dynamically changing the prices of goods based on a customer's purchasing power and willingness to pay [6]. Price discrimination is classified into three types [3]:

1. First-degree – the consumer is charged an individual price equal to his or her maximum willingness to pay, often in a form of a coupon.
2. Second-degree – pricing schemes in which the price of a good or service does not depend on the characteristics of the customer but on the quantity bought.
3. Third-degree – prices that differ between groups or types of buyers.

As surveillance, data collection, and IoT technologies become more invasive and common, companies collect immense amounts of personal data on customers. Recent research showed that more than 70% of companies collect personal data in the EU [7], whereas Google alone has stored on average 10 GB + of personal information, including demographics, searches, and geographical data, on each user [16].

Price discrimination, in the form of group discounts for pensioners or loyalty program discounts, is nothing novel or necessarily detrimental to the customer, however, with the emergence of big data, the role of the data collected has changed monumentally. New technologies make the cost of analyzing said data and creating unique and accurate online profiles of users lower than ever before. Individually tailored prices are soon to be a reality [6, 8, 9], thus erasing the boundary between first and third-degree price discrimination. As stated in [8], "*in the information age, the anonymity of the consumer, and the consumer's consequent safety in numbers, will disappear, and with it the last bulwark of the individual against the power of big business*".

At the moment, online profiling is used primarily for targeted marketing (73% of companies say having a comprehensive user profile is extremely important to them [15]) and a more personalized user experience. Despite many fears, there is limited evidence of systemic price discrimination [8]. For example, numerous independent studies have disproved the idea of price discrimination in online airline tickets, despite the very common belief of its existence [6]. On the other hand, it is argued that comprehensive research, and thus accurate findings, is impossible without full access to the data collected and practices by companies that are restricted from the public [10].

D. Paying for Privacy and Personal Data Economy

Online consumers deploy different self-help tactics to preserve their privacy [11]. Paying for Privacy (PFP) models and Personal Data Economy (PDE) models are different approaches that businesses use towards user data and privacy. Both models give rise to significant concerns for consumers, given that they're being used by companies to utilize new monetization methods.

PDE models are used by companies to buy data directly from people and are divided into two categories:

1. **Data-transfer model** offers consumers a platform where they can send their data either directly to PDE companies or to unrelated third parties.
2. **Data-insight model** offers consumers a marketplace to monetize their data as well as platforms to control, collect, combine, and acquire insights from their data.

Such models already exist with more products in the process of being patented. For example, a platform called "Cozy" falls under the data-insight model, providing users with a safe environment to control and protect their data [12]. The biggest issue brought up by PFP models is the continued transformation of privacy as a capital good. Under the use of PFP models, customers must pay extra costs to prohibit the collection and disclosure of their data for advertising purposes. PFP models encourage turning privacy into a luxury or tradeable good that is largely attainable by a selected group of people, which creates uneven access to privacy and makes predatory and discriminating behavior more likely.

A discount PFP product is a product where users can exchange their privacy and data for a discount. The benefits of exploiting consumer data mostly benefit businesses rather than users. Furthermore, different groups of consumers have distinct preferences for privacy [13]. Indeed, attitudes toward privacy are subjective, as the definition of sensitive information differs depending on various factors, such as socioeconomic background [4].

3 Survey Methodology Specifics

A. Participants

During the period starting November 14th, 2022, and ending December 19th, 2022, a total of 125 participants completed a survey on data privacy, of which 86% are currently students at the University of Nicosia. The majority of respondents were 17–25 of age (76.8%), 12.8% were in the 25–34 age group, and the rest 10.4% were older than 35, which was expected as the target group of the survey was university students.

B. Assessments and Measures

The assessment for this research effort was a quantitative approach using a survey questionnaire. After conducting a literature review, a questionnaire was designed to assess the opinions and how informed the respondents were on the topics of privacy and personal data. The questionnaire was anonymous. Responses were collected by sharing an online link or QR code to the questionnaire in person or through WhatsApp.

An initial questionnaire was drafted and tested by 5 respondents whose responses were not included in the final dataset used for analysis. Following the feedback, the survey was assessed and improved on clarity and understanding of the questions asked and additional questions were added. With improvements made, the final survey comprised of 4 sections and 33 questions (some with sub-questions), as shown in Table 1. All sections had both dichotomous questions with yes or no answers, a rating scale, and open-ended questions.

Table 1. Questionnaire Composition

Section	*Questions*	*Topics*
A – General	5	Demographics and personal data
B – Terms and Conditions	5	Cookies, Terms and Conditions, GDPR
C – Price Discrimination	14	Price discrimination awareness, benefits, and experience
D – Data and Third Parties	9	Opinions on Third Parties data sharing and data protection

4 Survey Findings and Assessment

Table 2 illustrates the responses to the Terms and Conditions section of the survey. While participants have attempted to read both Terms and Conditions and cookie policies, most do not complete reading the policies successfully. When asked to choose the reason why participants fail to complete reading the conditions (options being: Only to use of the app/website, It takes too long to read, I have trust in the "service provider"/company, Could not understand them, I am not concerned/I have no personal issues/I am indifferent/unconcerned), 51% are choosing to agree with the terms solely to use the app/website. 34% also stated that usually the terms are incomprehensive and 40% stated that they are somehow understandable, but not fully. Surprisingly, the length of the policies is not an important reason as respondents indicated that even if the policies were short in length, they still would not read them.

Table 2. Terms and Conditions

Question	*Percentage of positive answers*
Have you ever read the terms and privacy conditions for a website or a mobile app?	86
Have you ever read the cookies policy? *Cookies collect your data, such as clicks, shopping preferences, device specifications, location, and search history*	50
Have you ever accepted Terms and Conditions (T&C) or cookies without reading them fully?	92
Would you read the Terms and Conditions if it only took a few minutes?	42

A small percentage of 8% of the participants stated they always read the terms stated. Of that percentage, 30% decide not to agree with the conditions stated. This concludes that overall, only 2% of all participants decline the terms and conditions, after fully reading them. In addition, an unexpectedly substantial 50% of participants accept the terms without reading them, solely to use the app.

Table 3 exhibits participants' awareness and past encounters with price discrimination. According to the respondents' feedback, 82% delayed a purchase to wait for future personalized sales and 62% of those participants proceeded with a purchase, caused by a flash sale that came up afterward. Only 59% of the buyers were satisfied with the product they ended up purchasing.

Table 3. Price Discrimination

Question	*Percentage of positive answers*
Have you ever delayed a purchase because you expected a future sale?	82
Have you ever made an impulse purchase because of the "one-time offer"/"flash sale"/" limited-time offer"?	62
If 'yes', Did it meet your expectations and did the benefit match the price you paid?	59
Do you use any method to avoid price discrimination?	42
Do you think it is possible to regulate price discrimination?	73
Should price discrimination be illegal/regulated by law?	80
Would you say price discrimination is ethical?	20

According to Table 4, a significant percentage of 90% is aware of third-party data sharing. Nevertheless, 70% of all participants mistakenly believe that third-party data sharing is illegal/ regulated by law. Even though 85% stated that third-party sharing is unethical, only 24% are willing to pay for potential services that offer personal data protection methods. In addition, a surprising 34% stated that they would share their data for compensation such as money/ free services and discounts. Noteworthy results from open questions showed that numerous participants expect personalized ads/coupons or recommendations in exchange for their collected data.

When asked for additional comments, one participant noted *"Gathering our data shouldn't be a problem if companies use it mainly to advertise and other positive uses, it somehow lessens the time and stress of searching and finding some products since the advertisement brings it to your screen. Businesses just need to vigorously emphasize more on protecting our data and assuring users of how their data are being protected."*

Table 4. Data and Third Parties

Question	*Percentage of positive answers*
Are you aware that your online behavior and personal data are most likely shared with Third-Parties, for example, advertising agencies, without your consent?	90
Do you think sharing data with Third-Parties non-consensually is ethical?	14.4
Do you think sharing data with Third-Parties non-consensually is legal?	30
Would you consent to give/sell your data for a reward?	34
Would you be willing to pay more for a service that offers higher protection and/or no tracking of data?	24

5 Conclusion and Future Work

Personal data economy is a new trend, constantly changing and adopting to new conditions. Being completely anonymous in the 21st century comes at the cost of money (PFP models), effort, and often quality of life. Some even agree with Scott McNealy's quote "*You have zero privacy. Get over it*" [14].

The launch and enforcement of GDPR was a crucial step to standardize data protection in the European Union. However, the dynamic and innovative nature of digital technologies, such as Bitcoin and NFTs, highlight the need for further regulation and transparency in the domain. Price discrimination on its own, for example, group discounts for pensioners or loyalty program discounts, is not novel or necessarily detrimental to customers. Depending on the context it can add or subtract from societal welfare thus further emphasizing the demand for digital privacy education.

This work and findings could provide a strong basis methodologically (i.e., survey questions could be used in other populations) and a working hypothesis for further surveys and analysis in different populations with diverse backgrounds. Researching digital privacy is of utmost importance, as it can help shape the future of personal data use and protection. Understanding people's expectations and concerns regarding personal data is crucial in this effort.

Acknowledgment. We appreciate the University of Nicosia support throughout this research effort. We particularly extend our gratitude to the students who completed the survey. Without them, this research wouldn't have been possible.

References

1. Knudson, L.E.: Stalking in the Grocery Aisles: using section 5 of the FTC act to curtail big data driven price discrimination. Iowa Law Rev. **107**(3), 1283–1315 (2022)

2. Sharma, C., et al.: The economics of privacy and utility: investment strategies, CoRR, vol. abs/2208.10253, 2022. https://doi.org/10.48550/arXiv.2208.10253. Accessed Jan 2023
3. Zuiderveen Borgesius, F., Poort, J.: Online price discrimination and EU data privacy law. J. Consum. Policy **40**, 347–366 (2017). https://doi.org/10.1007/s10603-017-9354-z. Accessed Jan 2023
4. Acquisti, A., et al.: The economics of privacy. J. Econ. Liter. **54**(2), 442–92 (2016). https://www.jstor.org/stable/43966740. Accessed Jan 2023
5. Jacobi, T., Stonecipher, D.: A Solution for the third-party doctrine in a time of data sharing, contact tracing, and mass surveillance. Notre Dame Law Rev. **97**(2), 823–870 (2022). https://scholarship.law.nd.edu/ndlr/vol97/iss2/7. Accessed Jan 2023
6. Vissers, T., Nikiforakis, N., Bielova, N., Joosen, W.: Crying Wolf? On the price discrimination of online airline tickets. In: Proceedings of the 7th Workshop on Hot Topics in Privacy Enhancing Technologies (HotPETs 2014), Amsterdam, Netherlands (2014)
7. Statista, global companies collecting personal data by region, Statista (2021). https://www.statista.com/statistics/1172965/firms-collecting-personal-data. Accessed Jan 2023
8. Woodcock, R.A.: Big data, price discrimination, and antitrust. Hastings Law J. **68**(6), 1371–1424 (2017). https://repository.uchastings.edu/hastings_law_journal/vol68/iss6/5. Accessed Jan 2023
9. Esteves, R.-B.: Price discrimination with private and imperfect information. Scandinavian J. Econ. **116**(3), 766–96 (2014). https://www.jstor.org/stable/43673660. Accessed Jan 2023
10. Azzolina, S., Razza, M., Sartiano, K., Weitschek, E.: Price discrimination in the online airline market: an empirical study. J. Theor. Appl. Electron. Commer. Res. **16**, 2282–2303 (2021)
11. Elvy, S.: Paying for privacy and the personal data economy. Columbia Law Rev. **117**(6), 1369–1459 (2017)
12. Cozy Cloud: "About Cozy Cloud," Cozy Cloud. https://cozy.io/en/about/. Accessed Jan 2023
13. Notice of proposed rulemaking: protecting the privacy of customers of broadband and other telecommunications services, WC Docket No. 16–106, 142–47 (1 Apr 2016). http://apps.fcc.gov/edocs_public/attachmatch/FCC-16-39A1.pdf. Accessed Jan 2023
14. Sprenger, P.: Sun on privacy: 'Get over it', Wired. http://www.wired.com/politics/law/news/1999/01/17538. Accessed Jan 2023
15. SuperOffice: "Customer profiles: how to target your ideal customer". Customer Profiles: how to target your ideal customer. www.superoffice.com/blog/customer-profiles. Accessed Jan 2023
16. Curran, D.: "Are you ready? This is all the data facebook and google have on you". The Guardian, 30 Mar 2018 www.theguardian.com/commentisfree/2018/mar/28/all-the-data-facebook-google-has-on-you-privacy. Accessed Jan 2023
17. Office of the commissioner for personal data protection, Law 125(I) (2018). https://www.dataprotection.gov.cy/dataprotection/dataprotection.nsf/All/2B53605103DCE4A4C225826300362211. Accessed Jan 2023

Host IP Obfuscation and Performance Analysis

Charan Gudla[1(✉)] and Andrew H. Sung[2]

[1] Mississippi State University, Starkville, MS 39762, USA
gudla@cse.msstate.edu
[2] The University of Southern Mississippi, Hattiesburg, MS 39406, USA
andrew.sung@usm.edu

Abstract. Cyber-attacks happen every second, and we see in the news regarding compromised entities. The traditional defenses, techniques, and procedures still fail to protect the systems from cyber threats. There is a need for systems which are more resilient and prevent compromising themselves. Cyber security gaps can be filled with dynamic systems along with traditional ones. The static nature of the system configurations is one reason that paves the way for the threat actor to initiate an attack. Moving Target Defense shifts the attack surface to prevent cyber threats and break the cyber kill chain in the early stages. Host IP address obfuscation is one of the techniques to implement dynamic nature in the system's configuration. Implementing dynamic nature deteriorates the network controller performance more than anticipated, and the network can be in-operable at some point. This paper implements a simple IP obfuscation technique in Software Defined Networking, and the network controller performance is measured. In the end, we will discuss various network performance measurement metrics needed to be considered and benchmarked in future work.

Keywords: Moving Target Defense (MTD) · Software-Defined Network · Cyber-Attack · Threat Actor · Cyber Kill Chain

1 Introduction

Moving Target Defense (MTD) is a cybersecurity approach that aims to hinder or postpone attacks on a system by adjusting to the constantly changing network conditions. In the cyber kill chain [1], reconnaissance is the initial step, and the traditional static network structure provides attackers with ample time to gather information. Attackers can use this time to identify the network's vulnerabilities and potential exploits. MTD, on the other hand, seeks to disrupt the scanning attack phases by introducing dynamic elements into the network.

Software-Defined Networking (SDN) separates the control and data planes, enhancing network orchestration and management. By providing a more intelligent approach to configuring, controlling, and operating networks, SDN is designed to simplify network management, reduce resource utilization, lower operational costs, and drive innovation in network evolution and new services [2]. SDN decouples the control plane and

K. Daimi and A. Al Sadoon (Eds.): ICR 2023, LNNS 721, pp. 245–255, 2023.
https://doi.org/10.1007/978-3-031-35308-6_21

data plane entities, enabling network intelligence and a logically centralized state. By abstracting the underlying network infrastructure from the applications, SDN delivers on its promise.

There are multiple elements involved in software-defined networking. One of these is the SDN controller, which supplies APIs and protocols for managing network devices, services, and applications. The SDN controller functions as a centralized system for governing rules, policies, and control directions related to network infrastructure or applications. The northbound interface acts as a bridge between the controller and applications, enabling the introduction of policies and services into the network. Meanwhile, the southbound interface allows the controller to access networking hardware. When it comes to network communication protocols, TCP is connection-oriented and requires a three-way handshake for connection establishment. UDP, on the other hand, does not necessitate a connection establishment between hosts.

In this article, we implemented the MTD technique to evaluate traffic within a conventional SDN network. The dynamic nature of MTD causes frequent obfuscation of network parameters, such as IP address, MAC address, and ports, which can result in additional overhead on the controller. When obfuscation occurs, multiple flows are added to the flow table, which may lead to the loss of data packets during network reconfiguration. For TCP connections, lost packets are retained, but at the expense of maximum bandwidth usage. However, in UDP connections, lost packets are not recovered. To change the IP addresses of all hosts in the network, the controller assigns new IP addresses to all hosts simultaneously at random intervals. Alternatively, the IP address of each host is changed at discrete intervals, meaning each host's IP address is changed at random times rather than at the same time. We benchmarked the controller's performance for traditional, random, and discrete applications.

The paper is aligned as follows: the related work is described in Sect. 2. The experimental setup and the evaluations are discussed in Sect. 3. Finally, the paper is concluded in Sect. 4.

2 Related Work

In this segment, we will explore various MTD techniques and SDN overheads. One such technique is Dynamic Network Address Translation (DYNAT) [3, 4], where the attackers spend a considerable amount of time scanning the network. DYNAT replaces the data in the TCP/IP header to thwart malicious scanning attempts. Trusted users are provided with predefined vital parameters to ensure uninterrupted service. The extent of network overheads largely depends on the deployment and the fields that are obfuscated. For instance, if MAC addresses are obfuscated in a switched network, it could cause the switches to consume more memory and increase Address Resolution Protocol (ARP) traffic to determine the next switch port for routing packets. This may require additional hardware to manage the routing overheads.

Revere [5] is a methodology that entails the development of an open overlay, specifically an overlay network. Such a network is a dynamic network that can modify its routes, reconfigure itself, and react dynamically to nodes or links going offline. However, this does result in additional network traffic caused by transmitting control messages between nodes. Moreover, the network's reconfiguration and routing can lead to unanticipated network overheads.

The Randomized Intrusion-Tolerant Asynchronous Services (RITAS) [6] is a fault-tolerant consensus-based protocol designed to operate on top of TCP and IPSec. This protocol incurs an execution overhead that runs multiple services, requiring additional resources and time for the protocols to reach an agreement. Additionally, memory overhead is a necessary resource for running multiple services. IPSec adds an extra 24 bytes to each packet header, while protocols reaching an agreement generate additional network traffic. Furthermore, IPSec adds an average of 30% latency to each protocol.

Antonatos et al. proposed Network Address Space Randomization (NASR) [7] as a defense mechanism against worm attacks. It focuses on analyzing endpoints that are either infected or in the process of getting infected. By employing the DHCP protocol, the endpoint information is modified. However, the drawback is that IP address changes during interactions result in dropped connections, causing network overhead.

The Mutable Network (MUTE) [8] modifies the IP addresses and port numbers of network hosts without altering their original system information. It acts as a virtual overlay on top of the existing network, and traffic is routed independently over the virtual relay. To ensure secure communication, encrypted channels are utilized to synchronize IP address information. However, using MUTE may increase network infrastructure overhead, including routers and switches. This could potentially lead to network infrastructure failure due to additional routing overhead.

DynaBone [9], short for Dynamic Backbone, generates a multitude of inner virtual overlay networks within a larger outer virtual overlay network. These inner networks employ distinct routing protocols, networking, and hosts that offer diverse services or protocols to increase variety. Despite being part of a single network, the outer overlay network hosts are unaware of the inner networks. Performance and traffic are monitored using sensors positioned at the entry of internal overlays. Depending on the networking and routing protocols employed within the network, extra latency may be introduced, and bandwidth may decrease. Overheads, such as encryption and authentication protocols, add to the workload. The impact of additional routing and network infrastructure load is currently unknown.

ARCSYNE (Active Repositioning in Cyberspace for Synchronized Evasion) [10] is a technique that involves changing the IP addresses of hosts at VPN gateways, which are implemented in the kernel operating system of the gateway. The gateway shares a secret and participates in a hopping and clocking mechanism, where it computes a new IP address using the secret and clock at each clock tick. Similarly, the gateway also computes the IP addresses of other gateways in the same way. This IP address hopping does not disrupt the gateways or streaming services, and the gateways continue to accept data packets even after the IP address changes during a grace period. The grace period is measured by the time it takes for a data packet to travel from one gateway to another. However, changing the address information in data packets can impact delivery times and cause network overhead.

The system known as Random Host Mutation (RHM) [11] frequently changes the routable IP addresses of hosts. RHM achieves this by assigning short-lived virtual IP addresses that are randomly and consistently changed. A special gateway called the

MTG is used to translate the virtual IP addresses to the corresponding real IP addresses at the network edge. To reach the IP address changing hosts, hostnames are translated by DNS to the real IP address, which is then translated to the virtual IP address before being provided to the source hosts. Hosts can reach each other using the real IP address with authorization from the MT Controller, and sessions are maintained until existing flows are terminated. OpenFlow virtual switches [12] or TAP network kernel devices are used to adapt for address mapping. However, the multiple virtual IP addresses assigned to endpoints for maintaining sessions during mutations result in an overhead in address space. Frequent mutations also cause routing-update overhead, leading to an increase in the size of the routing table.

OF-RHM (OpenFlow Random Host Mutation) [13] is a technique that frequently changes the routable IP addresses of hosts, while keeping their real addresses unchanged. To achieve this, short-lived virtual IP addresses are created for the hosts, which are changed frequently and consistently. OpenFlow switches and controllers are used as RHM gateways and controllers, respectively, to coordinate the virtual IP mutations across the network. An OpenFlow controller is responsible for translating virtual IP addresses to real IP addresses and managing DNS messages and end-host address assignments.However, assigning IP addresses to end-hosts and maintaining the flows can cause address-space overhead. This overhead is directly proportional to the mutation rate - the higher the mutation rate, the higher the overhead. Additionally, the rate of mutation and flow termination also contribute to flow-table overhead.

The technique of spatio-temporal address mutation [14] involves dynamically mutating the IP addresses of hosts based on the time that other hosts use those addresses. This introduces a level of dynamism to the host and IP address bindings. However, executing this technique creates overhead for the controller as it must compute random mutations for each interval. Additionally, there is an address space overhead involved in maintaining sessions during mutation, which can be substantial if the mutation rate is high. Furthermore, the technique generates DNS traffic overhead due to queries being sent to the DNS server in shorter intervals than usual.

AVANT-GUARD [15] SDN includes two security mechanisms that safeguard the network. The first one protects the control-plane from saturation attacks by enabling connection migration. The second mechanism ensures the safety of the data plane by dynamically modifying flow rules in response to traffic indicating an attack. This technique is categorized as MTD, as it involves dynamic changes to flow rules. However, implementing this method increases the execution overhead on the data plane since evaluations are necessary, and it also requires additional storage for the rules. Additionally, there may be network overhead if the data plane communicates with the control plane through payload delivery or various trigger reports.

Dynamic Flow Isolation (DFI) [16] is a network technology that adapts to changing contexts by applying network access policies to systems. This context includes factors such as time of day and third-party tools alerts. DFI uses flow rules on switches to manage the rate limit and control of ingress and egress flows from endpoints. Policy decision points (PDPs) process sensor information and install new flow rules based on the current policy. However, when new flow rules are sent to the controller by the switch, a latency overhead occurs during the decision process by DFI. This latency is constant regardless of the size of the new flow rule and can be minimized if the rule already exists in the system.

3 MTD Experimental Setup and Evaluation

This section introduces benchmarking [17] analysis to measure SDN controller network stability in terms of performance, scalability, and reliability. The popular Leaf-Spine network topology is adopted and emulated in Mininet. IPerf traffic generators are initiated at the required nodes to generate the network traffic. The Leaf-Spine topology and parameters are shown below (see Figs. 1 and 2) and the configuration in Table 1. We used TCP Dump to capture the network traffic data and do further analysis. The number of switches and hosts from topology 1 to topology 5 are increased. Adding more resources to the network topology increases the load on the controller. As the load is increased from T1 to T5, the controller's performance is measured. The benchmarking analysis is performed on the random host address mutation technique, and discrete host address mutation technique against traditional software-defined network, and results are evaluated. We can observe from the experiment that the proposed MTD network outperformed the random MTD network. Each topology test is repeated ten times, and the average value is taken.

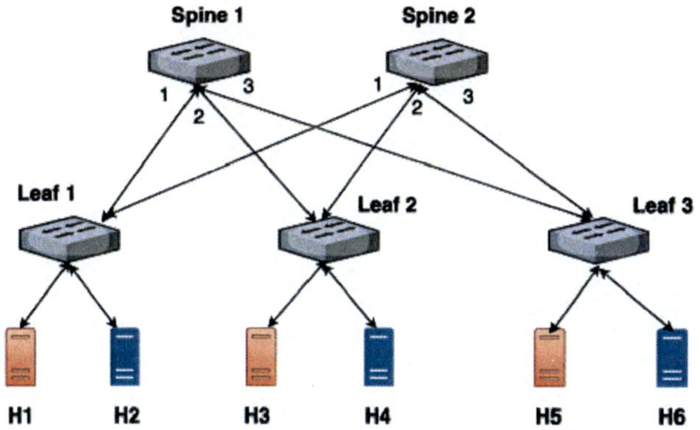

Fig. 1. Leaf-spine topology

Table 1. Topologies

Topologies	OVS Switches	Nodes
T1	16	200
T2	32	400
T3	48	600
T4	64	800
T5	80	1000

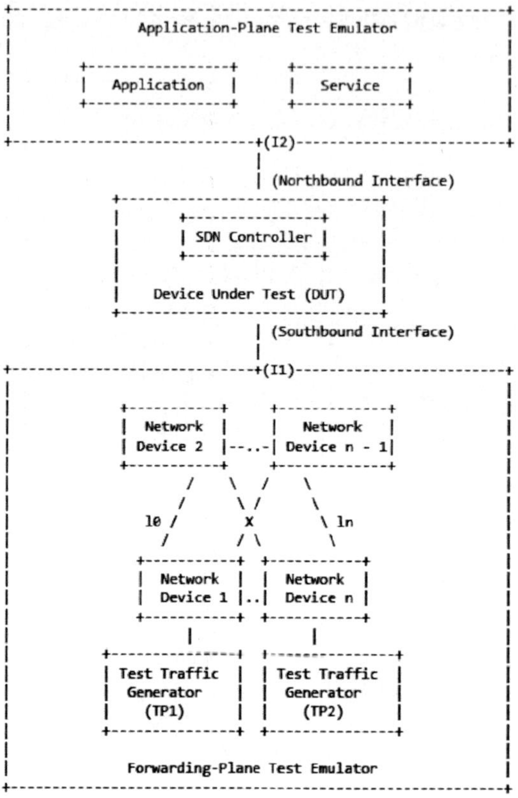

Fig. 2. Leaf-spine topology with controller

3.1 Benchmarking Performance

To measure the performance of the MTD network, we benchmarked network topology discovery time and network topology change detection time against traditional network.

Network Topology Discovery Time. The time taken to discover the network devices and determine the complete topology of the network. Link layer discovery protocol is used to determine the discovery time (see Fig. 3).

T_{m1} is the timestamp of the initial discovery message sent by the controller.
T_{mn} is the final discovery message sent by the controller.
The time for the last discovery message $= T_{mn}$
Topology Discovery Time $(\mathrm{D}_{\mathrm{T1}}) = \mathrm{T}_{\mathrm{mn}} - \mathrm{T}_{\mathrm{m1}}$.
The average of the topology discovery time is as follows:

$$(\mathrm{D}_{\mathrm{T1}}) = \mathrm{T}_{\mathrm{mn}} - \mathrm{T}_{\mathrm{m1}}$$

The network topology discovery time is measured for both random and discrete MTD techniques enabled networks against the traditional network. Traditional network took less time to discover the topology, and the random MTD network took greater time

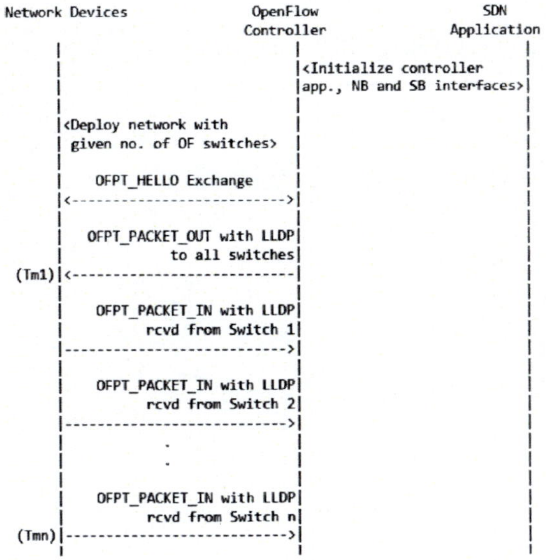

Fig. 3. Network topology discovery process

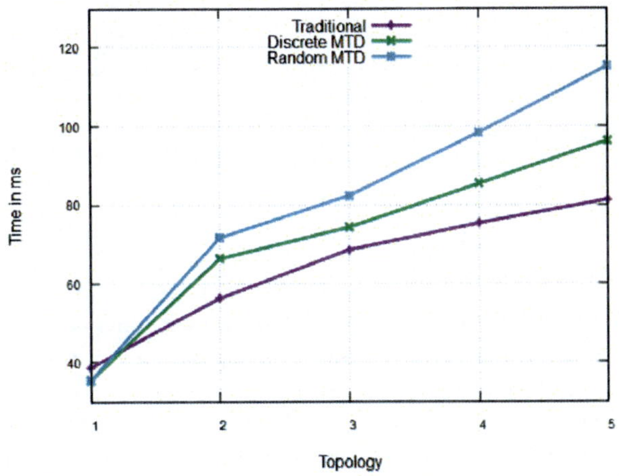

Fig. 4. Network topology discovery time benchmark

to discover the topology. The discrete MTD network discovery time is closer to the traditional network (see Fig. 4).

Network Topology Discovery Time. The time it takes for the controller to notice changes in the network topology. It is vital to test how quickly the controller can identify any network-state change events to provide fast network failure recovery.

T_{cn} is the time when the controller receives the first topology change notification.

T_{cd} is the time when the controller sends the initial topology rediscovery message.

$$(D_{T1}) = T_{\mathrm{mn}} - T_{\mathrm{m1}}$$

$$\text{Average Network Topology Change Detection Time} = \frac{\text{TDT1} + \text{TDT2} + \text{TDT3} .. \text{TDTn}}{\text{Total Trials}}$$

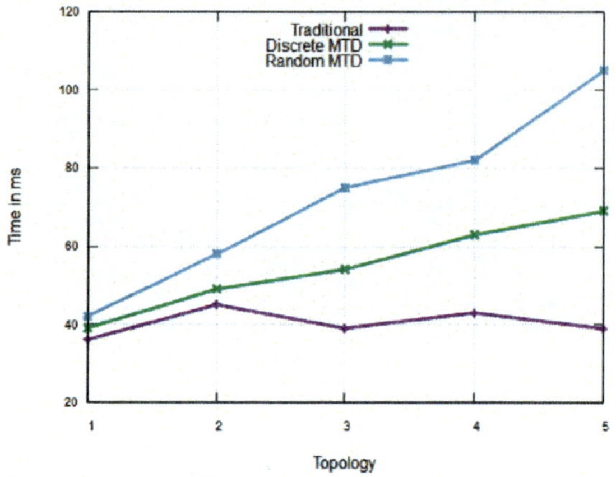

Fig. 5. Network topology change detection time benchmark

Discrete MTD network performed better than the random MTD network (see Fig. 5). The controller does not have additional operational cost in the traditional network to frequently mutate the host's IP address since the network is static. The random MTD network has more operational cost than the discrete MTD network, reducing the controller overhead.

3.2 Benchmarking Reliability

To measure the performance of the MTD network, we benchmarked controller failover time. When the controllers are in redundancy mode, and one of the active controllers fails, the time it takes to transition from the active controller to the backup controller. The time period begins when the active controller is turned off and ends when the new controller's southbound interface receives the first rediscovery message. When two controllers are paired together, and one of them fails, this benchmark assesses the impact of provisioning new flows. The Controller Failover Time is calculated as the difference between the final valid frame received before the traffic loss and the first valid frame received after the traffic loss.

The time taken by the backup controller to become active in a traditional network is very small when compared to the random and discrete MTD networks (see Fig. 6). The traditional network is static, and there is no IP address mutation. On the other hand, random and discrete MTD networks continuously change the IP address of the host. In dynamic networks, the controller has to synchronize data with the backup controller to avoid data loss. Data Synchronization is a limitation in this research, and synchronizing the data across the controllers is a costly operation and is considered future work. Since the dynamic networks change the IP addresses frequently, when the controller failed, it

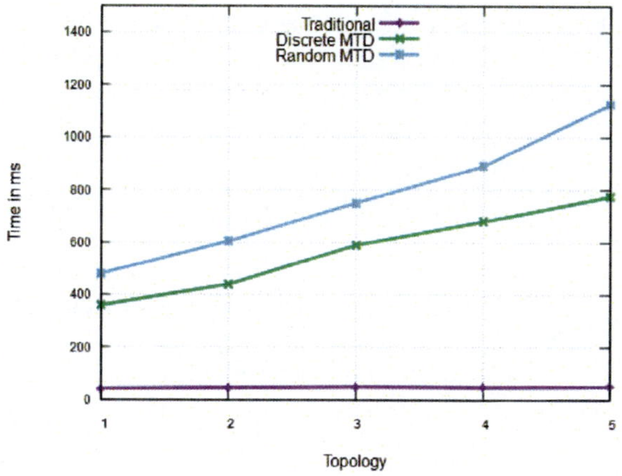

Fig. 6. Controller failover time benchmark

took more time to become active for the backup controller. However, the discrete MTD network performed better than the random MTD network.

4 Conclusion and Future Work

In this paper, MTD software-defined network and traditional topologies are emulated in Mininet, and Ryu is used as the external controller. The benchmarking framework is developed to measure the stability of the controller in terms of performance, and reliability. The discrete MTD network outperformed in all tests compared to random MTD network. The future work includes benchmarking processing, memory, communication, scalability and security overheads.

The processing overhead arises because the controller is responsible for processing and analyzing network traffic and making decisions based on the network policies and rules that have been programmed into it. Depending on the complexity of the network and the number of devices and flows, this processing overhead can be significant and can impact the performance of the controller. The processing overhead of the controller can be measured by monitoring its CPU usage and memory usage over time.

The controller needs to maintain various data structures such as flow tables, network topologies, and device information in its memory. As the size of the network grows, the amount of memory required by the controller also increases, which can become a limitation for some hardware or cloud-based deployments. This memory overhead can be measured by monitoring its memory usage over. This can help to identify if the controller is running out of memory and if additional resources need to be allocated.

The communication overhead arises due to the controller communication with network devices, such as switches and routers, to control the flow of traffic in the network. This communication can introduce latency and delay, which can affect network performance, particularly for time-sensitive applications such as voice and video. This overhead can be measured monitoring the latency and delay in response times.

As the network grows in size, the number of devices and flows that the controller needs to manage also increases leading to an increase in scalability overhead. This can make it challenging to maintain the required level of performance and responsiveness, which can impact the overall user experience. This can be measured by monitoring the performance of the network as it grows in size. This can be done by measuring metrics such as packet loss, latency, and throughput, and comparing them to the expected performance levels.

Since the controller is a central point of control for the network, it is a potential target for attacks. Therefore, additional security measures, such as encryption and access control, need to be implemented to protect the controller from unauthorized access or malicious attacks. The security overhead of the controller can be measured by monitoring access logs and security events, and analyzing them for any suspicious activity.

References

1. Ward, Bryan C.: Survey of Cyber Moving Targets Second Edition. (2018)
2. Underdahl, B., Kinghorn, G.: Software Defined Networking For Dummies, Cisco, Special John Wiley & Sons Inc, Hoboken, New Jersey (2015)
3. Kewley, D., Fink, R., Lowry, J., Dean, M.: Dynamic approaches to thwart adversary intelligence gathering. In: DARPA Information Survivability Conference & Exposition II, 2001. DISCEX'01. Proceedings, vol. 1, pp. 176–185. IEEE (2001)
4. Michalski, J.: Network security mechanisms utilizing dynamic network address translation (2002)
5. Li, J., Reiher, P.L., Popek, G.J.: Resilient self-organizing overlay networks for security update delivery. IEEE J. Sel. Areas Commun. **22**(1), 189–202 (2004)
6. Moniz, H., Neves, N.F., Correia, M., Verissimo, P.: Randomized intrusion-tolerant asynchronous services. In: Dependable Systems and Networks, 2006. DSN 2006. International Conference on, pp. 568–577. IEEE (2006)
7. Antonatos, S., Akritidis, P., Markatos, E.P., Anagnostakis, K.G.: Defending against hitlist worms using network address space randomization. Comput. Netw. **51**(12), 3471–3490 (2007)
8. Al-Shaer, E.: Toward network configuration randomization for moving target defense. In: Jajodia, S., Ghosh, A.K., Swarup, V., Cliff Wang, X., Wang, S. (eds.) Moving Target Defense: Creating Asymmetric Uncertainty for Cyber Threats, pp. 153–159. Springer New York, New York, NY (2011). https://doi.org/10.1007/978-1-4614-0977-9_9
9. Touch, J.D., Finn, G.G., Wang, Y.S., Eggert, L.: DynaBone: dynamic defense using multilayer internet overlays. In: DARPA Information Survivability Conference and Exposition, 2003. Proceedings, vol. 2, pp. 271–276. IEEE (2003)
10. AFRL resources: Personal communication
11. Al-Shaer, E., Duan, Q., Jafarian, J.H.: Random Host Mutation for Moving Target Defense. In: Keromytis, A.D., Di Pietro, R. (eds.) SecureComm 2012. LNICSSITE, vol. 106, pp. 310–327. Springer, Heidelberg (2013). https://doi.org/10.1007/978-3-642-36883-7_19
12. Luo, Y.B., Wang, B.S., Wang, X.F., Hu, X.F., Cai, G.L.: TPAH: a universal and multiplatform deployable port and address hopping mechanism. In: 2015 International Conference on Information and Communications Technologies, pp. 1–6. IET (2015)
13. Jafarian, J., Al-Shaer, E., Duan, Q.: Openflow random host mutation: transparent moving target defense using software-defined networking. In: Proceedings of the First Workshop on Hot Topics in Software Defined Networks, pp. 127–132. ACM (2012)

14. Jafarian, J., Al-Shaer, E., Duan, Q.: Spatio-temporal address mutation for proactive cyber agility against sophisticated attackers. In: Proceedings of the First ACM Workshop on Moving Target Defense, pp. 69–78. ACM (2014)
15. Shin, S., Yegneswaran, V., Porras, P., Gu, G.: AVANT-GUARD: scalable and vigilant switch flow management in software-defined networks. In: Proceedings of the 2013 ACM Conference on Computer and Communications Security, pp. 413–424. ACM (2013)
16. Skowyra, R., Bigelow, D.: Dynamic flow isolation: adaptive access control to protect networks, Cyber Security Division Transition to Practice Technology Guide (2016)
17. Vengainathan, B., Basil, A., Tassinari, M., Manral, V., Banks, S.: Benchmarking methodology for software-defined networking (SDN) controller performance. RFC **8456**, 1–64 (2018)

An Overview of Vehicle OBD-II Port Countermeasures

Abdulmalik Humayed(✉)

Jazan University, Jazan, Saudi Arabia
ahumayed@jazanu.edu.sa

Abstract. Vehicles' On-Board Diagnostics (OBD) is a standardized way to communicate with a vehicle's components for environmental and technical purposes. The OBD-II port allows such communication via plugging a cable into it and, more recently, OBD dongles with wireless capabilities. Because of the absence of message authentication in in-vehicle networks, there are significant security weaknesses when exploiting the OBD-II port by connecting with malicious devices. Regulators use ECUs and their data to test emission levels, whereas technicians use them to diagnose problems. On the other hand, the OBD-II port could be misused to attack vehicles and, eventually, passengers and their safety.

In this paper, we provide an overview of countermeasures capable of preventing attacks originating from the OBD-II port. We compare the countermeasures and discuss challenges and future directions.

Keywords: Automotive · Security · OBD-ii · OBD · Ecu · OBD-II Dongle · Attacks · On-Board Diagnostics · Countermeasures

1 Introduction

Modern vehicles have become complex, built of dozens of interconnected computers called Electronic Control Units (ECUs). ECUs ensure vehicles' safety and functionality. Due to the complex nature of modern vehicles, an approach to self-diagnose vehicles has come about to report problems and provide a way for regulators, mechanics, and owners to exchange data with vehicles' ECUs. Therefore, a standardized On-Board Diagnostics (OBD) interface was developed in 1988, and today OBD is deployed worldwide and mandated in the U.S. and Europe.

In 2010, security researchers demonstrated many attacks against modern vehicles via different attack surfaces [3,13]. Exploiting the OBD and its protocols was the most effective attack surface to realize things like updating the firmware of ECUs to perform unauthorized tasks. In addition, directly sending commands and fabricated data to ECUs was relatively easy because the OBD and the internal network are connected directly and indirectly.

Recently, OBD dongles became popular with insurance companies and vehicle owners. A dongle is plugged into a vehicle and communicates wirelessly with

K. Daimi and A. Al Sadoon (Eds.): ICR 2023, LNNS 721, pp. 256–266, 2023.
https://doi.org/10.1007/978-3-031-35308-6_22

manufacturers, insurance companies, or companion apps. Wen et al. [33] conducted a security analysis on 77 OBD dongles and revealed that all of them have vulnerabilities that threaten the deploying vehicle. Attackers could exploit vulnerabilities in these devices to perform attacks ranging from privacy invasion to complete control of a vehicle. In addition, Pareja et al. [22] found vulnerabilities in a Movistar OBD-II dongle that attackers could exploit to control a fleet of vehicles by using a vulnerability in the dongle's SMS API.

Significant research efforts have been devoted to vehicles' security in response to the vulnerabilities and attacks demonstrated in [3,13]. Solutions such as message authentication, intrusion detection [30,32], and firewalls [12,34] have been proposed to secure vehicles. Although the academic literature has plenty of surveys about vehicle security and countermeasures, there is a lack of surveys about countermeasures specific to the OBD-II port. Therefore, we aim to address this gap.

In this paper, we review the history of OBD and CAN. In addition, we present an overview of countermeasures designed to secure the OBD-II port and dongles. Finally, we discuss a few challenges and future directions.

The rest of the paper is organized as follows: we overview the CAN bus, OBD, OBD-II port, OBD dongles, and their security issues in Sect. 2, the related work in Sect. 3, and the attacker model in the context of the OBD-II port in Sect. 4. Then, we present OBD-II port's countermeasures in categorizing them based on their mechanism in Sect. 5, followed by a discussion about challenges and future directions in Sect. 6. Finally, we conclude the paper in Sect. 7.

2 Background

2.1 Controller Area Network (CAN)

CAN has been widely used in many distributed real-time control systems. While components differ, the main concepts and working mechanisms remain similar in all CAN applications. A CAN network consists of nodes interconnected by a bus. Each node is controlled by a microcontroller (MCU), a.k.a. ECU in automotive CAN networks.

All ECUs are connected to a bus network which consists of several subnetworks, namely Controller Area Network (CAN), Media Oriented Systems Transport (MOST), Local Interconnect Network (LIN), and FlexRay. Each subnetwork consists of a number of interconnected ECUs. Most modern vehicles have a central gateway that controls the traffic between the sub-networks as shown in Fig. 1.

The new advancements in modern vehicles resulted in the increase in the number of access channels to the in-vehicle network. The CAN bus can be accessed physically, through the On-Board Diagnostics (OBD-II) port, and wirelessly, through interfaces such as Bluetooth, WiFi, and cellular connections. The various access channels makes modern vehicles more heterogeneous and introduce potential security complications.

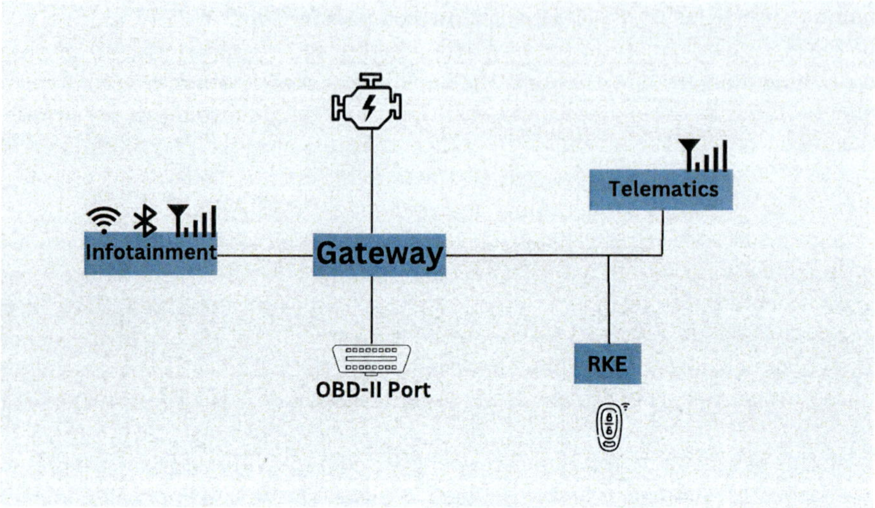

Fig. 1. The CAN Bus

2.2 OBD-II

The system for On-Board Diagnostics (OBD) stemmed from the requirement introduced by the California Air Resources Board (CARB) in 1988 to ensure that emission systems in vehicles perform according the specifications of the vehicle, or indicate otherwise to the driver or a mechanic when there is a problem in the vehicle [25]. In 1996, OBD-II specification (SAE J1962) was mandated for all vehicles sold in the U.S. so the OBD-II port, a.k.a. Diagnostic Link Connector (DLC), can exchange data with diagnostic tools. This gives repair shops the ability to connect with various systems to diagnose problems and acquire emission-related data.

Although OBD-II was intended to make emission-related data such as vehicle speed, engine RPM, engine temperature, and fuel injection accessible, other uses arise thanks to manufacturers "hidden" features that would allow reprogramming of ECUs' or disabling theft protection system [35]. In addition, the U.S. mandated all vehicles sold since 2008 to support ISO 15765 standard that defines Controller Area Network (CAN) standard through the OBD-II interface. It is even used by insurance companies to monitor the speed and fuel usage of a vehicle [33].

In most vehicles today, the CAN bus is directly connected to the diagnostic port under the steering wheel, where CAN bus messages can be received and transmitted. To carry diagnostic information, special OBD-II messages are defined, called PIDs (Parameter IDs), and are used by the protocol. These OBD-II PIDs are standardized, unlike CAN bus messages that are highly customized by vehicle manufacturers. Additionally, the PID message is similar to the CAN bus message. A PID for a query is identified by 0x7DF, and the data field contains a service number and a PID number. A manufacturer may also define private PIDs in addition to these universal PIDs.

2.3 OBD Dongles

The very nature of OBD-II is to make vehicles' internal data accessible by external entities, be it emission control authorities, insurance companies, or repair shops.

Traditionally, diagnostic tools are plugged into the OBD-II port by emission control authorities or repair shops. The other end of the cable is connected to a laptop equipped with suitable software for querying the vehicle's ECUs and displaying the results to the user.

Then things improved when OBD-II dongles came about recently, where cables are no longer needed. A dongle is equipped with a wireless interface that allows WiFi or Bluetooth connections through laptops or, more recently, mobile apps. Wireless dongles have gained popularity thanks to the low-cost convenience they offer.

2.4 Security Issues in CAN and OBD-II

Inherent Lack of Security in CAN. When CAN was initially developed, its nodes needed to be more technically ready to be connected to the external world and thus assumed to be isolated and trusted. As a result, CAN was designed without basic security features such as encryption and authentication that are now considered essential to communication networks [6,7].

The protocol's broadcast nature also increases the likelihood of attacks exploiting these security vulnerabilities. Therefore, a malicious message injected by a compromised electronic control unit (ECU) on the bus, if it conforms to CAN specifications, will be treated the same as a legitimate message from a benign ECU and broadcasted over the bus. Moreover, wireless communication capabilities have been added to CAN nodes for expanded functionality (e.g., TPMS, navigation, entertainment systems) without carefully examining the potential security impacts [8,23,26]. More recently, insurance companies and third parties have their OBD dongles equipped with wireless connections for monitoring and diagnostic purposes. Therefore, the attack vector becomes magnified for remote attacks by allowing some previously physically isolated units to connect to external entities through wireless connections.

Insufficient Security in OBD-II. Since CAN lacks basic security, a compromised OBD dongle poses a significant threat to a vehicle and its passengers.

ISO 14229-3 is a standard implemented in the Unified Diagnostic Services (UDS) protocol that builds on OBD. UDS makes it possible to communicate with various ECUs to perform things like reading and writing arbitrary memory locations, updating firmware, or even overriding I/O in safety-critical ECUs. UDS implements UDS SecurityAccess service to authenticate parties trying to perform potentially unsafe operations through a simple challenge-response mechanism. A value, called "seed", is generated by an ECU and sent to the requesting party to calculate a value based on the seed, called "key". If the resulting key is correct, the ECU allows the requester to perform the requested critical task. The problem with such a mechanism is its vulnerability to brute-force attack due to the small key size and algorithm's simplicity [4].

2.5 Security Issues in OBD-II Dongles

Wen et al. [33] tested 77 OBD dongles available in the market and concluded that all 77 dongles were vulnerable to at least two vulnerabilities. Other means of communication through the OBD-II create two types of threats: 1) remotely injecting malicious messages to the CAN bus and 2) potential personal data leakage when data OBD dongles send data [11]. In addition, Yan et al. [36] tested 20 OBD-II dongles and found that 50% of them vulnerable.

3 Related Work

There need to be more surveys of the countermeasures specifically designed to defend against attacks from the OBD-II port. However, there is a plethora of papers covering various areas of security in in-vehicle networks.

Some papers, such as [5,9], surveyed the work of cryptographic techniques used to add security and defend against various attacks on CAN. In addition, [16, 37] discussed anomaly- and signature-based Intrusion Detection Systems (IDS) for in-vehicle networks.

Researchers have conducted comprehensive research such as in [14,24], where they presented reviews of the security challenges of modern vehicles and corresponding countermeasures. They also presented the attack models and identified research challenges and future directions. One of the research gaps they identified in [24] was the need for a comparative study that surveys countermeasures built to address attacks originating from the OBD-II port, which is the primary purpose of this paper.

Sahana et al. [28] surveyed in-vehicle network countermeasures such as cryptographic techniques and IDS, focusing on firewalls and packet-filtering techniques. Most proposals state their ability to defend against attacks, including those originating from the OBD-II port.

4 Attacker Model

Attackers posing a threat to a vehicle exploiting the OBD-II port could be classified based on their proximity to the vehicle as follows:

1. Attackers with physical access: directly plugs into the OBD-II port.
2. Attackers with short-range wireless access: exploits short-range communication channels such as the Bluetooth wireless interface in an OBD-II dongle plugged into the OBD-II port.

3. Attackers with long-range wireless access: exploits long-range communication channels such as the cellular wireless interface in an OBD-II dongle plugged into the OBD-II port.

The classification of the attacker model stresses the importance of considering all types that could exploit the three attack surfaces.

5 Countermeasures

5.1 Improving Existing Countermeasures

The OBD-II uses the Unified Diagnostic Services (UDS) protocol on the CAN. UDS is an application-layer diagnostic protocol in the Open Systems Interconnection (OSI) model defined by ISO-14229.

As mentioned previously, UDS has a vulnerable *challenge-response* mechanism intended to authenticate any communicating device through the OBD-II port. Yadav et al. [35] proposed an additional authentication layer to improve the security of the seed-key mechanism.

5.2 Gateways and Firewalls

Luo and Hu [17] proposed a secure gateway that distributes keys to connected ECUs for message authentication and integrity verification. In addition, the gateway contains a firewall to filter incoming messages based on a whitelist.

Klement et al. [10,11] proposed arguably the first mechanism to filter incoming and outgoing traffic through the OBD-II port. Their firewall is located between the OBD-II port and external OBD dongles, so incoming and outgoing traffic can be filtered using rules. The rules give a high level of granularity to control the traffic by rejecting a CAN message, replacing its content selectively, or limiting its occurrences.

5.3 Intrusion Detection Systems (IDS)

Since the OBD-II port is used to diagnose the state of vehicles, it has to be connected to the internal network. Therefore, separating the port from the network seems counterintuitive. An IDS that recognize unacceptable messages such as malicious injection seems to be a logical solution [15]. Miller and Valasek [21] proposed using a device plugged into the OBD-II port to detect unusual messages and short-circuit the CAN bus, rendering the bus unusable. The authors did not define what constitutes unusual traffic. Although their solution might successfully thwart attacks originating from the OBD-II port, this comes with a very high cost, namely, disabling all CAN messages.

CANShield is a signal-based intrusion detection framework that uses deep learning techniques to detect various types of attacks [29].

5.4 Secure OBD Dongles

The authors of [19] evaluated the security of the Telia Sense, an IoT system consisting of an OBD-II dongle and a mobile application. They concluded that the system is secure due to its limited functionalities and the encrypted 4G connection to the server.

A role-based access control policy was proposed [18] using authentication certificates. The idea is that each OBD-II dongle needs to be certified by manufacturers before connecting to a vehicle. Once the vehicle verifies a device, it can communicate with specific ECUs based on its privilege. On the other hand, dongles that are not verified would only have permission to read the bus, whereas a certified mechanic's scan tool would have both read and write permissions.

Ammar et al. [2] proposed a gateway between the OBD-II port and the CAN network such that the gateway manages the authentication of connected devices through the port. The gateway is also responsible for establishing secure sessions through session keys. The authors utilized an end-to-end Role Based Access Control (RBAC) mechanism to protect the OBD-II port, making accessing the CAN network adhere to roles. The proposal could be installed on existing vehicles by software update without hardware modifications.

Alshaeri et al. [1] presented a set of security protocols for establishing authenticated secure connections between OBD-II dongles and their companion app with the OBD-II port. Their formal evaluation showed that the proposal is robust. However, it must be clarified if there will be delays when implemented on actual hardware.

5.5 New Standards

The SAE proposed a J3138 standard that is intended through a series of recommendations to improve security without impacting the ability of any off-board device connected to the vehicle's OBD-II port [27]. A test method that ensures the guidance is followed was introduced in [38] (Table 1).

6 Challenges and Research Opportunities

Lack of Information Sharing. As aforementioned, modern vehicle manufacturers often have gateways modules that separate the OBD-II port from other CAN subnetworks. These gateways are designed to only forward diagnostic traffic between a tester connected to the port and other CAN networks inside the vehicle. However, manufacturers do not usually publish information like the types of deployed countermeasures in the gateways. For example, know whether code signing is needed to reprogram ECUs and deploy IDS and firewalls. Sharing such information is beneficial for both other manufacturers and consumers. The former could learn different protection techniques, while the latter could make an informed decision on which vehicle is more secure [20].

Table 1. Summary of Countermeasures

Ref	Defense Objective	Placement	OBD-II Port Compatibility
[35]	Improve UDS challenge-response mechanism to prevent unauthorized access	Gateway	Yes
[17]	Whitelist filtering	Gateway	Yes
[10,11]	Traffic filtering	DLC	Yes*
[21]	Short circuit the CAN bus upon detecting abnormal traffic	DLC	Yes*
[29]	Signal-based detection	Gateway	Yes
[19]	Encrypted traffic	OBD dongle	Yes*
[18]	OBD dongles' verification	OBD dongles	Yes*
[2]	OBD dongles' verification	Gateway	Yes*
[1]	Secure connections between OBD dongles and their apps	OBD dongle & its mobile app	Yes*

***Specifically-built for the OBD-II port or dongles**

The Need for Network Redesign. Physical isolation of the OBD-II port and CAN bus is arguably the best way to protect the CAN bus. However, legislative requirements force vehicle manufacturers to have the OBD as mentioned in Sect. 2. This results in deploying gateways that separate the internal bus while keeping it available for legitimate diagnostic purposes. However, attacks that successfully bypass the OBD-II port and acquire access to the internal CAN bus could lead to devastating attacks.

Due to the strong physical connection between the OBD-II port and CAN network, it is costly to separate the two due to legislative and logistical reasons. However, a promising solution is to eliminate the wired connector and replace it with wireless technology. Subke et al. [31] describe a gradual 4-step approach to replacing the OBD-II port with a wireless 5G data link that involves replacing the port with an Ethernet link then a 5G modem.

Distrusted OBD. There are many OBD dongles and mobile apps anyone can easily plug into an OBD-II port to diagnose problems, track performance or location, or log activities. The problem with such devices is the lack of trust in the supply chain. The level of security of unknown in such devices. Wen et al. [33] showed that most OBD dongles have security flaws that could be exploited, rendering them attack vectors. Pham et al. [24] proposed that OBD devices must come from a trusted manufacturer. In addition, there should be a way to verify a device has been compromised. Furthermore, the privacy of collected data of the OBD devices should be used only by the intended parties. Finally, the OBD devices should be authenticated without introducing significant delays.

7 Conclusion

In this paper, we first review the history of OBD and CAN and their relevant security issues. OBD-II port poses many vulnerabilities to vehicles when exploited. The introduction of the OBD-II dongles worsened the security posture, magnified the attack vector, and made it possible for remote attackers thanks to wireless capabilities. Therefore, the attacker model emerged from an attacker with physical access only as a remote attacker. We follow that by reviewing the relevant automotive security surveys and finding a gap in OBD-II port security surveys. Additionally, we compared the existing OBD-II port countermeasures and highlighted those specifically built to secure the OBD-II port. Finally, one of the biggest challenges to securing the port is moving from the existing automotive internal architecture built on OBD-II and CAN to a new one.

References

1. Alshaeri, A., Younis, M.: Protocols for secure remote access to vehicle onboard diagnostic systems in smart cities. IEEE Intell. Transp. Syst. Mag. **14**(5), 209–221 (2022)
2. Ammar, M., Janjua, H., Thangarajan, A.S., Crispo, B., Hughes, D.: Securing the on-board diagnostics port (obd-ii) in vehicles. SAE Int. J. Transp. Cybersecurity Privacy (11-02-02-0009), 83–106 (2020)
3. Checkoway, S., et al.: Comprehensive experimental analyses of automotive attack surfaces. In: USENIX Security Symposium, vol. 4, p. 2021. San Francisco (2011)
4. Foster, I., Prudhomme, A., Koscher, K., Savage, S.: Fast and vulnerable: a story of telematic failures. In: 9th USENIX Workshop on Offensive Technologies (WOOT 15) (2015)
5. Gmiden, M., Gmiden, M.H., Trabelsi, H.: Cryptographic and intrusion detection system for automotive can bus: survey and contributions. In: 2019 16th International Multi-Conference on Systems, Signals & Devices (SSD), pp. 158–163. IEEE (2019)
6. Gupta, R.A., Chow, M.Y.: Networked control system: overview and research trends. IEEE Trans. Ind. Electron. **57**(7), 2527–2535 (2010)
7. Hoppe, T., Kiltz, S., Dittmann, J.: Security threats to automotive can networks — practical examples and selected short-term countermeasures. In: SAFECOMP (2011)
8. Humayed, A., Luo, B.: Cyber-physical security for smart cars: taxonomy of vulnerabilities, threats, and attacks. In: ACM/IEEE ICCPS (2015)
9. Jadoon, A.K., Wang, L., Li, T., Zia, M.A.: Lightweight cryptographic techniques for automotive cybersecurity. Wireless Communications and Mobile Computing (2018)
10. Klement, F., Pöhls, H.C., Katzenbeisser, S.: Change your car's filters: efficient concurrent and multi-stage firewall for obd-ii network traffic. In: 2022 IEEE 27th International Workshop on Computer Aided Modeling and Design of Communication Links and Networks (CAMAD), pp. 19–25. IEEE (2022)
11. Klement, F., Pöhls, H.C., Katzenbeisser, S.: Man-in-the-obd: A modular, protocol agnostic firewall for automotive dongles to enhance privacy and security. In: International Workshop on Attacks and Defenses for Internet-of-Things, pp. 143–164. Springer, Cham (2022). https://doi.org/10.1007/978-3-031-21311-3_7

12. Kornaros, G., Tomoutzoglou, O., Coppola, M.: Hardware-assisted security in electronic control units: secure automotive communications by utilizing one-time-programmable network on chip and firewalls. IEEE Micro **38**(5), 63–74 (2018)
13. Koscher, K., et al.: Experimental security analysis of a modern automobile. In: 2010 IEEE Symposium on Security and Privacy, pp. 447–462. IEEE (2010)
14. Limbasiya, T., Teng, K.Z., Chattopadhyay, S., Zhou, J.: A systematic survey of attack detection and prevention in connected and autonomous vehicles. Vehicular Communications, p. 100515 (2022)
15. Liu, J., Zhang, S., Sun, W., Shi, Y.: In-vehicle network attacks and countermeasures: challenges and future directions. IEEE Network **31**(5), 50–58 (2017)
16. Lokman, S.F., Othman, A.T., Abu-Bakar, M.H.: Intrusion detection system for automotive controller area network (can) bus system: a review. EURASIP J. Wirel. Commun. Netw. **2019**, 1–17 (2019)
17. Luo, F., Hu, Q.: Security mechanisms design for in-vehicle network gateway. Tech. rep, SAE Technical Paper (2018)
18. Markham, T.R., Chernoguzov, A.: A balanced approach for securing the obd-ii port. SAE Int. J. Passenger Cars-Electron. Electr. Syst. **10**(2) (2017)
19. Marstorp, G., Lindström, H.: Security testing of an obd-ii connected iot device. E2B: IOT Hacking (2017)
20. Miller, C.: Lessons learned from hacking a car. IEEE Design Test **36**(6), 7–9 (2019)
21. Miller, C., Valasek, C.: A survey of remote automotive attack surfaces. Black Hat USA **2014**, 94 (2014)
22. Pareja Veredas, R., Mehaboobe, Y.: Scalable attacks on connected vehicles (2022)
23. Petit, J., Shladover, S.E.: Potential cyberattacks on automated vehicles. IEEE Trans. Intell. Transp. Syst. **16**(2), 546–556 (2015)
24. Pham, M., Xiong, K.: A survey on security attacks and defense techniques for connected and autonomous vehicles. Comput. Secur. **109**, 102,269 (2021)
25. Rizzoni, G., Onori, S., Rubagotti, M.: Diagnosis and prognosis of automotive systems: motivations, history and some results. IFAC Proc. Vol. **42**(8), 191–202 (2009)
26. Rouf, I., et al.: Security and privacy vulnerabilities of in-car wireless networks: a tire pressure monitoring system case study. In: USENIX Security Symposium (2010)
27. SAE: J3138_202210: Diagnostic link connector security (2018). https://www.sae.org/standards/content/j3138_202210/
28. Sahana, Y., Gotkhindikar, A., Tiwari, S.K.: Survey on can-bus packet filtering firewall. In: 2022 International Conference on Edge Computing and Applications (ICECAA), pp. 472–478. IEEE (2022)
29. Shahriar, M.H., Xiao, Y., Moriano, P., Lou, W., Hou, Y.T.: Canshield: Signal-based intrusion detection for controller area networks. arXiv preprint arXiv:2205.01306 (2022)
30. Studnia, I., Nicomette, V., Alata, E., Deswarte, Y., Kaâniche, M., Laarouchi, Y.: Survey on security threats and protection mechanisms in embedded automotive networks. In: 2013 43rd Annual IEEE/IFIP Conference on Dependable Systems and Networks Workshop (DSN-W), pp. 1–12. IEEE (2013)
31. Subke, P., Mayer, J.: The future of obd: Enhanced on-board diagnostic system with remote access. Tech. rep, SAE Technical Paper (2022)
32. Taylor, A., Leblanc, S., Japkowicz, N.: Anomaly detection in automobile control network data with long short-term memory networks. In: 2016 IEEE International Conference on Data Science and Advanced Analytics (DSAA), pp. 130–139. IEEE (2016)

33. Wen, H., Chen, Q.A., Lin, Z.: {Plug-N-Pwned}: Comprehensive vulnerability analysis of {OBD-II} dongles as a new {Over-the-Air} attack surface in automotive {IoT}. In: 29th USENIX Security Symposium (USENIX Security 20), pp. 949–965 (2020)
34. Wolf, M., Weimerskirch, A., Paar, C.: Security in automotive bus systems. In: Workshop on Embedded Security in Cars, pp. 1–13. Bochum (2004)
35. Yadav, A., Bose, G., Bhange, R., Kapoor, K., Iyengar, N., Caytiles, R.D.: Security, vulnerability and protection of vehicular on-board diagnostics. Int. J. Secur. Appl. **10**(4), 405–422 (2016)
36. Yan, W.: A two-year survey on security challenges in automotive threat landscape. In: 2015 International Conference on Connected Vehicles and Expo (ICCVE), pp. 185–189. IEEE (2015)
37. Young, C., Zambreno, J., Olufowobi, H., Bloom, G.: Survey of automotive controller area network intrusion detection systems. IEEE Design Test **36**(6), 48–55 (2019)
38. Zachos, M., Subke, P.: Test method for the sae j3138 automotive cyber security standard. Tech. rep, SAE Technical Paper (2020)

Health Informatics and Biomedical Imaging

Novel Deep Learning-Based Technique for Tuberculosis Bacilli Detection in Sputum Microscopy

Lara Visuña(✉), Javier Garcia-Blas, and Jesus Carretero

Computer Science and Engineering Department, University Carlos III of Madrid, Leganes, Spain
lvisuna@pa.uc3m.es, {fjblas,jcarrete}@inf.uc3m.es

Abstract. Nowadays, tuberculosis is one of the more deadly diseases. Nevertheless, an accurate and fast diagnosis has a great influence on disease prognosis. The research goal of this work is to speed up the time to diagnosis, as well as to improve the sensibility of sputum microscopy as a tuberculosis diagnosis tool. This work presents a novel deep learning technique for automatic bacilli detection in Ziehl Neelsen (ZN) stain sputum microscopy. First, the microscopy images are enhanced and completely fragmented. Then a single deep convolutional network indicates which image fragments include bacilli or not. Results demonstrate the effectiveness of our framework, obtaining a 92.86% recall and 99.49% precision, along with a significantly decreasing detection time. Finally, this research compared the results with previous works in bacilli detection, showing a considerable improvement in the results, illustrating the feasibility of our results.

Keywords: CNN · Deep Learning · Computer Vision · Tuberculosis · ZN stain

1 Introduction

Nowadays, tuberculosis (TB) is one of the deadliest diseases. It is a contagious disease caused by the bacteria called Mycobacterium Tuberculosis, spread by infected people through the air. In 2021, there are estimations of over 1.6 million tuberculosis deaths, leading to the cause of death from a single infectious agent until the coronavirus (COVID-19) pandemic outbreak [1]. Despite this great number of deaths, about 85% of people can be cured with proper diagnosis and treatment [1].

Despite the technology and medical advances, the World Health Organization (WHO) reported reductions in the total number of people diagnosed with TB in 2020 and 2021, which according to them, it could reflect an increase in the number of undiagnosed cases. Fast and accurate diagnosis enables breaking the transmission of the disease and an early treatment. Multiple diagnosis techniques are available such as culture, molecular test, etc. One of the widely used diagnosis

K. Daimi and A. Al Sadoon (Eds.): ICR 2023, LNNS 721, pp. 269–279, 2023.
https://doi.org/10.1007/978-3-031-35308-6_23

methods is sputum smear microscopy, a well-known technique that permits the detection of the disease but also treatment monitoring and the infection evolution. Sputum smear microscopy is an inexpensive and rapid diagnosis technique, which makes it the first diagnostic tool in middle, low-income countries. Sputum microscopy is a manual process that requires observation through a microscope to locate bacillus. This technique is error prone, its sensitivity is about 55-95 % depending on the experience of laboratory technicians but also depending on the burden of infection [2].

One of the more extended Sputum smear microscopy techniques is Ziehl Neelsen (ZN) stain, in which the acid-fast bacilli (AFB), like Mycobacterium Tuberculosis, turns the color to red or hot pink. The bacillus can be seen in the microscopy slides in different forms: singles bacillus, V-shapes, clumps, or bacilli fragments. The number of bacillus reported is related to the level of infection and how infectious a patient is [3]. In addition, even fragments must be reported.

A correct diagnosis and monitoring of the disease requires multiple microscopy images that have to be analyzed. If not AFB are found in 100 microscopy fields of study, the test is reported as negative. If nine or fewer bacillus are reported in 100 microscopy fields, the result is scanty. With a higher reported bacillus amount, the grading must be 1+ to 3+, following the indications depicted in Table 1. The sensibility of ZN microscopy decreases if the bacillus amount is less than 1000/ML of sputum, then, only 10% of the slide shows the presence of AFB [3].

Table 1. Tuberculosis grading and diagnosis based on the AFB count in microscopy images [3,4].

AFB found	Microscopy fields	Grading
0	Reported in 100 microscopy fields	Negative
1-9	Reported in 100 microscopy fields	Scanty
10-99	Reported in 100 microscopy fields	1+
1-10	Reported for every microscopy field	2+
>10	Reported for every microscopy field	3+

These situations makes it important to detect all the bacillus in the microscopy slides. With the objective of avoiding the dependence on the human factor, and increasing the sensibility, this paper designed and implement an automatic bacilli detector in sputum smear microscopy using deep learning techniques. The deep learning-based detector is designed emphasizing the locating of single, V-shape, and fragments of bacillus, due to its greater difficulty when it comes to being seen in the microscope images. The main contributions of the paper are as follows:

- Design and develop a novel approach to detect bacilli with one stage deep learning algorithm. In the system, microscopy images are preprocessed and fragmented. Then, they are introduced into the Convolutional Neural Network (CNN), which decides the areas in the image reported as bacillus.

- We present multiple evaluation metrics compared with previous works, showing a significant improvement detecting Acid fast bacilli in microscopy images. The system showed a 92.86% recall and 99,49% precision.
- This approach accelerates the process of AFB recount, reducing the diagnosing time, and also, enhancing sensibility versus manual bacilli searching.
- The one stage CNN algorithm is highly generalizable and could be trained for locating other bacteria and germs in microscopy images.

We present literature review in Sect. 2, where analyze previous techniques to detect AFB. In Sect. 3 our framework is presented, as well as, all the materials and procedures implemented. Sections 4 and 5 show the experimental results and discussions, respectively. Finally, the main conclusion are introduced in Sect. 6.

2 Literature Review

There are several research projects that have reported remarkable results for automatic bacilli detection using segmentation and deep learning techniques.

A segmentation technique taking advantage of AFB color was presented by Raof et al. [5]. The segmentation was made through color pixel study and image enhancement techniques. More preprocessing methods were presented by Li et al. [6], where a fusion multi-frame method is applied followed by a single layer perceptron to filter the background. Then, a neural network classifier is trained for the automatic classification of bacillus, into single, two, and three bacillus.

For touching and single bacillus, Panicker et al. [7] developed an automatic bacillus detector. This solution was evaluated with 22 smear microscopic images, achieving 97.13% recall and 78.4% precision. The proposed method used a simple segmentation approach to classify the foreground and background of the image, after that, the foreground is classified by a CNN into bacilli and non-bacilli. Also in 2018, a full deep learning algorithm presented by Kant et al. [8] proposed to extract (20×20) pixels patches from the original image, then two cascade CNN decided between positive and negative bacillus. Another full deep learning technique was proposed by El-Melegy et al. [9], where a faster R-CNN architecture was used for bacilli detection. The faster R-CNN combines a Region proposal network (RPN), which generate regions of interest, and a CNN (VGG16, in this case), achieving an 89.7% F-score.

In 2021, V. Shwetha et al. [10] proposed another two stage algorithm. First, after a preprocessing stage k-means clustering is used for segmentation. Then, a pretrained CNN classifies the previous patches into bacilli or another cell. SqueezeNet achieves 97% accuracy, differencing cells of bacillus.

Given that the number of bacilli is related to the infection level, there are works diagnosing tuberculosis according to the number of bacillus detected. The authors in [11] presented an automatic mycobacterium identification algorithm to detect the infection level. After noise reduction, an area threshold algorithm for segmentation is developed. Later, the bacilli features are extracted using local oriented histogram to feed a deep learning algorithm achieving an accuracy of

97.55 classifying the disease infection level. In [12] a DenseNet CNN architecture is used over 2200 sputum images, to detect the presence or absence of the tuberculosis disease. Achieving an accuracy of 99.7%.

Existing literature presents previous algorithms and methods available for AFB detection. However, this research line continues to be a challenge. The standard practice for TB bacillus detection is as follows: after preprocessing, a first algorithm proposes region candidates or discards the background, followed by the classification algorithm. With this scheme, some bacillus can be miscounted or labeled as background. We can observe there is a lack of a one stage algorithm in the literature. In this work, we propose a deep learning-based one stage algorithm for AFB detection, avoiding the phase of proposing regions. This scheme prevents false negatives and accelerates AFB detection and tuberculosis diagnosis.

3 Material and Methods

The automatic tuberculosis bacilli detection system proposed are based on microscopy ZN stain images, which can be inserted in the deep learning-based system alone or in batches. The microscopy images are enhanced and fragmented in patches of 80 pixels height and 80 pixels wide following the scheme presented in Sect. 3.1.

Microscopy images patches are the input of the CNN architecture, which is trained following the procedures described in Sect. 3.2. The deep learning-based bacilli detector architecture is composed of a CNN followed by a deep neural network.

A predesigned NasNetmobile architecture is introduced as the CNN element in the detection system. NASNetMobile architecture was proposed by Google Brain [13]. NASNet is automatically designed by a Neural architecture search (NAS) with a controller Recurrent neural network (RNN), which samples different neural architectures. NASNetMobile was designed with the aim of high accuracy and low inference latency. After the convolutional element, a deep neural network is implemented to end the detection process.

The deep neural network is composed of a hidden layer with 128 neurons and an ELU (shown in Eq. 1) as an activation function. Then, the output layer includes 2 neurons and a Softmax (shown in Eq. 2) as an activation function. The two output neurons differentiate into background and bacillus patches. Between the two layers, a dropout is included to avoid overfitting. The complete detection system architecture is presented in Fig. 1.

$$f(x) = \begin{cases} x, x > 0 \\ \alpha(e^x - 1), x \leq 0 \end{cases} \tag{1}$$

$$S(x_i) = \frac{e^{x_i}}{\sum_{j=1}^{n} e^{x_j}} \tag{2}$$

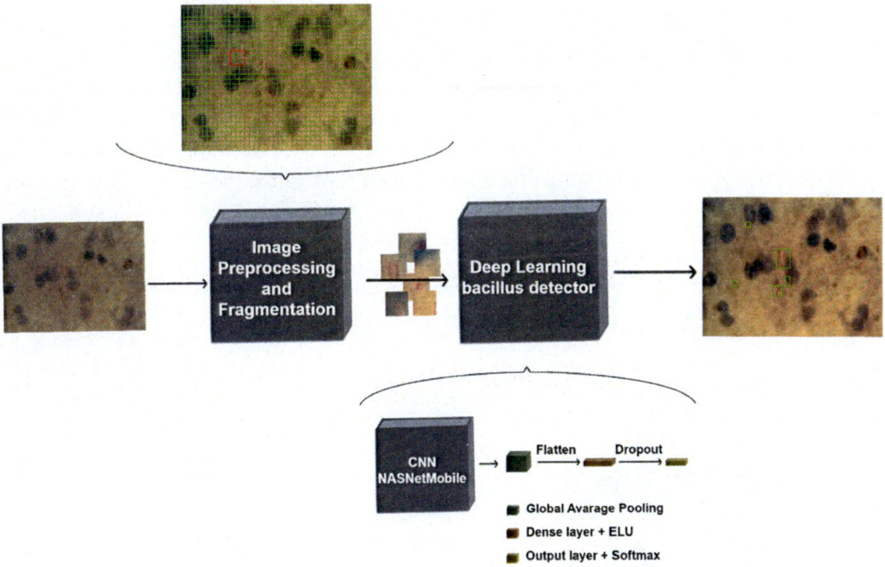

Fig. 1. System block architecture of deep learning-based technique bacilli detection.

The patches including bacilli information are classified by the network as bacilli. Even when the presence of bacillus is detected by the network, not all the patch areas have to include bacilli information. In order to make a fit bounding box and avoid reporting imprecise information only the center area of the patch will be reported as bacilli. Since the central area of the image includes the more relevant information for the CNN analysis. Once all the patches are analyzed by the system, the sputum image is reported with all the identified bacillus.

3.1 Data Acquisition and Preprocessing

For the development of this project, 200 sputum ZN microscopy images were employed. The microscopy images were collected by the AI Research and Automated Laboratory Diagnostics and are available in Kaggle [14]. All the images are in *jpg* format with (1.124×1.636) pixels size. The dataset also includes bounding boxes framing the bacillus.

Table 2. Database division into train, validation, and test.

	Train	Validation	Test	Total
Images	120	40	40	**200**
Annotated bacilli	436	235	188	**859**

For training, validation, and testing, the microscopy images were categorized as shown in Table 2. In addition, the table resumes the amount of annotated bacilli included in the dataset. These annotated bacilli are reported by bounding box, a mean of 4 bacillus are reported by image. The distribution of labels by microscopy image is plotted in Fig. 2. During the data preparation stage, the bounding boxes of the training images were corrected to enhance the CNN training.

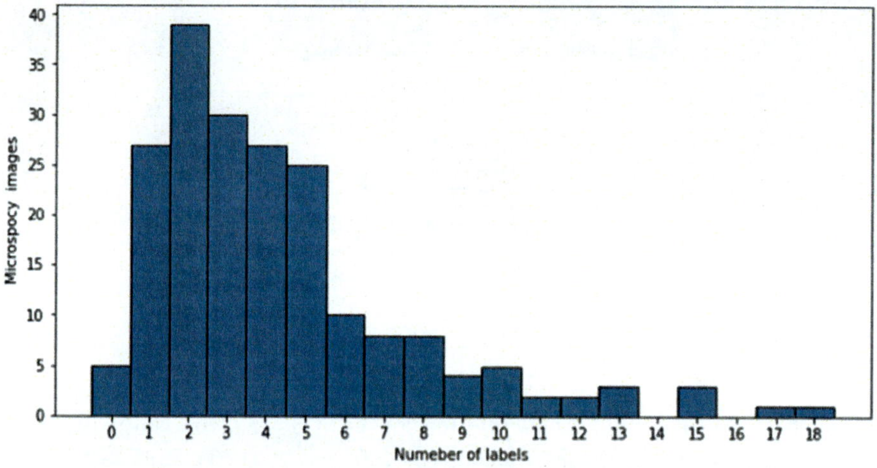

Fig. 2. Annotated bacillus distribution.

The microscopy images of the dataset present different light intensities, biological structures, and backgrounds. Figure 3 shows a sample of the training images. The images include mostly AFB fragments, single bacillus, or small clumps of bacillus, due to there are more difficult to locate by a manual procedure.

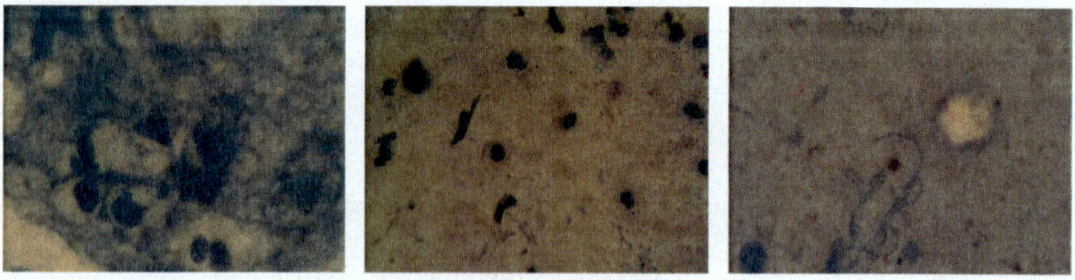

(a) (b) (c)

Fig. 3. Training microscopy images examples.

A normalization scheme is applied to the sputum images, in order to homogenize them. The values of all the images are also scaled into 0-1 values. Then, the enhanced images are completely fragmented into patches of 80 pixels height and 80 pixels width. Patches are formed with a sliding window, with steps of 40 pixels, until cover all the microscopy image area. This method allows every patch to share pixels with the previous and next patch, as well as, with the upper and downer patch, thus achieving that all the bacillus are captured by the fragments of images for their subsequent classification.

3.2 Training Procedures

Training is the most important stage to neural network learning. For training the CNN, only the train-set was used. The 120 microscopy images were transformed into patches, so after preprocessing and fragmentation, 130180 patches resulted.

According to the reported bounding box, the patches were labeled as bacilli or background. The final training data is strongly unbalanced, in the 130180 patches, only 995 were labeled as bacilli. Based on these findings, the Poisson loss function was selected (shown in Eq. 3).

$$L_{poisson} = \sum_{i=1}^{n} y_{pred_i} - Y_i * log(y_{pred_i}) \tag{3}$$

To avoid overfitting and to take advantage of previous strong training sessions, a transfer learning scheme is applied followed by soft training. We explode NASNetmobile with the previous ImageNet challenge training [15]. The complete deep learning system was trained in 50 epochs, a batch size of 32 images was selected, and a low learning rate of 1,00E-04 in the Adam optimizer. The hyperparameters were selected based on validation results, in order to optimize several metrics like accuracy, recall, precision, and F1-score.

4 Results

In this section, we present the training and performance results of our model. The experiments were performed with Jupyter Notebooks and implemented using Python 3.6.9, TensorFlow 2.5.0 and Keras 2.5.0. The training was executed with an NVidia RTX 3090. The system was trained during 4.5 h until reach the 50 epochs.

The accuracy and loss curves are depicted in Fig. 4. They show a final accuracy of 99.98% for test images and for 99.06% validation images.

We used 40 test images to assess our system and the output result was computed in 50.76 s for the full test set. The detection system achieved a classification patch accuracy of 99.34%. It is important to note that, patches are imbalanced as there are about 100 times more background patches than bacillus patches. So, the bacilli level result is presented in Table 3, where the recall, precision, and F1-score are computed by analyzing the bacillus detected in the microscopy images

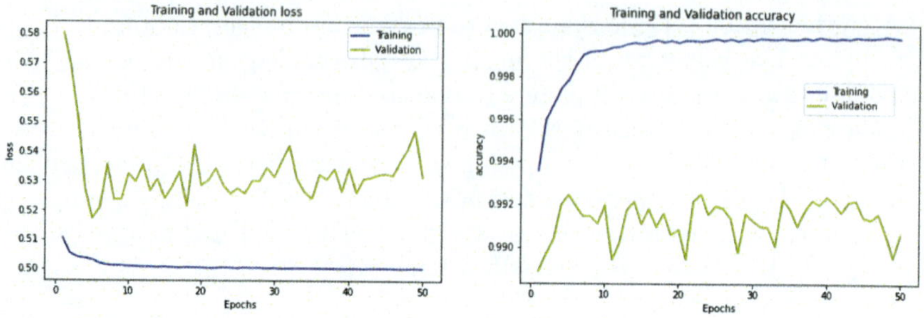

Fig. 4. Loss and accuracy curves for training and validation subsets.

versus the actual bacillus in the microscopy image. The system scored 92.86% recall and 99.49% precision detecting bacillus in sputum ZN stain microscopy images.

Table 3. Detection performance at bacilli level.

	Recall	**Precision**	**F1-score**
Result with Test-set	92.86%	99.49%	96.06%

Figure 5 shows the deep learning-based bacilli detection system results. Every column shows pictures for three different microscopies including: the input image, the original manual bounding box, and the system output.

5 Discussion

This paper introduced the implementation of a deep learning-based automatic bacilli detector. The detector works with ZN stain microscopy images. The system is trained focus on the detection of AFB in microscopy images with low bacilli amount, due to their higher complexity of detection in a manual search.

The system was trained with 120 microscopy images, with the bacilli previously pointed by bounding boxes. These bounding boxes were manually indicated and only points out singles bacillus. Even though the proposed system was trained with this information, analyzing the test result proved, the deep learning system reached abstract this knowledge to point out singles bacillus but also overlaps bacillus. This performance can be seen in the second and third columns of Fig. 5, where clumps of two bacillus are detected by the presented system.

The system can also detect bacillus fragments or partially visible bacillus, as illustrated in the first column of Fig. 5. The original box points out two bacillus locations versus the three pointed out by the system. The original bounding box miscounted the third bacilli since it is under blue pigment.

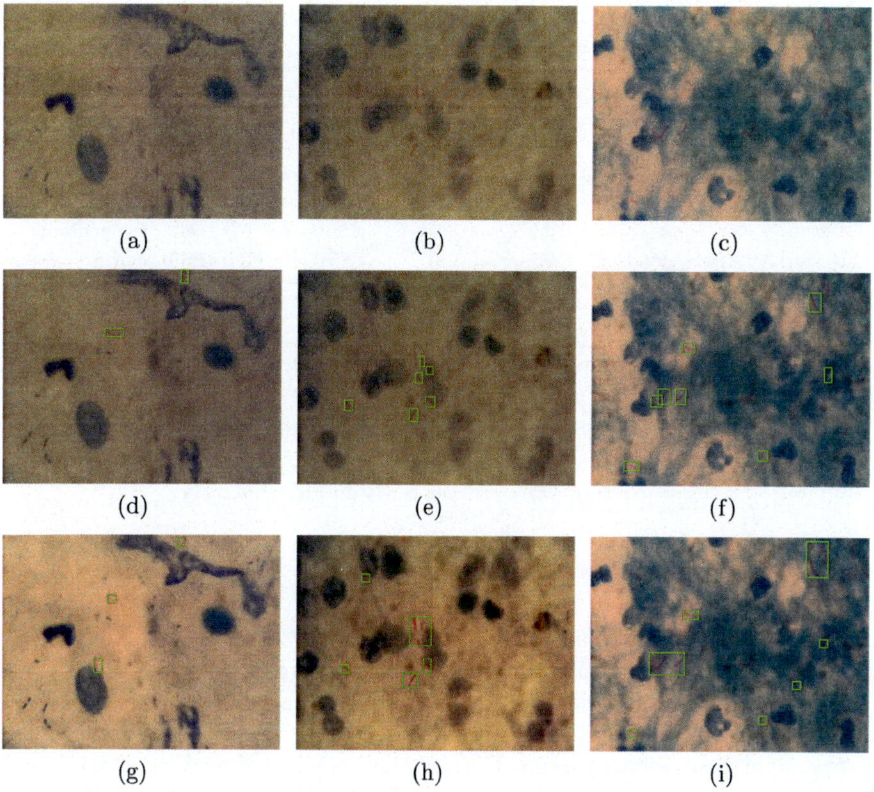

Fig. 5. Detection results on the ZN sputum microscopy images. Original images (a-c), reported bounding boxes (d-f), and system output (g-i).

Following the analysis of the test results, the system presents some miscounted bacillus. This event occurs in blurred images of the dataset, further, they were also miscounted by the original bounding box. This suggests that by improving the training bounding boxes and by increasing the training images, the system would be enhanced and this issue is avoided.

This study presented a literature review related to the topic. In Table 4, the proposed system was compared with previous deep learning-based bacillus detectors models. The table shows, different dataset sizes, preprocessing techniques, and deep learning algorithms.

All the previous studies show a two stage algorithms insight, in which the first stage selects bacillus candidates, then a classificator decides which of them are truly bacillus. In the presented approach the detector architecture is an one stage algorithm. Even dispensing with the first stage, the system shows reliable results, reaching the best precision reported. Concerning inference time, there are no reports in the consulted literature.

Table 4. Deep learning techniques and performance in bacilli detection reported in previous literature.

	Recall	Precision	F1-score	Test-set	Detection Technique
[10]	97.00%	98.00%	97.50%	298	Thresholding segmentation + CNN
[7]	97.13%	78.40%	86.77%	22	Binarization segmentation + CNN
[8]	83.78%	67.55%	74.79%	40	Two cascade CNN
[9]	98.30%	82.60%	89.77%	300	Faster R-CNN (Data Augmentation)
This work	**92.86%**	**99.49%**	**96.06%**	**40**	**Single CNN architecture**

The presented results reported an acceleration of the process of AFB recount, thus, reducing tuberculosis diagnosing time. According to results, the detector is also able to increase the sensibility of the ZN stain microscopy as a diagnostic tool avoiding unnoticed bacillus due to lack of experience of laboratory technicians,the big burden of work, or partially hidden bacillus.

6 Conclusions

In this paper, we proposed a one stage deep learning-based bacilli detector that automatically localizes AFB in ZN stain sputum microscopy images.

Sputum images are enhanced and fragmented, the deep learning network uses these fragmented patches as input. During the training more the 95% of patches as labeled as background. Despite the imbalanced dataset, the method reports a precision 99.49% and a recall of 92,86% finding AFB in the Test-set. The proposed system outperforms the original manual detection, detecting even overlapping bacillus.

Our results were compared with a significant number of previous literature research, showing the method's feasibility. The results reported enhance the previous solutions avoiding the candidate proposal stage in the system, reaching the higher precision reported in the literature. The method can provide precise and fast AFB detection, thus, aiding tuberculosis diagnosis and prognosis.

Our current efforts focus on the train phase of our deep learning-based bacilli detector. We plan to use optical microscopy time-lapse videos to report the bacilli tuberculosis growth rate under different conditions. Our goal is to prove that the one stage method can be trained with different microscopy techniques, maintaining the current accuracy. Finally, future work will attend to further compare this work with another CNN architectures.

Acknowledgments. This work was supported by the Innovative Medicines Initiative 2 Joint Undertaking (JU) under grant agreement No 853989. The JU receives support from the European Union's Horizon 2020 research and innovation programme and EFPIA and Global Alliance for TB Drug Development non-profit organisation, Bill & Melinda Gates Foundation and University of Dundee.

DISCLAIMER. This work reflects only the author's views, and the JU is not responsible for any use that may be made of the information it contains.

References

1. World Health Organization (WHO) (2022). Global Tuberculosis Report 2022. https://www.who.int/publications/i/item/9789240061729
2. Das, P.K., Ganguly, S.B., Mandal, B.: Sputum smear microscopy in tuberculosis: it is still relevant in the era of molecular diagnosis when seen from the public health perspective. Biomed. Biotechnol. Res. J. (BBRJ) **3**(2), 77 (2019)
3. Deka, B.C., Saikia, D., Pratim Kashyap, M.: Diagnosis of tuberculosis. Europ. Jo. Molecular Clin.Med. **9**(07) (2022)
4. Global Laboratory Initiative (GLI). Laboratory Diagnosis of Tuberculosis by Sputum Microscopy (2013)
5. Raof, R.A.A., Mashor, M.Y., Ahmad, R.B., Noor, S.S.M.: Image segmentation of Ziehl-Neelsen sputum slide images for tubercle Bacilli detection. Image Segmentation, pp. 365–378 (2011)
6. Li, Z., Ling, J., Wu, J., Luo, N., Tan, M., Zhong, P.: Research on preprocessing method for microscopic image of sputum smear and intelligent counting for Tubercule Bacillus. IOP Conf. Ser. Mater. Sci. Eng. **466**(1), 012112 (2018). IOP Publishing (2018)
7. Panicker, R.O., Kalmady, K.S., Rajan, J., Sabu, M.K.: Automatic detection of tuberculosis bacilli from microscopic sputum smear images using deep learning methods. Biocybern. Biomed. Eng. **38**(3), 691–699 (2018)
8. Kant, S., Srivastava, M.M.: Towards automated tuberculosis detection using deep learning. In: 2018 IEEE Symposium Series on Computational Intelligence (SSCI), pp. 1250–1253. IEEE (2018)
9. El-Melegy, M., Mohamed, D., ElMelegy, T.: Automatic detection of tuberculosis Bacilli from microscopic sputum smear images using faster R-CNN, transfer learning and augmentation. In: Morales, A., Fierrez, J., Sánchez, J.S., Ribeiro, B. (eds.) IbPRIA 2019. LNCS, vol. 11867, pp. 270–278. Springer, Cham (2019). https://doi.org/10.1007/978-3-030-31332-6_24
10. Shwetha, V., Prasad, K., Mukhopadhyay, C., Banerjee, B., Chakrabarti, A.: Automatic detection of Bacilli bacteria from Ziehl-Neelsen sputum smear images. In: 2021 2nd International Conference on Communication, Computing and Industry 4.0 (C2I4), pp. 1–5. IEEE (2021)
11. Mithra, K.S., Sam Emmanuel, W.R.: Automated identification of mycobacterium bacillus from sputum images for tuberculosis diagnosis. SIViP **13**(8), 1585–1592 (2019). https://doi.org/10.1007/s11760-019-01509-1
12. Panicker, R. O., Soman, B., Sabu, M.K.: Tuberculosis detection from conventional sputum smear microscopic images using machine learning techniques. In: Hybrid Computational Intelligence, pp. 63–80. CRC Press (2019)
13. Zoph, B., Vasudevan, V., Shlens, J., Le, Q.V.: Learning transferable architectures for scalable image recognition. In: Proceedings of the IEEE Conference on Computer Vision and Pattern Recognition, pp. 8697–8710 (2018)
14. Uddin, S.: Tuberculosis Image Dataset. https://www.kaggle.com/datasets/saife245/tuberculosis-image-datasets. Accessed March 2023
15. Russakovsky, O., et al.: ImageNet large scale visual recognition challenge. Int. J. Comput. Vis. **115**, 211-252 (2015)

Real Time Remote Cardiac Health Monitoring Using IoT Wearable Sensors - A Review

Pawan Sharma[1], Javad Rezazadeh[2](✉), Abubakar Bello[3], Ahmed Dawoud[4], and Ali Abas Albabawat[5]

[1] Study Group Australia, Darlinghurst, Australia
Suad1941@yahoo.com.au
[2] Crown Institute of Higher Education (CIHE), North Sydney, Australia
Javad.rezazadeh@cihe.edu.au
[3] Western Sydney University, Penrith, Australia
a.bello@westernsydney.edu.au
[4] University of South Australia, Adelaide, Australia
ahmed.dawoud@unisa.edu.au
[5] Computer Science Department, University of Duhok, Duhok, KRG, Iraq
ali.abas@uod.ac

Abstract. Many heart patients in rural areas are unable to get the appropriate emergency treatment on time due to the limitations of the IoT wearable sensor connections with a reliable and accurate network. This paper provides a review that aimed to analyze Connectivity, Scheduling and Backup (CSB) components of IoT wearable sensors for smart healthcare. The IoT technology helps to connect the remote patients reliably by establishing the best network connection. This study compares important techniques with different IoT sensors used to detect the vital situations for remote cardiac health monitoring. In IoT health monitoring, Smartphones will be of capable classifying the collected data from the sensors and generate two different signals as emergency and normal for the accurate data transmission. Moreover, Bluetooth Low Energy (BLE) is used to connect the sensor and smartphone whereas 3,4G/WI-Fi is used to connect to the health caregivers with reliable connections. Finally, suitable algorithms will be taken for filtering the data before forwarding to a health center database. This review provides appropriate analysis for network connection, data accuracy with scheduling and backup module for IoT health monitoring.

Keywords: IoT · Wearables · heart patients · Smart Healthcare · Smartphone

1 Introduction and Literature Review

The Internet of Things (IoT) [1] is included 4 components, smart sensors [3], cloud computing [2, 28], wireless networks [18] and analytic software. The past years have witnessed for the gradually increased of the people suffering from chronic diseases; heart disease that needs urgent treatment [4]. Although there are many health clinics to check up for those patients, the health clinic is not able to check all high growing

K. Daimi and A. Al Sadoon (Eds.): ICR 2023, LNNS 721, pp. 280–291, 2023.
https://doi.org/10.1007/978-3-031-35308-6_24

population which number hits the high level that is reaching 2 billion in 2050 includ-ing 80% in developing countries [7]. The cost of hospitalization and the treatment on time may face a big issue all over the countries. The patients who need emergency treatment may face difficulties in coming years [30]. In such problem, most remote patients are attracted to the implementation of the Telemedicine; that is being updated with different solutions and time saving mechanisms [4]. The monitoring could be for the elderly people, different patients like heart patients, patients who had done surgery etc. [30]. The wireless sensor in the hospital network architecture for monitoring health and also activities of the patient is described on [5]. In [6] The next Linear acceleration-based transmission duty cycling decision control (LA-TDC) algorithm with the accelerometer sensor are efficiently used and reduced the false alarm occurrence [5]. Leu, Ko (2018) focused on Wireless Body Sensor Network (WBSN) and Mobile Physiological Sensor System (MoPSS) which use to measure the body parameters to determine accuracy in terms of the packet loss rate of the heart patients [7]. This is done using a high tech MoPSS technique. Earlier the filtering technique [8] is used to classify the data to develop the alarm if emergency is detected [8]. A real time approach is applicable on [9] the Hilbert adaptive beat identification technique for the indication of the heart-beat timings where combined signal passed through the band pass filter which gives the accuracy of the data in the detection of emergency. In [21] introduced accuracy in terms of the data acquisition method to monitor cardiac patients for early warning [10]. They offer a solution as mobile devices collect Electrocardiography (ECG) and Seism CardioGraphy (SCG) data to monitor the cardiac patients efficiently for early warning. An adaptive persistent m data (APMD) transmission protocol [11] is proposed to reduce delay with reliability guarantee for pervasive sensing data communication systems. Also, the adaptive streaming method integrating Content Centric Networking (CCN) [12] which transfer 300Mbps which is higher than the previous one and improved delay. In [13] proposed the localized wrist sensor for reliability in terms of minimizing the body sensors of the patients. The work introduced in [14] investigates the Opportunistic Smartphone-based Gateway as a solution of excessive use of excessive use of hardware resources in terms of CPU and memory on heart patients. The Respiratory sinus arrhythmia (RSA) algorithm [15] and dual work technique of the Smartphone helps to minimize the computational needs on the server in terms of processing bio-signals for patients.

2 Factors for IoT Healthcare System

Figure 1 describes the general structure of the components or users connecting with each other.

The first mechanism is the connection between sensors and Smartphone where the sensors are sending data using the Bluetooth connectivity. After that the Smartphone is not only act as a gateway to forward the signal but also to process some raw information into meaningful data or information [30]. In the next part we explain Connectivity, Scheduling and Backup (CSB) components. The first factor Connectivity includes all the connection type used in the system. Connectivity refers to the metric how all the parts of the network are connected. It refers to the strength or structure of the network. Second, we describe the Scheduling technique, where algorithms are generated as the

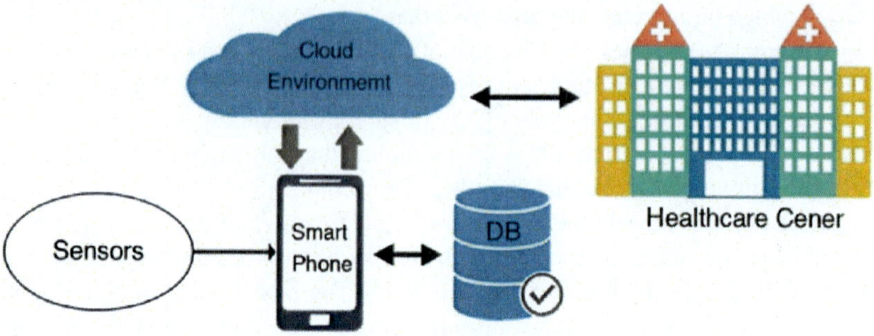

Fig. 1. General flow diagram for IoT Healthcare System

threshold or used to create red or green signal of the parameters. Lastly, we describe the backup plan for the data that are used as a log by the health personnel. These three factors, sub-factors and their connections and relations are demonstrated on Table 1.

Table 1. Main attributes, Description of attributes and instances of the CSB Components

Factors/Class	Main attributes	Attributes description	Instances
Connectivity:	Interconnection between sensors, Smartphone, and health center		
Bluetooth	Bluetooth Low Energy (BLE)	cheaper installation cost, less hardware, and high compatibility	Bluetooth, BLE
Cellular Network:	Data transfer speed, data delay	speed from beginning to the end of download	3G, 4G, 5G
Wi-Fi	Gateway, Networking bandwidth	good bandwidth to transfer data to the cloud and datacenter	WAN
Scheduling:	Implementation of a new traffic network for queuing the data as their priority		
Priority Basis:	Non-preemptive priority queue Data acquisition time	The data that carry the vital parameters of the heart patients which helps to treat immediately in the emergency condition	Data Filtering Technique Threshold algorithm
Non- Priority Basis:	Normal model	The real time continuous normal data, emergency data are sending regularly	Simple transfer algorithm with threshold,
Backup:	Stored data defines the condition of the heartbeat		
End time Data Backup	Once backup	Data backup is one time at the end of the day or any processes	Less time consuming
Segmented Data Backup	Multiple data backup technique	Data backup is done when needed	Multiple copy Storage of data

2.1 Connectivity

Connectivity illustrates the strength process of maintaining various parts of a network to the others. Connectivity refers to the metric how all the parts of the network are connected [27]. We provide different types of connectivity used in the care of heart patients in Table 2.

Table 2. Classifying the features on different network types

Network types	Features
Wireless Wide Area Networks (WWAN)	Extends over a large area like cities or country 3G, 4G, GSM
Wireless Local Area Network (WLAN)	For a small area like a Home, School or University. It uses Radio waves signals. It follows IEEE 802.11standard
Wireless Metropolitan Area Network (WMAN)	It has range from 30 to 50 km. It is also known as Wima
Wireless Personal Area Network (WPAN)	It follows IEEE 802.15.1 for instance Bluetooth and IEEE 802.15.4 for instance ZigBee. They are suitable Power efficient, short ranging
Wireless Body Area Network (WBAN)	It follows IEEE 802.15.6

Most of the papers uses wireless medium to transfer the sensor data to the Smartphone [1–4]. Bluetooth has been the most reasonable one due to its cheaper installation cost, less hardware, and high compatibility [4]. That's why; substantial research work has been done on developing Bluetooth integrated health care systems on different papers [16]. Further we can use the Ultra-Wideband (UWB) technology which can operates between 3.1 GHz to 10.6 GHz for certain short-range communication [26]. Ultra-Wide Band and WMTS (Wireless Medical Telemetry Service) are another technology that could be used for body monitoring system as they operate in low transmission power [17].

Table 3. Classification of connectivity with their range, bandwidth

	MICS	WMTS	IEEE 802.15 .6 (UWB)	IEEE 802.15.4 (ZIGBEE)	IEEE 802.15.1 (BLUETOOTH)	802.11B/G (WLANS)
Frequency Band	402–405 MHz	608–1432 MHz	3–10 GHz	2.4 GHz	'2.4 GHz	2.4 GHz
Bandwidth	3 MHz	6 MHz	>500 MHz	1 MHz	1 MHz	20 MHz
Data Rate	19 or 76 kbps	76 kbps	850 kbps–20 Mbps	250 kbps (2.4 GHz)	721 kbps	>11 Mbps
Range	0–10 m	>100 m	1,2 m	0–10 m	10,100 m	0–100 m

The Table 3 clearly describes the bandwidth, data rate in general. According to the different papers most of them used 3G networks to communicate [31]. Although, 3G speeds rise up over time, 4G speeds is mostly constant fast from beginning to the end of download. In real scenario 4G is ten time faster than 3G. 4G technology is slowly replacing 3G in regional area [20]. The Table 4 describes the cellular network for remote areas. The cloud environment [2, 28] allows medical staff to visualize and analyze the patient's data. This environment [19] helps to identify and raise alerts when the patients require urgent observations.

Table 4. Classification of main factor Connectivity

Connectivity	Technique/Device used	Strength of connectivity	Limitations
Bluetooth	A Smartphone, and wearable wireless sensors connected	Cheaper installation cost, less hardware, and high compatibility	It is only for short ranges
Ultra-Wideband (UWB)	Wearable sensors are connected with Smartphone using high speed	operates between 3.1 GHz to 10.6 GHz for certain short range, operate in low transmission power	It should be integrated in both systems
Cellular Network	Smartphone is connected with the health center	The connection is easily available in remote areas	May have low bandwidth
Wi-Fi (WAN)	Smartphone is connected with the health center	Speed is significantly more than the cellular network. It is mostly applicable for the real time monitoring	The network traffic may occur

2.2 Scheduling Basis

The collected data from the sensors are classified on the priority and non-priority based. The data can be compressed using compressing techniques. Also, the filtering technique is another part of the scheduling techniques. Network coding based dynamic retransmit/rebroadcast decision control (NC-DRDC) [5] algorithm improves throughput by an average of more than 2.25 times and reduces network traffic by 27.8% than existing network coded communication. Gundogdu and Calhan, (2016) describes the priority basis transmission of the data from the connector node [20]. Non-preemptive priority queue model is used in this analysis [23]. In this paper we analyzed a signal driven approach as it can transfer faster in low bandwidth. We are also explain filtering method technique with this priority method for best accuracy.

2.3 Data Backup

Heart patient data are very important to backup as the stored data defines the condition of the heartbeat. The logs of the heart-beat record help to the doctor to analyze and refer for further treatment process. The medical care givers can maintain independence to data, and the data will give continuous feedback for handling heart patients. We further divided the backup policy into segmented backup and one-time backup. The backup through the network should be done with the help of a gateway app in the normal form having end-to-end encryption for security and also another appropriate solution for data security is blockchain [29]. The data can be stored in different databases according to the category. This type of backup used to all the patients whose data are normal [25]. This backup saves time for both health care givers and patients.

As classified in the above Table 5, most of the papers, Connectivity is done through the Bluetooth from sensors to the Smartphone of the heart patients. After that some are using Cellular networks, and some are using Wi-Fi network to connect with the health centers.

Table 5. Classification and analysis based on the three main factors: Connectivity, Schedule and Backup

Ref	Type of patients	Vital signs	Network connectivity	Schedule basis	Data backup	Technique used
			Bluetooth 3G/4G, Wifi	PS /NPS	1B/SB	
(Kakria et al. 2015)	Cardiac	HR	Bluetooth, WiFi, 3G	PS	SB	Android listening port
(Wang et al. 2016)	General	ECG	Bluetooth, Zigbee	NPS	NA	Compressed Sensing (CS) Android App
(Gundogdu and Calhan 2016)	Heart	ECG, heart sound, temperature	3G, Wifi, Bluetooth	PS	SB	Time Division Multiple Access (TDMA), Riverbed Modeler
(Tadi et al. (2016)	Heart	ECG, SCG	NA	NPS	1B	Hilbert transform tri-axial microelectromechanical accelerometer
(H. Lee et al. 2017)	Cardiac	HR	Bluetooth, Wifi	NA	NA	Wearable cardiac sensor (WiSP), Holter monitor
(Sahoo et al. 2017)	Heart	ECG, SCG	Bluetooth, Wifi	PS	1B	Data Acquisition Module, Warning System
(Golzar 2017)	Cardiac	ECG, HR	Bluetooth	PS	SB	Amplifier, Filter

(continued)

Table 5. (*continued*)

Ref	Type of patients	Vital signs	Network connectivity	Schedule basis	Data backup	Technique used
			Bluetooth 3G/4G, Wifi	PS /NPS	1B/SB	
(Dosinas et al. 2017)	General	HR, temperature, Pressure	Bluetooth, GPRS	NPS	SB	Data transmission unit (DTU), Filtering
(Baig et al. 2017)	Chronic, Ageing	HR, temperature, Pressure	Bluetooth, Wifi	PS	SB	Wearable Patient Monitoring (WPM)
(Crema et al. 2017)	General	Electrocardiogram (ECG), respiratory rate	Bluetooth, Wifi Internet	PS	SB	Bodyguardian (BG) Heart Monitor, Dedicated Smartphone
(Aloi et al. 2017)	Heart and Others	HR	Zigbee, Bluetooth, Ant +,NFC, Wifi	NA	NA	Interoperability, Smartphone-centric Computing, Smart Object
(Jay Mourya 2017)	Heart	HR, Temperature	Bluetooth, Wifi	PS	SB	AVR ATMMega32 IC, crystal oscillator
(Fajingbesi et al. 2017)	Heart	BP, HR, Temperature	Bluetooth, Wifi	PS	SB	Geo-location feature, Fuzzy logic Server
(Lee SP et al. 2018)	General	HR	Bluetooth	NPS	1B	Dedicated Wearable Sensor for cardiac rehabilitation (DCRW)
(Leu et al. 2018)	General	ECG, HR, BP, and SpO2	Bluetooth, Wifi	NPS	SB	WBSN Healthcare cloud Multi-threading

Abbreviations:
3G: Third Generation; HR: Heart Rate; SCG: Seismocardiography; NA: Not Applicable; 1B: One-time backup,
4G: Fourth Generation; RR: Respiratory Rate; SpO2: Blood Oxygen Saturation; PS: Priority Scheduling; SB: Segmented Backup,
Wi-Fi: Wireless Fidelity; ECG: Electrocardiogram; WBAN: Wireless Body Area Network; NPS: Non-Priority Scheduling.

3 Validation and Evaluation

In most of the papers, Connectivity is done through the Bluetooth from sensors to the Smartphone of the heart patients. After that some are using Cellular network, and some are using Wi-Fi network to connect with the health centers. For many types of the connectivity, the Smartphone is main gateway to transfer and capable to classify the data as emergency or normal. After the Smartphone for not only act as a gateway to forward the signal but also to process some raw data into meaningful information. This system may compare the threshold of the particular vital parameters of the body to classify if there is any emergency situation or normal situation on body. Connectivity is the connection medium with the strength of data rate of the devices and wearable sensors. Different types of connectivity are available in the market, but we choose the

Bluetooth with low energy. Bluetooth has been the most reasonable one due to its cheaper installation cost, less hardware, and high compatibility. That's why; substantial research work has been done on developing Bluetooth integrated health care systems on different paper [16]. In this system evaluation we analyse Bluetooth connection between wearable sensors and Smartphone. Also, we preferred the cellular connectivity in the remote areas using the latest 4G technology to connect Smartphone with the health care giver. The 4G technology can upload the real data to the cloud environment too. The connectivity from the health center may use the Wi-Fi technology to connect with the database in the cloud environment. The speed of the network is significantly more than the cellular network. It is applicable for the real time monitoring. Another factor to be considered is Scheduling technique for the accuracy of the data of the heart patients. The scheduling-based algorithm is developed according to forward the emergency signal at priority. The data queuing technique is only activated after finalizing the data classification and filtering to avoid noise. Thus, we recommended the threshold technique with the filtering technique to forward the real data of the heart patient. At first the data is compared with the threshold given in the system. The data then classified as the emergency data or normal data. After that the processed data are again passed through the filter where most of the noise is reduced to send the real data. This helps us to increase the accuracy in terms of data loss. The data is now calculated, and two red and orange signals are generated. The red signal denotes the emergency situation and the orange signal classify that significant change is occurred and should be checked by the health care giver. The Smartphone is able to forward the signals to the doctor and cloud respectively. The third factor we considered in the research is data backup for the reliability of the data. The data log of the heart patients defines the condition of the body. The patient can easily monitor for his regular checkup without visiting to the doctors. The continuous data backup helps to minimize the time-consuming process for the patient to visit the doctors.

In considering the most relevant factors of the CSB system, we also determined the co-factors which must be evaluated and validated to clarify whether there are any added benefits in using the system. We classify the differences between evaluation and validation in the following ways: evaluation clarifies the value of the system with its usefulness whereas validation proves that the right system was built with the accuracy of the system and techniques used in that system. In the given Table 6, we consider the components in the selected journals are validated or evaluated. This Table 6 summarizes these validations and evaluations with the technique used. Many of the papers described some area of validation or evaluations of their recommended systems. Most of the papers, they focused on validation in terms of accuracy. A number of papers are focused on the data transmission accuracy in terms of clean signal reached at the destinations. Also, some of the papers are considered in the techniques to send the clean signal and accuracy of the patient's scheduling technique of the system. The signal of the emergency patient data is important to transfer data with accuracy in the emergency situation of the heart patients.

Qualitative results showed that the threshold technique is used to classify the data. In [20] investigated the new traffic queuing model to classify the data from the sensors as their priority of the patients using Riverbed Modeller simulation and TDMA technique for the queuing of the data into three levels; emergency, on-demand and normal as their

Table 6. Validation and Evaluation

Ref	Type of patients	Vital signs	Technique used	Validation and evaluation	Study criteria	Results
(Kakria et al. 2015)	Cardiac	HR	Android listening port	Accuracy in wireless data transmission	Alarm detection technique	Decrease the transmission time by 22% than 3G
(Tadi et al. 2016)	Heart	ECG, SCG	Hilbert transform tri-axial accelerometer	Accuracy of the data	Heart beat interval measurement	
(Wang et al. 2016)	General	ECG	Compressed Sensing(CS) Android App, 1-bit Bernoulli	Data and Power efficiency	Data and Power efficiency of sensor is increased	22% increase in Data and Power efficiency of sensor
(Gundogdu and Calhan 2016)	Heart	ECG, heart sound, temperature	Time Division Multiple Access (TDMA), Riverbed Modeler	Classification of the data	Priority based signal	Red, Orange and green signal are generated
(Golzar 2017)	Cardiac	ECG, HR	Amplifier, Filter	Accuracy measurement	Decrease in delay time	An accuracy of 91.62% is from the wireless ECG system
(H. Lee et al. 2017)	General	HR	Dedicated Wearable Sensor for cardiac rehabilitation (DCRW)	Accurate HR measurements	Use of Multichannel photo sensors for HR measurements	Clean signal is generated
(Sahoo et al. 2017)	Heart	ECG, SCG	Data Acquisition Module, Warning System	Accuracy in early warning	Data Acquisition Module	88% accuracy and effectiveness
(Dosinas et al. 2017)	General	HR, temperature, Pressure	Data transmission unit (DTU), Filtering	Accuracy on the wearable equipments	Threshold measurements	Increase 1% accuracy in heart patients and 2% in respiration
(Baig et al. 2017)	Chronic, Ageing	HR, temperature, Pressure	Wearable Patient Monitoring (WPM)	Data filtering	Only instant data are forward	Decrease the traffic in the network
(Crema et al. 2017)	General	ECG, respiratory rate	Bodyguardian (BG) Heart Monitor, Dedicated Smartphone	Dual Computation by the Smartphone	Data Classification	Improve data accuracy by sending emergency data
(Aloi et al. 2017)	Heart and Others	HR	Interoperability, Smartphone-centric Computing, Smart Object	IoT Interoperability	Smartphone centric computing	Decrease the 75% CPU and memory utilization

(*continued*)

Table 6. *(continued)*

Ref	Type of patients	Vital signs	Technique used	Validation and evaluation	Study criteria	Results
(Jay Mourya 2017)	Heart	HR, Temperature	AVR ATMMega32 IC, crystal oscillator	Real time monitoring	Inbuilt microprocessor technique	Decreases in different sensors attachment
(Fajingbesi et al. 2017)	Heart	BP, HR, Temperature	Geo-location feature, Fuzzy logic Server	Accuracy on data transmission	Wrist localized Sensor	87% data transfer accuracy. Decrease
(Leu et al. 2018)	General	ECG, HR, BP, and SpO2	WBSN, Healthcare cloud Multi-threading	Accuracy in terms of the packet loss rate	Mobile Physiological Sensor System	Decrease packet loss of 2%
(S. P. Lee et al. 2018)	Cardiac	HR	Wearable cardiac sensor (WiSP), Holter monitor	Data transmission through	Encrypted cardiac data wirelessly to a cloud server	

priority compared to [22] Wearable Patient Monitoring (WPM) for the heart patients. So, the evaluation is needed to ensure the use in the real time monitoring of the heart patients.

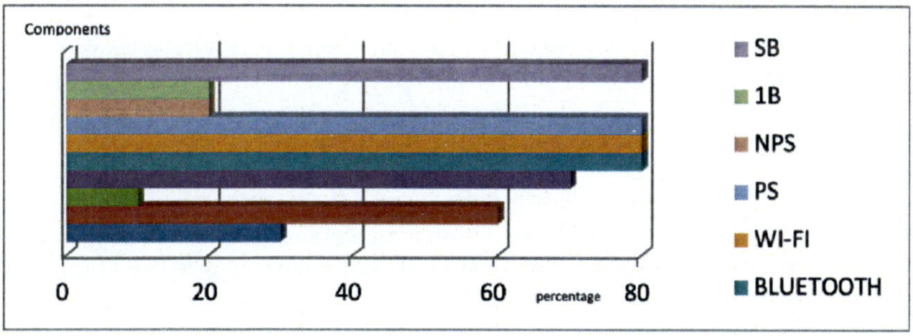

Fig. 2. Graph showing the percentage of components described in the selected publications.

For example, the connectivity terms Bluetooth is found in most papers that is 80% in total. The chart in Fig. 2 illustrates all the components used in the selected articles.

4 Conclusion

Remote health monitoring using IoT wearable sensors has emerged as a promising technology that can revolutionize healthcare delivery. The use of wearable sensors provides a convenient and cost-effective means of monitoring patients' vital signs and other health-related data in real-time. In this review paper we analyzed and compared real time health monitoring systems which are developed with suitable accuracy. This helps to connect the remote patients reliable by establishing the best network connection. The purpose of the study is to assess time-consuming process for the treatment of the heart patients and evaluates highlighted IoT health monitoring systems which are designed to help the patients who are far from the health center. Several studies have highlighted the potential of IoT wearable sensors to improve healthcare outcomes, particularly in the management of chronic diseases such as Cardiac. However, there are still some challenges that need to be addressed include issues related to data security, patient privacy, and data management. There is also a need to establish clear guidelines for the use of IoT wearable sensors and to ensure that healthcare providers are adequately trained in their use.

References

1. Mousavi, M., Rezazadeh, J., Sianaki, O.A.: Machine learning applications for fog computing in IoT: a survey. Int. J. Web Grid Serv. **17**(4) (2021)
2. Farhadian, F., Rezazadeh, J., Farahbakhsh, R., Sandrasegaran, K.: An efficient IoT cloud energy consumption based on genetic algorithm. Digit. Commun. Netw **150**, 1–8 (2019)
3. Rezazadeh, J., Moradi, M., Ismail, A.S., Dutkiewicz, E.: Superior path planning mechanism for mobile beacon-assisted localization in wireless sensor networks. IEEE Sens. J. **14**(9), 3052–3064, September 2014
4. Farrokhi, A., Rezazadeh, J., Farahbakhsh, R., Ayoade, J.: A decision tree-based smart fitness framework in IoT. SN Comput. Sci. **3**(1) (2022)
5. Prakash, R., Balaji Ganesh, A., Sivabalan, S.: Network coded cooperative communication in a real-time wireless hospital sensor network. J. Med. Syst. **41**(5), 1–14 (2017). https://doi.org/10.1007/s10916-017-0721-8
6. Kakria, P., Tripathi, N.K., Kitipawang, P.: A real-time health monitoring system for remote cardiac patients using smartphone and wearable sensors. Int. J. Telemed. Appl. 2015 (2015)
7. Leu, F., Ko, C., You, K.K.R., Ho, C.L.: A smartphone-based wearable sensor for monitoring real-time physiological data. Comput. Electr. Eng. **65**, 376–392 (2018)
8. Dosinas, A., et al.: Sensors and signal processing methods for a wearable physiological parameters monitoring system. Elektronika Ir Elektrotechnika **23**(5), 74–81 (2017)
9. Jafari Tadi, M., Lehtonen, E., Hurnanen, T., Koskinen, J., Eriksson,: A real-time approach for heart rate monitoring using a Hilbert transform in seismocardiograms. Physiol. Meas. **37**(11), 1885–1909 (2016)
10. Sahoo, P.K., Thakkar, H.K., Lee, M.Y.: A cardiac early warning system with multi channel SCG and ECG monitoring for mobile health. Sensors (Switzerland), **17**(4) (2017)
11. Liu, Y., Liu, A., Li, Y., Li, Z., Choi, Y., Sekiya, H., Li, J.: APMD: a fast data transmission protocol with reliability guarantee for pervasive sensing data communication. Pervasive Mobile Comput. **41**, 413–435 (2017)
12. Wang, Y., Doleschel, S., Wunderlich, R., Heinen, S.: Evaluation of digital compressed sensing for real-time wireless ECG system with bluetooth low energy. J. Med. Syst. **40**(7), 1–9 (2016). https://doi.org/10.1007/s10916-016-0526-1
13. Fajingbesi, F.E., Olanrewaju, R.F., Rasool Pampori, B., Khan, S., Yacoob, M.: Real time telemedical health care systems with wearable sensors. Asian J. Pharm. Res. Health Care **9**(3), 138 (2017)
14. Aloi, G., et al.: Enabling IoT interoperability through opportunistic smartphone-based mobile gateways. J. Netw. Comput. Appl. **81**, 74–84 (2017)
15. Crema, C., Depari, A., Flammini, A., Vezzoli, A., Bellagente, P.: Virtual respiratory rate sensors: an example of a smartphone-based integrated and multiparametric mHealth gateway. IEEE Trans. Instrum. Meas. **66**(9), 2456–2463 (2017)

16. Nag, A., Mukhopadhyay, S.C., Kosel, J.: Wearable flexible sensors: a review. IEEE Sens. J. (2017)
17. Arefin, Md.T., Haque, A.K.M.: Wireless body area network: an overview and various applications. J. Comput. Commun. **5**, 53–64, 17 May 2017
18. Rezazadeh, J., Moradi, M., Ismail, A.S.: Mobile wireless sensor networks overview. Int. J. Comput. Commun. Netw. **2**(1), 17–22 (2012)
19. Abawajy, J.H., Hassan, M.M.: Federated internet of things and cloud computing pervasive patient health monitoring system. IEEE Commun. Mag. **55**(1), 48–53 (2017)
20. Gündoğdu, K., Çalhan, A.: An implementation of wireless body area networks for improving priority data transmission delay. J. Med. Syst. **40**(3), 1–7 (2016). https://doi.org/10.1007/s10916-016-0443-3
21. Lee, H., Chung, H., Ko, H., Jeong, C., Noh, S.E., Kim, C., Lee, J.: Dedicated cardiac rehabilitation wearable sensor and its clinical potential. PLoS ONE **12**(10) (2017)
22. Baig, M.M., GholamHosseini, H., Moqeem, A.A., Mirza, F., Lindén, M.: A systematic review of wearable patient monitoring systems – current challenges and opportunities for clinical adoption. J. Med. Syst. **41**(7), 1–9 (2017). https://doi.org/10.1007/s10916-017-0760-1
23. Golzar, M., Fotouhi-Ghazvini, H., Zakeri, F.S.: Mobile cardiac health-care monitoring and notification with real time tachycardia and bradycardia arrhythmia detection. J. Med. Sig. Sens. **7**(4), 193–202 (2017)
24. Lee, S.P., et al.: Highly flexible, wearable, and disposable cardiac biosensors for remote and ambulatory monitoring. NPJ Dig. Med. **1**(1), 2 (2018)
25. Gogate, U., Marathe, M., Mourya, J., Mohan, N.: Android based health monitoring system for cardiac patients. Int. Res. J. Eng. Technol. (IRJET) **6**(8) (2017)
26. Fotros, M., Rezazadeh, J., Sianaki, O.A.: A survey on VANETs routing protocols for IoT intelligent transportation systems. In: Proceedings of the Workshops of the International Conference on Advanced Information Networking and Applications, pp. 1097–1115 (2020)
27. Rezazadeh, J., Moradi, M., Ismail, A.S.: Message - efficient localization in mobile wireless sensor networks. J. Commun. Comput. **9**(3) (2012)
28. Sahraei, S.H., Kashani, M.M., Rezazadeh, J., FarahBakhsh, R.: Efficient job scheduling in cloud computing based on genetic algorithm. Int. J. Commun. Netw. Distrib. Syst. **22**, 447–467 (2018)
29. Sharifinejad, M., Dorri, A., Rezazadeh, J.: BIS-A Blockchain-based Solution for the Insurance Industry in Smart Cities. arXiv 2020, arXiv:2001.05273 (2020)
30. Mozaffari, N., Rezazadeh, J., Farahbakhsh, R., Ayoade, J.A.: IoT-based activity recognition with machine learning from smartwatch. Int. J. Wirel. Mob. Netw. **12**, 15 (2020)
31. Fotros, M., Rezazadeh, J., Ayoade, J.: A timely VANET multi-hop routing method in IoT. In: 20th Parallel and Distributed Computing, Applications and Technologies, pp 19–24. IEEE (2019)

Taxonomy of AR to Visualize Laparoscopy During Abdominal Surgery

KC Ravi Bikram[1], Thair Al-Dala'in[2], Rami S. Alkhawaldeh[3](✉), Nada AlSallami[4], Oday Al-Jerew[5], and Shahad Ahmed[6]

[1] Study Group Australia, Sydney, Australia
Suad1941@yahoo.com.au
[2] Western Sydney University, Sydney, Australia
t.aldalain@city.westernsydney.edu.au
[3] Department of Computer Information Systems, The University of Jordan, Aqaba, Jordan
r.alkhawaldeh@ju.edu.jo
[4] Computer Science Department, Worcester State University, Worcester, MA, USA
[5] Asia Pacific International College, Parramatta, Australia
[6] Department of Computer Science, The University of Duhok, Duhok, KRG, Iraq

Abstract. The augmented reality (AR) is the latest technology in laparoscopy and minimally invasive surgery (MIS). This technology decreases post-operative pain, recovery time, difficulty rate, and infections. The main limitations of AR systems are system accuracy, the depth perception of organs, and real-time laparoscopy view. The aim of this work is to define the required components to implement an efficient AR visualization system. This work introduces Data, Visualization techniques, and View (DVV) classification system. The components of DVV should be considered and used as validation criteria for introducing any AR visualization system into the operating room. Well-designed DVV system can help the end user and surgeons with a clear view of anatomical details during abdominal surgery. This study validates the DVV taxonomy and considers system comparison, completeness, and acceptance as the primary criteria upon which the proposed DVV classification is based upon. This work also introduces a framework in which AR systems can be discussed, analyzed, validated and evaluated. State_of_the_art solutions are classified, evaluated, validated, and verified to describe how they worked in the domain of AR visualizing laparoscopy during abdominal surgery in the operating room. Finally, this paper states how the proposed system improves the system limitations.

Keywords: Augmented reality (AR) · Minimally invasive surgery (MIS) · laparoscopy · 3D image · classification · Operating Room (OR)

1 Introduction

AR visualization has become a promising technology in the medical field for surgical guidance, training, diagnosis and planning [1,13]. Introducing AR to

K. Daimi and A. Al Sadoon (Eds.): ICR 2023, LNNS 721, pp. 292–302, 2023.
https://doi.org/10.1007/978-3-031-35308-6_25

laparoscopic surgery proved to be a feasible solution to reduce intervention which causes loss of direct vision and tangible feedback on the spot for the surgeons. The main purpose of the technology is to help the surgeon eliminate most of the shortcomings of open surgery like proper depth perception, less operating time, real-time laparoscopic view and high-quality image during surgery [11]. This is typically achieved by proper registering pre-operative datasets like CT images, MRI, X-ray, etc. to intraoperative datasets and the patient in the operating room (OR) [16]. Due to the use of AR in image-guided surgery, and in pre and intra-operative surgical plans, the patient's anatomical representation and graphical models of the surgical instruments are localized in real-time which guides the surgeons during surgical procedures [2]. In abdominal surgery where non-rigidity of abdominal tissues and organs remains challenge, the AR visualization system provides the surgeon more extensive view beyond the visible anatomical surface of the patient thereby reducing patient's trauma and improving clinical outcomes. Thus, the researcher has to focus on DVV components of AR systems to achieve high-quality visualization during abdominal surgery that helps surgeons in operation room. Numerous AR systems and visualization techniques have been proposed but few systems are occasionally used for image-guided surgery and even fewer are developed for commercial use. Previous AR visualization classification and framework have usually focused on only one or two aspects of the visualization [14]. *The main purpose of this study is to introduce a framework in which the components of AR system can be discussed, analysed, validated and evaluated. It allows a better comparative understanding of the most relevant and important components and sub-components of this technology. It also shows how the system accuracy, image quality and real-time view can be improved in AR visualization systems.*

The remaining of this paper is organized as follows: The literature survey is given in Sect. 2. In Sect. 3, we have introduced the components of the DVV system. We evaluate and validate the DVV classification in Sect. 4 and Sect. 5 gives the discussion and explores the components which are not explained clearly in the chosen publications and point out future research efforts. Finally, conclusions are given in Sect. 6.

2 Literature Review

Bernhardt et al. [2] explained the primitive AR visualization technique used in laparoscopy during abdominal surgery known as surface rendering. The technique displays the surface representing the interfaces between two separate structures like lung/air or vessel/lumen using different methods like marching cubes, statistical atlases, geometrical priors and random forest. It helps to enhance the realism with a frame rate of 10 f/s or 25 f/s for continuous motion perception and ease interpretation of the surface with an average latency of 250m at that time. But it miserably fails to visualize complete surface reconstruction, invisible and inner critical structures, high resolution of the organs and tissues and could not produce a reliable result which affects the accuracy of the system.

Rowe, et al. [14] proposed a complex lighting model to produce the photorealistic image considering CT images, eliminating the shadowing effect. It helps to visualize complex anatomy and soft tissues during surgery differentiating the operative organs, vacuum and other organs in terms of opacity. But, the image quality was affected by noise interference reducing the efficiency of the system. Cheung et al. [5] proposed a new algorithm other than the primitive one known as the intraductal dye injection technique with an indocyanine green (ICG) fluorescence imaging system using a camera head to detect a bile leak and bile duct during the liver and adrenal gland surgeries. The proposed system reduces the complication rate to 15%, and survival and accuracy were increased to 90% but were time-consuming and cumbersome which fail to explain the distribution variation of covariates among individuals. Zhao, et al. [15] proposed 3D reconstruction algorithm for accurate and real-time measurement of intra-operative data into 3D geometric CAD model and 3D mesh patient model for clear visualization of the abdominal organs during surgery. The system recognized the deformation distance using the root mean square of the coordinates, spot detection higher than 0.99mm and image quality to 0.9 f/s, and finally increasing the accuracy of the system. But failed to increase image quality in overexposed areas or distortion of normal anatomy. Bourdel, et al. [3] explained the use of AR software to view a tumor in the kidney and uterus. The AR approach provides a clear orthographic projection of a tumor with high accuracy of resection with less difficulty level (0.87). Zou, et al. [17] proposed a spectral imaging technique using deformable modelling on the animal model. The system uses image detection to reduce the processing time and refreshment rate with high accuracy but they are not sure that the same output can be maintained if the system is applied to humans. Kenngott, et al. [17] proposed marker based visualization system using CT image registration on liver resection preventing blood clots using a hand port or trocar. The system helped for good visualization of the liver (2.8 mm) and bleeding point (minimal) from the CT image providing better tactile feedback. Ganni, et al. [9] proposed a markerless AR visualization system where the 2D operative image (CT images) obtained from angular movement by endoscope are superimposed on the 3D autostereoscopic image. The false discovery rate (0.04s), the relative distance between the operative organ(0.1mm), and the false negative rate (0.08s) were reduced, increasing the true positive rate (0.9s) and positive predictive value (0.85s) by the system. But the operative organ detection in bright light reduces the system efficiency. Chen, et al. [4] proposed a novel simultaneous localization and mapping algorithm (SLAM) based on all data stages (input datasets, analytical abstraction, visualization abstraction and view) and transformation operators (data transformation, visualization transformation and visualization mapping transformation) that maps data between all stages. The algorithm superimposed 2D intra-operative images (i.e. CT images and MRI) on the 3D autostereoscopic image considering tissue deformation without changing data structures at any stage of the process. Chen's algorithm helps in-depth perception and error variation using root mean square distance through coordinate points which is based on the surface area of operative abdominal organs. This method provides a good result; 90% accuracy in organ recognition and 0.1 mm RMSD, but real-time processing was high (0.6 s).

3 Proposed System Components

Based on our literature review and prior knowledge of the technology and domain, we believe in increasing system accuracy, giving a clear depth perception during the surgery, and having a real-time laparoscopy view. Therefore, first, we must find out what available data must be used in the surgery. Second, we must figure out how these related data can be effectively merged and visualized. Lastly, we must know how the analyzed data can be displayed. This information helps the end user in successful abdominal surgery. The main components of robust AR system for visualizing laparoscopy during abdominal surgery are data, visualization techniques and view. Table 1 summarizes the features of the selected research on three components.

Data: The purpose of using data as part of classification is to pinnacle the significance of determining which accessible data should be displayed to the end user. Different type of data is presented, but we considered only a few data classes to lessen viewer or end user confusion. Only the raw data obtained from the sensor or endoscopic camera or endoscope is considered which helps to produce the analyzed imaging data that combines with prior knowledge to form derived imaging data.

Majority of the paper describes the surface representation of the modality data. Kenngott et al. [12], Cheung et al. [5], and Bernhardth et al. [2] used a simple representation of the surfaces using CT images. Volume data were used in some of the systems like Rowe, et al. [14], Bourdel, et al. [3], and Ganni, et al. [9]. Image intensity is defined in all the paper that uses volumetric data which helped in processing speed and depth perception. Rowe, et al. [14] used a cinematic rendering technique and Bourdel, et al. [3] used AR software to calculate the image intensity. Whereas, Ganni, et al. [9] used 3D reconstruction algorithm, volumetric rendering, spectral imaging technique and motion tracking to determine the image quality of the data. Bernhardt et al. [2] and Christiansen et al., (2018) used both surface and volume models, whereas Zhao et al. [15] used 3D mesh patient model using mesh data and Zou, et al. [17] used point patient model to increase the image quality of the output. Bernhardt et al. [2], Bourdel, et al. [3], Bernhardth et al. [2], and Chen, et al. [4] described the visualisation of prior knowledge data that too in terms of tool depiction. Bernhardt et al. [2], Chen, et al. [4], and Zhao et al. [15] described the visualization of derived data. The image quality of the output is mostly determined by this data in these systems.

Visualization Techniques: The visualization techniques component highlights the proficiency of using the data to provide the foremost statistical information for a specific task at a given surgical step. The primary purpose of using visualization techniques as part of classification is to determine which techniques are used to analyse the data. With help of visualization techniques, the analyzed imaging data, derived data, and prior knowledge data are transformed into visually processed data that interact with the interaction tools of the view to give the output to the viewer using display devices.

Most visualization techniques have dealt with the visualisation of anatomical data. Recent papers have used 3D imaging techniques whereas intraoperative images are transformed into 3D models for the visualisation process. Bernhardt et al. [2] system described surface and volume rendering techniques. Bourdel, et al. [3], and Cheung et al. [5] described AR software as visualization techniques. Ganni, et al. [9], and Kenngott et al. [12] described different visualization techniques which are motion tracking, video-based techniques, marker-based algorithm, Monochrome channel filtering algorithm and spectral imaging techniques. However, chen, et al. [4] described a new markerless visualization technique known as simultaneous localization and mapping algorithm (SLAM) which helps in error variation and depth perception.

View: The main purpose of using the view as part of classification is to spotlight how the analyzed data are displayed to the end user through output media. The visually processed data that are obtained from the perception location like patients, real environment, display devices etc. interacts with interaction tools of the view to produce the output in display devices. The display device helps to give output to the end user with a clear view and high-quality images. Monitor, endoscope, monocular and laparoscope are used as 2D display; 3D glasses, augmented microscope and polarized glasses are used as binocular stereoscopic 3D display and as autostereoscopic 3D display; autostereoscopic lenticular LCD, 3D endoscope MATLAB and video display are also used, as shown in Fig. 1.

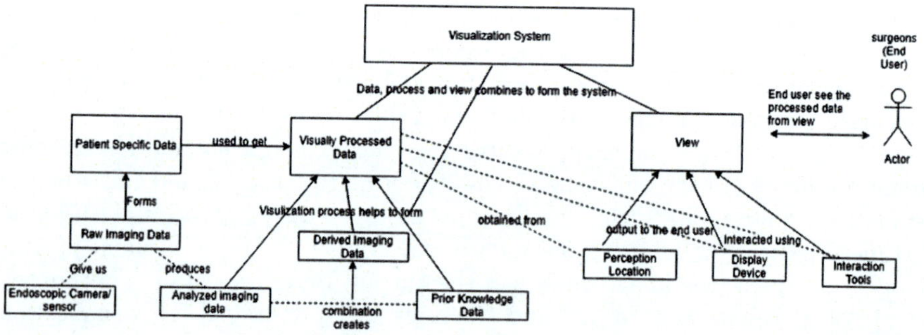

Fig. 1. The DVV classification (Data, visualization process and View), their classes and subclasses (solid-line arrow).

The perception location and display device were specified, whereas the interaction component has less attention from researcher. Kenngott et al. [12], Zou, et al. [17] and Chen, et al. [4] system perception location was patient whereas the remaining 20 paper system perception location was either the patient or a monitor. Bernhardt et al. [2] used an endoscopic camera or digital computer monitor as a display device whereas other paper system consists of a digital computer monitor as a display device. The scope of the interaction tools in the taxonomy is limited to hardware and virtual interaction tools. Some systems didn't specified interaction tool for the view like: Bernhardt, et al. [2], Bourdel et al. [3], Zhao, et al. [15], Cheung et al. [5], Zou, et al. [17], and Kenngott et al. [12] used marker position as interaction tools. However, Chen, et al. [4] used SLAM rendering to dense the surface mesh as the interaction tool.

4 Proposed System Components Evaluation and Validation

The accuracy of the system and depth perception of anatomical organs is proved by the validation and helps to build the right system, while evaluation provides usefulness and value of the system. Table 1 shows these validations and evaluations features.

The accuracy of the system was the focus of validation of most of the papers: Cheung et al. [5], Bourdel, et al. [3], Ganni, et al. [9] and Kenngott et al. [12]. Several papers looked at processing time (speed): Bernhardt et al. [2], Zou, et al. [17]. Few papers focused on the opacity of the system: Rowe, et al. [14] focused on sampling error. Bourdel, et al. [3], and Chen, et al. [4] evaluated and validated their system based upon the component with defined formula and compared those with others. Chen, et al. [4] used the whole system as the component and compared different factors of the output which would affect the accuracy of the system. Bourdel, et al. [3] described the accuracy of the system through segmentation and registration method. Bernhardt et al. [2], Zou, et al. [17], and Rowe, et al. [14] evaluated the system with the theory without any validation using the Vivo model describing the accuracy and processing speed of the system. Bernhardt et al. [2] evaluated all the visualization techniques used but didn't validate his claim in the paper. Another paper analysed the data in vivo model and draw the conclusion without validation. Zhao et al. [15], Ganni, et al. [9], and Kenngott, et al. [12] validated the accuracy of the system with help of phantom and animal models. To get the result as described they used camera movement without proper system evaluation same with the case of Bourdel, et al. [3] where validation of the system using the Vivo model was done in terms of accuracy without evaluation.

System Verification: Evaluation of the framework is the main task in the review report. Chen et al. [4] defined simultaneous localization and mapping (SLAM) algorithm for 3D reconstruction of anatomy structures using both quantitative and qualitative evaluation processes to assess the performance of the SLAM tracking error and quality of the proposed framework. Markerless model helps in increasing the visualization accuracy of abdominal organs. The 3D image construction is built based on the point cloud with the Poisson surface reconstruction algorithm. Bourdel, et al. [3] suggested that the classification can be

Table 1. DVV classification table of augmented reality visualization system

Author	Type of Surgery (Marker base or Marker less)	Domain	Data			Visualization Techniques	View			Component Validated or Evaluated	Study Criteria	Validation/Evaluation method and/or Data Set	Results
			Raw	A	Visually Processed		PL	DD	INT				
Bernhardt, et al. [2]	MB	N/S	MRI CT	S V	A: surface and volume model D: Image intensity, resolution & rigidity PK: Endoscope	Surface rendering & Volume rendering	P/M	EC/M	N/S	Whole system	Anatomical deformation, breathing and heartbeat and processing time.	Direct Measurement	Liver volume variation from 13% to 24%. Liver shift of 28mm whereas kidney shift of 46mm. Discrepancy rise to 44mm. Good frame rate (10fs or 25 for continuous motion perception). latency (up to 300ms or average 250 ms).
Rowe, et al. [14]	MB	Heart	CT	V	A: Volume rendered model D: image intensity PK: N/S	Cinematic rendering using complex lightning model	P/M	M	Transfer function	Image Detection	Opacity	Vivo Model	Clear view of left and right pulmonary arteries, branches of the main coronary artery and aortic arch.
Bourdel et al. [3]	ML	Uterus	MRI	V	A: 2D intraoperative image superimposed on endoscopic image D: recurrence rate PK: monocular laparoscope	AR software using dense structure from motion.	P/M	M	Multiple view using monocular laparoscope	Segmentation and Registration Method	Accuracy	Vivo Model	Laparoscopic myomectomy reaches 50% or more in 5 years. Accuracy is higher in AR group then control group and score difficulty level in between 0 to 4. 2.4 for control group and 0.87 for AR group.
Cheung et al. [5]	N/S	Liver	CT	S	A: monochromatic fluorescence imaging using near infrared light D: operation time PK: near infrared diode, camera and working port	Fluorescence imaging using indocyanine green (ICG)	P/M	M	Move and rotate camera head for multiple view	Image Registration Method	Accuracy	Vivo Model	Less complication rates (15%) and higher survival rates (95%) then open group surgery.
Kenngott et al. [12]	MB	N/S	CT	S	A: 2D CT images are superimposed on video camera images D: N/S PK: N/S	Marker based technique depending on ray casting model	P	M	Markers position determine the view.	Registration method	Accuracy	Phantom model and porcine model	Phantom model: N=10 84% visualization feasibility. 2.8 ± 2.7 mm 95th percentile= 6.7 mm Porcine model: N=5 79% visualization feasibility. 3.5 ± 3.0 mm 95th percentile= 9.5 mm
Zhao, et al. [15]	N/S	N/S	CT	ME	A: 3D mesh patient model D: image quality and effectiveness PK: N/S	3D printing algorithm	P/M	M	N/S	Whole System	Accuracy	Animal model	Root mean square of coordinates defer by 0.598mm. Point cloud coordinates at 60%.
Chen, et al. [4]	ML	N/S	CT	ME	A: 2D intra operative image superimposed on 3D autostereoscopic image D: error variation and depth perception PK: endoscopic camera and endoscope	Simultaneous localization and mapping algorithm using moving least squares	P	M	End user uses SLAM to dense surface mesh	Whole system	Accuracy	Phantom model	Low RMSD value that determines correct visualization of the surfaces.
Ganni, et al. [9]	MB	Gall Bladder	MRI CT	V	A: pre-operative and intra operative image are superimposed in endoscopic images D: scaling and tracking method PK: laparoscopic camera	Motion Tracking	P/M	M	Control view of laparoscopic camera.	Whole system	Accuracy	Phantom model	Clear discrimination between expert and novice performance with no extra instruments.
Zou, et al. [17]	N/S	N/S	CT	PO	A: volume render model. D: operating time PK: computer	Deformable modeling technique	P	M	N/S	Image Detection	Processing time (Speed)	Vivo Model	Less execution and calculation time and low refreshment rate.
Fucentese, et al. [8]	ML	knee	CT	V	A: 2D intra-operative image superimposed on 3D autostereoscopic image D: N/S PK: Computer	Motion Tracking	P/M	M	Move and rotate smart glasses for multiple view	3-dimensional of the ligaments	Accuracy	Direct Measurement	Smart glasses and integrated sensors improves the efficiency of a novel AR-based surgical guidance system
Golse, et al. [10]	ML	Liver	CT	ME	A: 3D mesh patient model D: image quality and effectiveness PK: N/S	green rendered mesh	P/M	M	RGB-D camera	non-rigid registration method	Accuracy	Vivo Model	The vivo AR tests achieved a fast and agile setup installation (<10 min) and ex vivo quantification demonstrated a 7.9 mm root mean square error for the registration of internal landmarks.
Collins, et al. [7]	ML	uterus	MRI CT	V	A: pre-operative and intra operative image are superimposed in endoscopic images D: scaling and tracking method PK: laparoscopic camera	Deformable modeling technique	P/M	EC/M	End user uses SLAM to dense surface mesh and Control view of laparoscopic camera.	Whole system	Accuracy Speed	Vivo Model	3D reconstruction and registration take around 10 min proposed approach for tracking is robust and responsive.
Giselle, et al. [6]	N/S	Myelomeningocele	MRI	S V	A: 3D mesh patient model D: image quality and effectiveness PK: smartphone and tablets	ray casting target object rendering	P	M	Screen capture using smartphone	Whole system	Accuracy Processing time	Direct Measurement	Developing a virtual model for planning fetoscopy repair for myelomeningocele carries out preoperative and postoperative procedures.

PL: Perception location, DD: Display device, INT: Interaction tool, N/S: Not specified, A: Analyzed data, D: Derived data, PK: Prior knowledge, S: Surface(s), V: Volume(s), P: Patient, M: Monitor, EC: Endoscopic camera, PO: Point(s), ME: Mesh(s), ML: Marker less Surgery, MB: MarkerbaseSurgery evaluated and validated using a "system acceptance" measure considering the accuracy of the system in terms of registration and segmentation method.

System Acceptance: To evaluate the DVV classification, We concentrated on the anatomical deformation and sampling error that either boost or reduce the system efficiency. The verification system was not a standard since most of the publications did not consider soft tissue deformation in anatomical deformation during pre-operative and intra-operative data. However, these methods used to find anatomical deformation and sampling error, while checking the accuracy of the system can be an effective way to judge the proposed system. The proposed system's accuracy depends on soft tissue deformation consideration as the registration process may fail due to anatomical deformation. To determine whether this method is acceptable to the user, we thus examined the significance of anatomical deformation and sampling error while making it feasible and reliable in specified publications.

System Completeness: For verifying the completeness of the proposed system, we analyzed the existence and non-existence of most fundamental components and subcomponents in state-of-the-art papers. Table 1 summarizes the components to determine the completeness of the system. For completeness of a system, all the components and subcomponents of DVV classification must be included that support the objectives of the system as shown in Fig. 2.

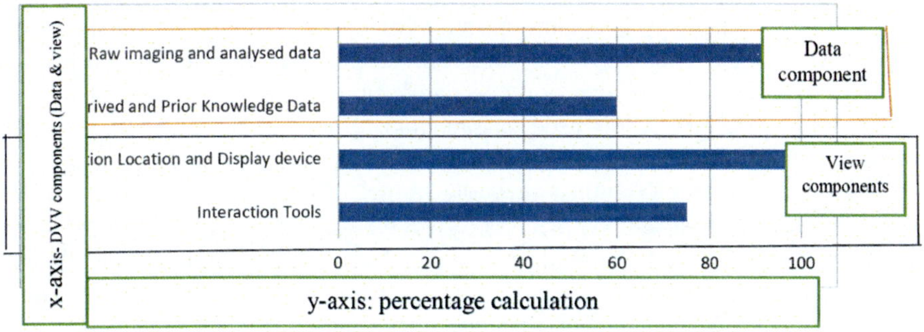

Fig. 2. Represent the percentage of sub factors of main DVV classification that has been described in the selected publications, the bar graph shows 100% and the sub factors which aren't explained in all the papers like derived data, prior knowledge data and interaction tool represents part in the bar graph.

System Comparision: To understand the grasp of the proposed system, we analyzed the components by comparing our paper to other works. The proposed classification can be compared with other recent classifications of similar topics, that is anatomical deformation, with proper evaluation and validation. However, the other works classified the system into data types, perception location and display device without interaction tools factors and evaluated the system on basis of anatomical deformation with direct measurement. According to Chen et al. [4], the system would be failed for initialization of the monocular images coordinates. If the surface coordinate datasets are wrongly initialized, then the accuracy of the system will be penalized. As the AR object can be placed anywhere on the patient's surface for correct depth perception, but if the endoscope moves rapidly it may cause a false reading of the analyzed intraoperative data or image. It just reduces the system accuracy and increases the sampling error. If the system fails to address the class or sub-class of the classification, then only the typology should be punished. *So, we believe that these limitations and failing criteria of previous papers must be the focus of current and future research, and these components and subclasses to be integral parts of the classification. Thus, each factor and sub-factors of our proposed system are specified in at least one publication.*

5 Discussion

The discussion is divided into three parts to focus more on each component as follows:

Data: Derived data helps in image intensity in most of the system and sometimes helps in processing time and depth perception. How surgical tools were visualized for navigation purposes is determined by the prior knowledge data. However, in a real surgical environment, sensors are used to track the location of a tool. These tools are visualized as surface and volume models which may be a problem for depth perception or soft tissue deformation cases. Chen, et al. [4] suggested a new algorithm to represent surgical tools which will improve rather than confuse the localization and navigation of the tools. All publications have described only the tools used for navigation but miserly fail to explain the system accuracy and surgery roadmaps on behalf of prior knowledge data. The surgical roadmap isn't explained properly in any of the papers. Chen, et al. [4] explained surgical roadmap as prior knowledge data in the paper describing the soft tissue deformation but couldn't explain clearly and validated their claims. All the common instances of derived data are explained in all the publications, but few works explored the visual representation of derived data.

Visualization Techniques: All chosen publications described different visualization techniques used in the AR visualization systems. Most of the papers described the complex light modelling method: Rowe, et al. [14] doesn't have a clear description for that modelling method. The transfer function stated by the author isn't evaluated or validated by other works. Image opacity obtained using the transfer function has a high sampling error which may be problematic, especially in our case where AR is being used.

View: All the publications had perception location and display device, but few only had interaction tools. Without analyzed data being interacted with the interaction tools, the result is obtained based on the theory. How the manipulated tools help to obtain the output is determined by the interaction tool of the view which isn't mentioned in most of the paper. Most of the paper failed to explain the interaction tools as explained in the above sections. Some papers considered hardware interaction tools neglecting virtual interaction tools and vice versa. Chen, et al. [4] considered both interaction tools to produce high accuracy of the system. The lack of prior knowledge and derived data and interaction tools in our classification suggested that shouldn't be considered in this type of data to classify the system. However, we believe that without the prior interaction tools, analyzed data can't be accurately visualized in the display device for the end user and the surgeon's expertise. Therefore, these components need further study for a proper AR visualization system.

6 Conclusion

AR visualization system is a great innovation in the medical field which overcomes the surgeon's limited visual view during surgical procedures. The development of AR visualization systems in image-guided surgery helped to reduce surgeons' limited visual field of view with 3D perception. We have described DVV classification based on data type, visualization techniques and view. This visualized data helps to interact with the user in terms of manipulation on screen as well as hardware device interaction. The nomenclature and proposed system in our diagram help to explain the main points of the AR visualization system. The DVV classification shows the classification, evaluation, validation, comparison and verification. The taxonomy was useful for finding the gap between current research and suggesting a new methodology for future study in the field. Our examination showed that few of the components of the system are evaluated, even fewer are validated and least are verified. Therefore, evaluation, validation and verification of the new system must eradicate the absence of such a system in clinical procedures and the operating room. We believed that DVV classification is useful for comparing, analyzing and consistently evaluating the system.

References

1. Barcali, E., Iadanza, E., Manetti, L., Francia, P., Nardi, C., Bocchi, L.: Augmented reality in surgery: a scoping review. Appl. Sci. **12**(14), 6890 (2022)
2. Bernhardt, S., Nicolau, S.A., Soler, L., Doignon, C.: The status of augmented reality in laparoscopic surgery as of 2016. Med. Image Anal. **37**, 66–90 (2017)
3. Bourdel, N., et al.: Use of augmented reality in laparoscopic gynecology to visualize myomas. Fertility Sterility **107**(3), 737–739 (2017)
4. Chen, L., Tang, W., John, N.W., Wan, T.R., Zhang, J.J.: Slam-based dense surface reconstruction in monocular minimally invasive surgery and its application to augmented reality. Comput. Methods Programs Biomed. **158**, 135–146 (2018)
5. Cheung, T.T., et al.: Pure laparoscopic hepatectomy with augmented reality-assisted indocyanine green fluorescence versus open hepatectomy for hepatocellular carcinoma with liver cirrhosis: a propensity analysis at a single center. Asian J. Endoscopic Surge **11**(2), 104–111 (2018)
6. Coelho, G., et al.: The potential applications of augmented reality in fetoscopic surgery for antenatal treatment of myelomeningocele. World Neurosurg. **159**, 27–32 (2022)

7. Collins, T., et al.: Augmented reality guided laparoscopic surgery of the uterus. IEEE Trans. Med. Imaging **40**(1), 371–380 (2021)
8. Fucentese, S.F., Koch, P.P.: A novel augmented reality-based surgical guidance system for total knee arthroplasty. Arch. Orthop. Trauma Surg. **141**(12), 2227–2233 (2021). https://doi.org/10.1007/s00402-021-04204-4
9. Ganni, S., Botden, S.M.B.I., Chmarra, M., Goossens, R.H.M., Jakimowicz, J.J.: A software-based tool for video motion tracking in the surgical skills assessment landscape. Surg. Endosc. **32**(6), 2994–2999 (2018). https://doi.org/10.1007/s00464-018-6023-5
10. Golse, N., Petit, A., Lewin, M., Vibert, E., Cotin, S.: Augmented reality during open liver surgery using a markerless non-rigid registration system. J. Gastrointest. Surg. **25**(3), 662–671 (2021)
11. Ivanov, V.M., et al.: Practical application of augmented/mixed reality technologies in surgery of abdominal cancer patients. J. Imaging **8**(7), 183 (2022)
12. Kenngott, H.G., et al.: Mobile, real-time, and point-of-care augmented reality is robust, accurate, and feasible: a prospective pilot study. Surg. Endosc. **32**(6), 2958–2967 (2018). https://doi.org/10.1007/s00464-018-6151-y
13. Kersten-Oertel, M., Jannin, P., Collins, D.L.: DVV: a taxonomy for mixed reality visualization in image guided surgery. IEEE Trans. Visual Comput. Graphics **18**(2), 332–352 (2011)
14. Rowe, S.P., Johnson, P.T., Fishman, E.K.: Cinematic rendering of cardiac CT volumetric data: principles and initial observations. J. Cardiovasc. Comput. Tomogr. **12**(1), 56–59 (2018)
15. Zhao, S., Zhang, W., Sheng, W., Zhao, X.: A frame of 3d printing data generation method extracted from CT data. Sens. Imaging **19**(1), 1–13 (2018)
16. Zhao, Z., et al.: Augmented reality technology in image-guided therapy: state-of-the-art review. Proc. Inst. Mech. Eng. Part H. J. Eng. Med. **235**(12), 1386–1398 (2021)
17. Zou, Y., Liu, P.X.: A high-resolution model for soft tissue deformation based on point primitives. Comput. Methods Programs Biomed. **148**, 113–121 (2017)

An XAI Integrated Identification System of White Blood Cell Type Using Variants of Vision Transformer

Shakib Mahmud Dipto[1], Md Tanzim Reza[1], Md Nowroz Junaed Rahman[1], Mohammad Zavid Parvez[2,3,4,5](✉), Prabal Datta Barua[6,7,8], and Subrata Chakraborty[7]

[1] Department of Computer Science and Engineering, BRAC University, Dhaka, Bangladesh

[2] Information Technology, APIC, Melbourne, Australia
zavidparvez@gmail.com

[3] Information Technology, Torrens University, Melbourne, Australia

[4] Peter Faber Business School, Australian Catholic University, Melbourne, Australia

[5] School of Computing, Mathematics, and Engineering, Charles Sturt University, NSW, Australia

[6] School of Business (Information System), University of Southern Queensland, Darling Heights, QLD 4350, Australia
prabal.barua@usq.edu.au

[7] School of Science and Technology, Faculty of Science, Agriculture, Business and Law, University of New England, Armidale, NSW 2351, Australia
subrata.chakraborty@une.edu.au

[8] Cogninet Australia Pty Ltd., Level 5, 29-35 Bellevue Street, Surry Hills, NSW 2010, Australia

Abstract. White Blood Cells (WBCs) serve as one of the primary defense mechanisms against various diseases. Therefore, in order to detect blood cancer as well as many other disorders, routine WBC monitoring may be necessary. Numerous studies have proposed automated 4 types of WBC detection through Machine Learning and Deep Learning based solutions. However, transformers based applications, which primarily originated from the field of Natural Language Processing, are very scarce. Our proposed study showcases the applications of Vision Transformers (VTs) for WBC type identification. Firstly, a pre-augmented dataset of nearly 12,500 images was taken. Afterward, two variants of VTs were trained and evaluated on the dataset. Our analysis revealed that the accuracy for all the models ranged from 83% to 85%, making the performance of the VTs equivalent to that of the standard Deep Learning models. Meanwhile, VTs have demonstrated significantly faster learning symptoms during the training phase, which can be useful when one wants to maximize learning through fewer epochs, for example, in a federated learning environment. Finally, the application of Explainable AI (XAI) was visualized on the VTs using Gradient-weighted Class Activation Mapping (GradCam).

Keywords: Vision Transformer · GradCam · Blood Cell · White Blood Cell · Transformer · Eosinophil · Neutrophil · Lymphocyte · Monocyte

K. Daimi and A. Al Sadoon (Eds.): ICR 2023, LNNS 721, pp. 303–315, 2023.
https://doi.org/10.1007/978-3-031-35308-6_26

1 Introduction

Blood cells hold a great deal of significance for the health of the body because they make up the majority of the human physique. Red blood cells (RBCs), white blood cells (WBCs), and platelets are the three main types of blood cells that circulate throughout the body's many organs. These cell types are distinct in terms of their purposes and functionalities. For instance, RBCs carry oxygen to various parts of the body, platelets help to stop bleeding, and WBCs act as a defense mechanism against diseases. Since an irregular distribution of the WBC elements can cause disruption in bodily functions, a thorough inspection of the WBC components is essential because they ensure the welfare of health. Our proposed study is based on the automated inspection of four types of WBC types; namely Eosinophil, Neutrophil, Lymphocyte, and Monocyte. The majority of earlier studies illustrated the automation process using machine learning (ML) and deep learning (DL) methods. However, transformers-based approaches, which are primarily from the domains of Natural Language Processing and relatively new in the subject of computer vision, have received very little to no research.

The proposed study demonstrates the application of two alternative variants of Vision Transformers (VTs), one is the standard version while the other one includes a locality self-attention mechanism, which allegedly helps to provide better performance on small datasets [1]. In addition, by integrating Explainable AI (XAI) leveraging Gradcam [2], the study attempts to display the interpretation of the transformers. The research questions that this partucular experiment tries to address are:

- Is the performance of the VTs on par with that of standard CNNs in terms of WBC classification?
- Can specialized VTs created for training on smaller datasets perform better than regular VTs, which are known to perform well on large datasets?
- Can XAI frameworks for transformers, such as GradCam, perform accurate saliency mapping?

These are the research questions we have addressed through the empirical analysis provided in the paper. Meanwhile, the proposed study's main contributions include:

- Demonstration of the usefulness of VTs compared to popular Convolutional Neural Network (CNN) methods in automated WBC identification. As per the authors' knowledge, there haven't been many studies on this topic.
- A comparison of the effectiveness of conventional VTs with self-attention-based VTs
- Utilization of Gradcam to demonstrate the understandability of the transformers based approaches

The paper is broken down into five principal sections. The review of literature is discussed in chapter two after this introductory chapter. The exposition of the proposed model, the analysis of the results, and the conclusion are covered in detail in sections three, four, and five respectively.

2 Literature Review

Computer vision related research on blood cells covers a wide range of topics, including disease identification and subcellular element detection. Although the utilized tools and methodologies also vary widely, most of them could be generally grouped as Machine Learning (ML) and Deep Learning (DL) based studies. This particular section provides some insight into some of these earlier works and methodologies.

Speaking of general ML based studies, Habibzadeh et al. proposed in their work to apply Dual-Tree Complex Wavelet Transformation to extract wavelet based features [3]. Support Vector Machine (SVM) was then applied to the reduced feature set to identify several types of white blood cells using shape, intensity, and texture data. Even with poor-quality samples, the method produced considerably accurate results. Meanwhile, to carry out feature selection, Gupta et al. recommended utilizing the Optimized Binary Bat algorithm, an evolutionary algorithm that is an enhanced version of the original Bat algorithm [4]. The authors of this study achieved very high accuracy by using algorithms like Logistic Regression, Decision Tree, KNN, and Random Forest on the chosen features. In another work, Benomar et al. concentrated on offering a system for differentiating WBC counts [5]. In this work, WBCs were identified using a noble color transformation technique. Afterward, utilizing color, texture, and morphological traits, the nucleus and cytoplasm of WBCs were segmented using the controlled watershed algorithm and then classified using the Random Forest algorithm. As we can see, the ML-based approaches generally consist of utilizing two subsequent methods, one for feature extraction and the other for deriving the results based on the extracted features.

The DL based research simplifies the process of feature extraction by automating it, making it popular for research and deployment. Cheque et al. presented an approach of using the Faster R-CNN network along with two parallel Convolutional Neural Networks (CNNs) to classify white blood cells [6]. In this method, mononuclear and polymorphonuclear WBCs were initially separated into two groups using Faster R-CNN. Following the aforementioned procedures, the dataset was divided into two cell groups. For each of the groups, two MobileNet architecture based CNNs leveraging transfer learning were developed and applied for classification. An interesting technique was proposed by Liang et al., where they used a combination of pre-trained CNN with Recurrent Neural Network (RNN) to classify Blood Cell Images [7]. They fed the training data to both the pre-trained CNN and RNN. The resultant extracted feature was then put through a softmax layer to categorize various types of white blood cells. There are more DL-based works that leverage existing popular architectures such as the utilization of VGGNet by Sahlol et al. [8], utilization of VGGNet, Inception V3, LeNet, and XeceptionNet by Sharma et al. [9], segmentation of WBCs using YOLO v3 by Praveen et al. [10], and so forth. There are also works that make use of custom CNN models. For instance, Akram and his co-researchers introduced a novel CNN architecture called multi-scale information fusion network (MIF-Net) for WBC segmentation [11]. They described this architecture as shallow in shape and it can combine internal along with external spatial information to enhance the segmentation process.

A few studies combined ML and DL-based methodologies to maximize their benefits in terms of WBC classification. In these scenarios, the DL component mostly comprises of CNNs that automatically extract features, which the ML classifiers then use for segmentation or classification. The work by Zhang et al. that combines adversarial residual networks with linear Support Vector Machine (SVM) [12] and the combination of AlexNet/GoogleNet with SVM by Cinar et al. [13] are some noteworthy ones.

As the reviews listed above demonstrate, Traditional ML and DL techniques dominate the field of WBC type detection from blood cell images. Transformers, which newly arrived in the realm of computer vision, have not been employed very often to categorize WBC types. The work by Choe et al. on the image transformer is one the most notable of the few works that were discovered [14]. In their work when Vision Transformer was pitted against ResNet in terms of WBC classification, it was able to outperform ResNet. There is also a dearth of research on the interpretability of the working procedures on WBC classification by these transformer based approaches. The lack of data on transformer based analysis combined with the recent domination of the approach in the field of computer vision has led us to research further on it, resulting in the proposed study.

3 Proposed Model

Taking input images, pre-processing, training the models, evaluation and comparison are the five main pillars of the proposed work. Initially, we trained the vision transformer models using the blood cell images. Afterward, necessary metrics were calculated and compared against the results of traditional DNN architecture. Given that our dataset is not particularly large, we opted for the VGGNet designs as traditional DNNs because they are simple to understand, extremely powerful, and better suited for small datasets than some of the deeper architectures. From the VGGNet family, the most popular two architectures, VGG16 and VGG19 were used. A quick introduction to the employed models is given in the following subsection.

3.1 Architecture Details

Vision Transformer [15]: The basic Vision Transformers (VTs) work by dividing images into small patches that are flattened. The flattened patches are next transformed into lower dimension embeddings, which are then sent through a transformer encoder. The encoded information is then passed through a Multilayer Perceptron (MLP) head consisting of numerous fully connected layers. This MLP based head helps to classify the images. In general, this architecture requires a large number of images for training from scratch. Fortunately, pretrained architectures are available which can be fine-tuned on smaller datasets.

Our version of VT is pre-trained on ImageNet-21k dataset, consisting of more than 14 million images. We took the model from Keras libraries, kept the default configurations except for the output layer to match the number of classes, and fined tuned on our small blood cell dataset.

Since the first iteration in 2020, VTs have gone through various modifications. One of these modifications incorporates the addition of Shifted Patch Tokenization (SFT) and Locality Self Attention (LSA) [16]. The incorporation of SFT and LSA makes the VT consider the local correlation between image pixels as opposed to regular VTs and hence, reduces the requirements for massive datasets. In our study, we experimented on both the regular VT and the SFT-LSA incorporated VT.

VGGNet [17]: Due to their popularity, power, and simplicity, VGG architectures are among the most widely used CNN architectures currently available. VGG architectures are a combination of convolution and max pool layers sequentially arranged, and the architectures are numbered based on the number of layers. The two most popular VGG variants, with 16 and 19 convolution layers, are VGG16 and VGG19 respectively. We have used these two architectures to provide a comparative performance analysis against the VTs.

3.2 Dataset Description

The blood cell image dataset consists of microscopic images of the blood tissues. The original dataset is hosted in Github [18]. Meanwhile, a pre-augmented variant is provided in Kaggle, resulting in close to 12,500 images after augmentation [19]. The augmented variant in Kaggle comes in train and test set only, we further created the validation set by splitting the test set and taking nearly 10% of images from it. The overall train-test-validation distribution is provided in Table 1.

Table 1. Dataset Train-Test-Validation Distribution

WBC Type	Train Distribution (No. of Images)	Validation Distribution (No. of Images)	Test Distribution (No. of Images)
Eosinophil	2497	66	557
Neutrophil	2499	62	562
Lymphocyte	2483	58	562
Monocyte	2478	58	562

Images from blood tissues spread out on slides were used to create the dataset. Therefore, RBCs, WBCs, and platelets are all represented in a single image. However, the WBCs can be clearly identified thanks to their distinctively large appearance and unique color. In Fig. 1, a few image samples are provided.

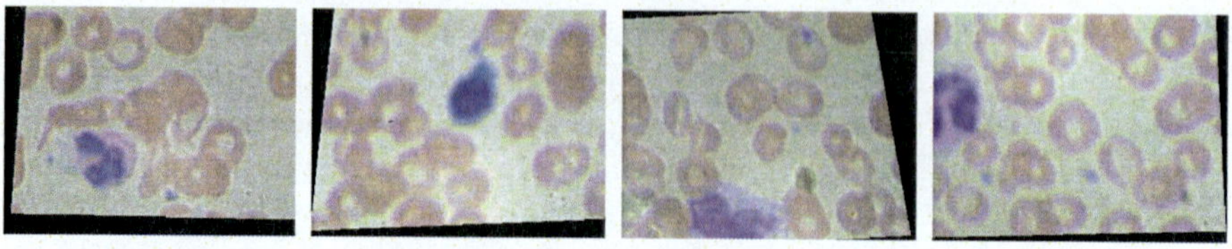

(a) Eosinophil (b) Lymphocyte (c) Monocyte (d) Neutrophil

Fig. 1. Sample images from the dataset

3.3 Model Description

The diagram in Fig. 2 gives a detailed summary of our study.

In our study, blood cell images were collected and preprocessed. The preprocessing steps include augmenting, scaling, and resizing the images. Initially, the input images were divided into three parts: training, testing, and validation sets. The train-test-validation distribution is done according to Table 1. Afterward, input images were passed through in 112×112 resolution and the preprocessing layer resized it up to 224×224 resolution. We normalized the pixel values within a range between 0–1, augmented the input images through horizontal flipping, zooming in between 20%, and rotating by 2% randomly. Afterward, the two variants of VTs were trained, validated, and tested on the corresponding data. Finally, an attempt to interpret the results has been made using GradCam.

Afterward, both the standard VT and the VT with SFT-LSA integration were applied to the input images. For each VT, the training simulation was run for 100 epochs, and the accuracy results, as well as precision, recall, F1 metrics, and other data, were extracted. Following that, the same metrics were extracted using 100 epochs of training on the VGG models. The retrieved metrics from all

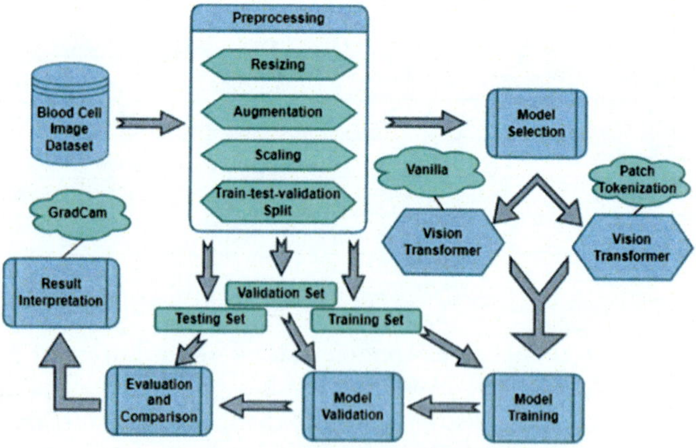

Fig. 2. Proposed Model

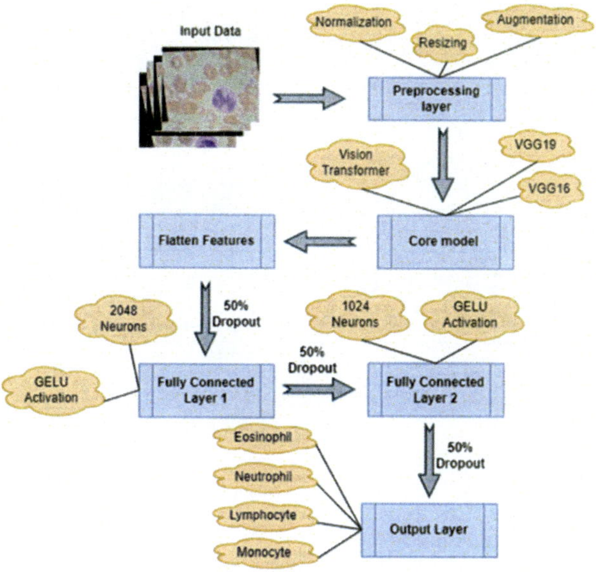

Fig. 3. Experimental Setup

the models were then examined and compared. For the fairness of comparison, we kept the experimental setups and the overall architectures of the models exactly the same. For our experiment, we performed analysis on a workstation consisting of a 3.9 GHz AMD Ryzen 9 5950X 16-core processor, 64 GB ram, and RTX 3090 24 GB. The overall model setups are provided in Fig. 3.

4 Result Analysis

50 epochs of training through vanilla VT and SFT-LSA incorporated VT show gradual improvement of training performance. As visible in Fig. 4, The validation loss reaches a plateau after around 15 epochs and no notable improvement was observed after that. The spikes in the validation loss curve are perhaps caused by the small validation set, where small variations in classification-misclassification scores caused big differences in terms of scores.

Overall, in terms of training performance, the two variants of VT show very few differences. Rather, we noticed the SFT-LSA incorporated variant taking more time to train, approximately 10 s per epoch in contrast to the 8 s per epoch for the regular VT. Therefore, SFT-LSA incorporated VT did not serve any major advantage for our case.

Additionally, the confusion matrices generated by the VTs are provided in Fig. 5.

As noticeable in Fig. 5, the matrices generated by the two variants of VTs show quite similar patterns. Both the models struggle to classify Monocyte and

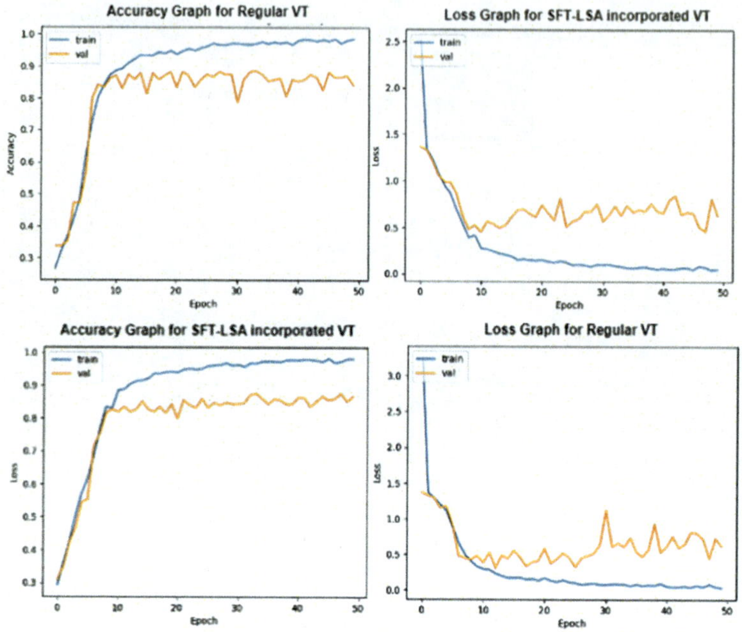

Fig. 4. Accuracy and loss graph for the two variants of VTs

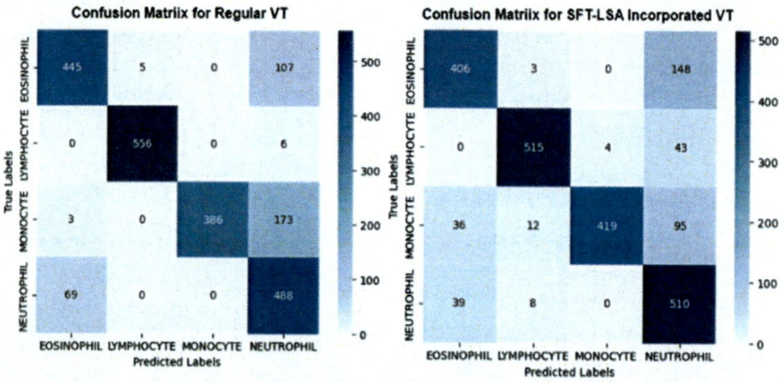

Fig. 5. Confusion matrices for the two variants of VTs

Eosinophil labeled images compared to the Lymphocyte and Neutrophil labeled images. A lot of Monocyte and Eosinophil images are classified as Neutrophils. As a result, it appears that the patterns of monocyte-eosinophil and monocyte-neutrophil pairings overlap. This circumstance is reflected in the results metrics generated by the VTs which are given in Fig. 6.

As we can see in Fig. 6, the recall score and the precision score for the labels Monocyte and Neutrophil are quite low respectively, showing the difficulty in Monocyte identification and high false positive for Neutrophil detection.

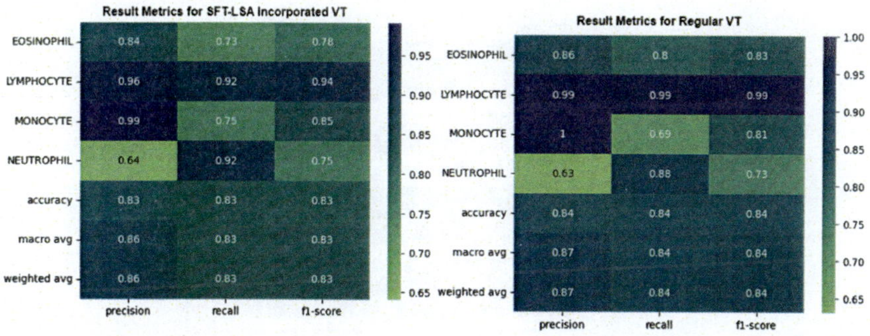

Fig. 6. Result metrics from the two variants of VTs

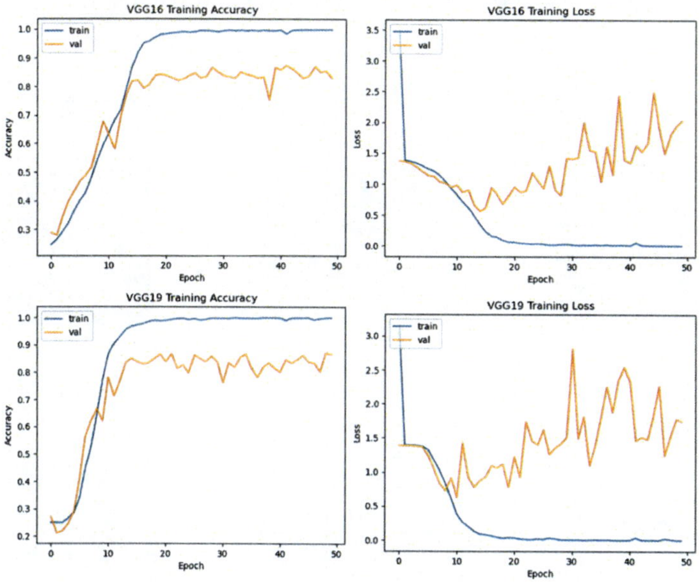

Fig. 7. Accuracy and loss graph for VGG16 and VGG19

Meanwhile, a comparison against the regular VGGNet models against VT shows similar performance in terms of min loss and max accuracy. However, as visible in Fig. 7, VGG models reach the max training plateau late compared to the VT models. The loss and accuracy fluctuation is also quite higher compared to what we can see in the training graphs of the VTs.

Finally, we analyzed the scores of the used architectures on the test set. For our trial case, VGG19 achieved the highest accuracy score of 85%, VGG16 scored the lowest of 82%, and both variants of the VTs scored in the middle.

The difference between the scores themselves, however, is very little and the order of performance may easily vary due to tumbling into different local maxima

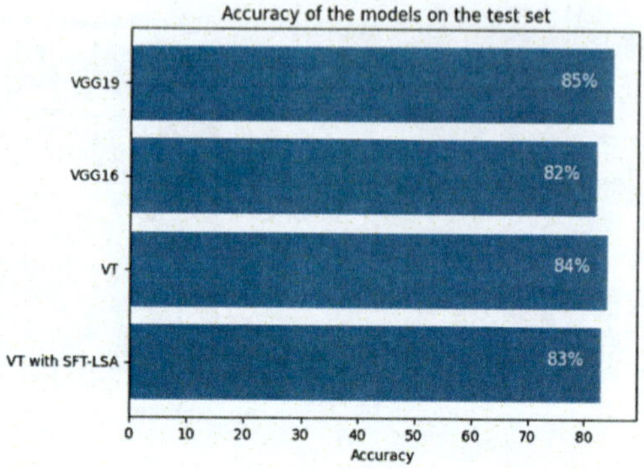

Fig. 8. Comparison of the performance on the test set

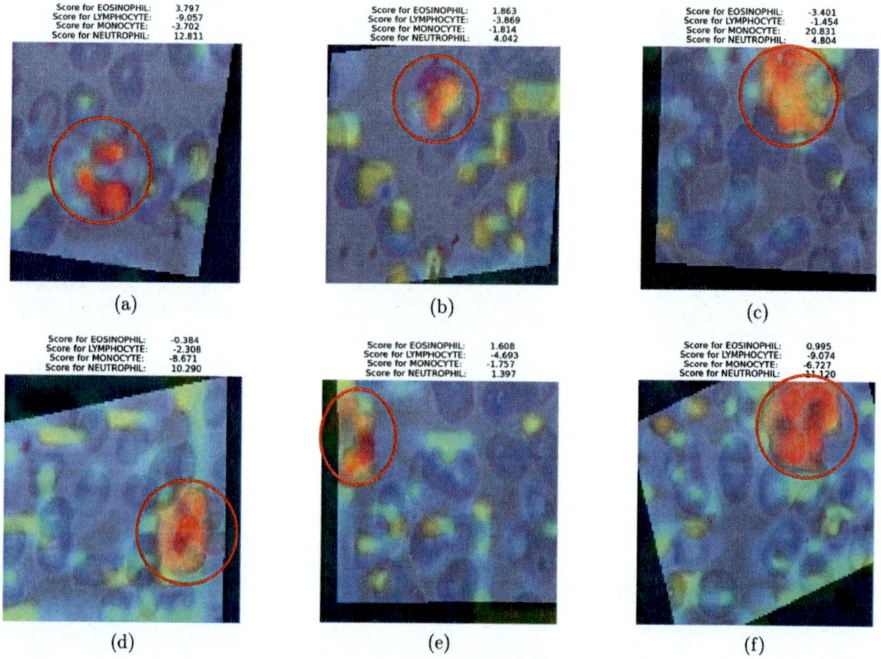

Fig. 9. GradCam activation maps for regular VT (Top) and SFT-LSA incorporated VT (Bottom)

at each trial case. Therefore, we can conclude that in terms of test results, all the models perform fairly close to each other.

Finally, we applied GradCam on the dataset in an attempt to visualize the attention map of the VTs. Some of the resultant maps from the correctly classified images are given in Fig. 9.

As visualized in Fig. 9, the gradient weighted class activation mapping for the transformers can be quite sparsely mapped throughout the images. There are still traces of correct activation mapping where the WBC gets highlighted but there are also sparsely distributed activation mapping around the platelets. Generally, this sparse distribution of attention maps is caused by the fact that the mapping only tells about the areas the network paid attention to, but not taking into account the areas that were actually used to make the final classification. Thus, resulting in sparse mapping all around the images. This can be improved by removing the lowest attention values using min fusion [20]. However, that particular implementation is outside of the scope of the current study. After all the analysis and evaluation, our overall findings are as follows:

- Even on a small dataset of 12,500 images, fined-tuned VTs performed quite competitively against regular CNNs. If the dataset was larger, the performance of VTs would have likely outperformed that of conventional CNNs due to the massive volume of data that VTs usually require
- Pre-trained VTs typically approach the maximum validation accuracy fairly quicker than regular CNNs, albeit having similar overall performance. The VTs converged on the validation set in only 9–10 epochs as opposed to 17–18 for the VGG models. When models have a limited number of learning iterations from a set of data, this rapid convergence might be extremely helpful. For instance, in a federated setting or during few-shot learning
- The SFT-LSA incorporated VT could not show better performance compared to the vanilla pre-trained VT, despite having slightly larger training time. Perhaps the dataset needed to be even smaller for proper utilization of the SFT-LSA incorporated VT
- GradCam results on VTs can be serviceable but sporadic. The GradCam results can be improved as suggested by other articles [20].

We have also arrived at the research problems' solutions thanks to these results. The research questions mainly involved the performance of the VTs and the results of the GradCam. As we can see, pre-trained VTs perform fairly well compared to regular CNNs. Meanwhile, GradCam can produce useful results despite its irregularity.

5 Conclusion

In conclusion, it is fair to state that VTs hold a lot of promise in the field of computer vision-based medical picture analysis. The application of VTs in image classification is still fairly new, with new variants being introduced on a regular basis. Our proposed study demonstrates that, despite VTs' inherent need for large amounts of data, fine-tuning a pre-trained VT can still yield decent results even on smaller datasets. There are also other variants of transformers that have proven to be performing better, swin transformers and Multi-axis vision transformers for instance. In general, our aim was to analyze the VTs to see how it performed against regular CNN, and we have successfully demonstrated it through our empirical analysis. In further work, we plan to apply the other variants of transformers to analyze their performance. In addition, we also wish to improve the performance of Explainable AI by modifying the process of activation mapping. The suggested improvements should provide a broader analysis of the application of transformers on WBC type classification.

References

1. Lee, S.H., Lee, S., Song, B.C.: Vision transformer for small-size datasets, arXiv preprint arXiv:2112.13492 (2021)
2. Selvaraju, R.R., Cogswell, M., Das, A., Vedantam, R., Parikh, D., Batra, D.: Grad-cam: visual explanations from deep networks via gradient-based localization. In: Proceedings of the IEEE International Conference on Computer Vision, pp. 618–626 (2017)
3. Habibzadeh, M., Krzyżak, A., Fevens, T.: Comparative study of shape, intensity and texture features and support vector machine for white blood cell classification. J. Theor. Appl. Comput. Sci. **7**(1), 20–35 (2013)
4. Gupta, D., Arora, J., Agrawal, U., Khanna, A., de Albuquerque, V.H.C.: Optimized Binary Bat algorithm for classification of white blood cells. Measurement **143**, 180–190 (2019)
5. Benomar, M.L., Chikh, A., Descombes, X., Benazzouz, M.: Multi-feature-based approach for white blood cells segmentation and classification in peripheral blood and bone marrow images. Int. J. Biomed. Eng. Technol. **35**(3), 223–241 (2021)
6. Cheuque, C., Querales, M., León, R., Salas, R., Torres, R.: An efficient multi-level convolutional neural network approach for white blood cells classification. Diagnostics **12**(2), 248 (2022)
7. Liang, G., Hong, H., Xie, W., Zheng, L.: Combining convolutional neural network with recursive neural network for blood cell image classification. IEEE Access **6**, 36188–36197 (2018)
8. Sahlol, A.T., Kollmannsberger, P., Ewees, A.A.: Efficient classification of white blood cell leukemia with improved swarm optimization of deep features. Sci. Rep. **10**(1), 2536 (2020)
9. Sharma, M., Bhave, A., Janghel, R.R.: White blood cell classification using convolutional neural network. Soft Comput. Signal Process.: Proc. ICSCSP **1**(2019), 135–143 (2018)
10. Praveen, N., Punn, N.S., Sonbhadra, S.K., Agarwal, S., Syafrullah, M., Adiyarta, K.: White blood cell subtype detection and classification. In: 2021 8th International Conference on Electrical Engineering, Computer Science and Informatics (EECSI), pp. 203–207 (2021)
11. Akram, N., et al.: Exploiting the multiscale information fusion capabilities for aiding the leukemia diagnosis through white blood cells segmentation. IEEE Access **10**, 48747–48760 (2022)
12. Zhang, C., et al.: Hybrid adversarial-discriminative network for leukocyte classification in leukemia. Med. Phys. **47**(8), 3732–3744 (2020)
13. Çınar, A., Tuncer, S.A.: Classification of lymphocytes, monocytes, eosinophils, and neutrophils on white blood cells using hybrid Alexnet-GoogleNet-SVM. SN Appl. Sci. **3**(4), 1–11 (2021). https://doi.org/10.1007/s42452-021-04485-9
14. Cho, P., Dash, S., Tsaris, A., Yoon, H.-J.: Image transformers for classifying acute lymphoblastic leukemia. In: Medical Imaging 2022: Computer-Aided Diagnosis, vol. 12033, pp. 633–639 (2022)

15. Dosovitskiy, A., et al.: An image is worth 16×16 words: transformers for image recognition at scale, arXiv preprint arXiv:2010.11929 (2020)
16. Lee, S.H., Lee, S., Song, B.C.: Vision transformer for small-size datasets, arXiv preprint arXiv:2112.13492 (2021)
17. Simonyan, K., Zisserman, A.: Very deep convolutional networks for large-scale image recognition, arXiv preprint arXiv:1409.1556 (2014)
18. BCCD Dataset. https://github.com/Shenggan/BCCD_Dataset. [Retrieved 14 Nov 2022]
19. Moony, P.: Blood Cell Images. https://www.kaggle.com/datasets/paultimothymooney/blood-cells. [Retrieved 14 Nov 2022]
20. jacobgil: Explainability for Vision Transformers. https://github.com/jacobgil/vit-explain. [Retrieved 15 Nov 2022]

Computer Science and Engineering Education

Data Management in Industry–Academia Joint Research: A Perspective of Conflicts and Coordination in Japan

Yuko Toda(✉) and Hodaka Nakanishi

Advanced Comprehensive Research Organization, Teikyo University, Tokyo, Japan
{y.toda,nakanishi}@med.teikyo-u.ac.jp

Abstract. This paper aimed to identify and organize issues that emerge due to interinstitutional differences when handling data in industry–academia collaborations. To achieve this, we interviewed personnel affiliated with companies that were conducting joint research with universities. The interviews revealed three main findings. First, issues related to data management can be classified into three types according to the differences in data creation and handling between collaborators. Second, the medical industry handles data using different methods from those employed by other industries. Third, given the expansion of data distribution opportunities, an increasing number of cases in industry–academia joint research cannot be handled under the conventional contract pattern. It is necessary to establish a new scheme for data management in industry-academia collaboration to cope with these issues.

Keywords: Data management · Industry–academia collaboration · Joint research · Data ownership · Data contract

1 Introduction

Data sharing is recognized as contributing to scientific development and innovation (National Research Council 1985; Roman et al. 2018) and is mentioned in the 2021's Science, Technology, and Innovation Basic Plan by Japanese government (Government of Japan 2021) as well. However, the practice of data sharing does not come without challenges, many of which emerge due to issues between stakeholders (Enders et al. 2021). In this context, collaborations such as industry–academia joint research often involve data sharing between companies and universities, which must therefore find ways to handle data together. To clarify the nature of this process, this study interviewed personnel affiliated with companies engaged in industry–academic joint research to identify and organize common issues that emerge due to interinstitutional differences.

The remainder of this paper is organized as follows: Sect. 2 provides a review of the literature on data management, focusing on industry–academia collaborations. Section 3 describes the employed interview methods, while Sect. 4 summarizes the results. Based on this, Sect. 5 organizes the identified issues and discusses future directions in data management. Finally, Sect. 6 provides a brief conclusion.

K. Daimi and A. Al Sadoon (Eds.): ICR 2023, LNNS 721, pp. 319–331, 2023.
https://doi.org/10.1007/978-3-031-35308-6_27

2 Literature Review

The effective use of research data has become an important issue, and multiple studies have shown that companies can use research data to enhance productivity (such as Bakhshi et al. 2014; Brynjolfsson and McElheran 2019). Data has a lifecycle which includes the stages of creation, utilization, storage, and annulment (Hitachi, n.d.) and companies can maximize the value of the data by managing them at each stage (IBM, n.d.).

Recently, industry-academia collaboration has been promoted with government support to achieve progress in innovation (O'Dwyer et al. 2022; Government of Japan 2021). However, the existence of different data handling approaches between companies and universities may create conflicts if the rights to the data are not clarified prior to the start of research activities (Northern Illinois University, n.d.). Some previous studies have investigated these occurrences. For example, a Finnish case study by Päällysaho et al. (2021) found a variety of issues related to data utilization at each stage of R&D, thus pointing out the importance of data ownership and sharing. However, conditions tend to vary depending on the national context. Japan's Ministry of Internal Affairs and Communications (2020) conducted a survey aimed at overall data utilization issues, reporting that many companies in the United States and Germany were aware of "data collection and management cost issues" in addition to problems with "distinction from personal data," but that a large percentage of companies in Japan did not see any problems, thus suggesting lagging data use. This is important, as problems will increasingly become apparent as use progresses.

Some scholars have suggested preemptive ways to resolve problems between industrial and academic institutions, including (1) the use of an intermediary organization to coordinate rights between parties (Perkmann 2015) and (2) consulting with researchers who will produce the data to clarify the nature of rights between the funding company and university at the beginning of the project (Northern Illinois University, n.d.). However, universities and companies may have widely different degrees of involvement during the data generation stage depending on the specifics of the project, which makes it difficult to clarify how rights will be held in advance. Many other issues are also highly possible, including discrepancies when calculating the value of the data. Despite their common emergence, few studies have examined these problems, and there is sufficient evidence on the situation in the field where data are actually generated. In this study, we addressed this gap by identifying and organizing a wide range of issues based on information obtained through interviews with personnel from relevant companies.

3 Methods

We took an inductive approach using the thematic analysis method, which is designed to decompose and organize qualitative data by tagging individual observational data with appropriate codes to facilitate the discovery of important themes. This method is highly suitable for identifying and clarifying issues in exploratory surveys. We chose this method because the purpose of this study is to identify issues industry-academia collaboration.

3.1 Subject of Analysis

As noted, this study identified and organized issues that emerged due to interinstitutional differences between companies and universities when handling data in industry–academia joint research. For this purpose, we visited and interviewed personnel at 16 companies that had conducted this type of collaboration (Table 1). At each location, we interviewed persons who were involved in the data handling process (e.g., positions that oversaw the research project or managed research contract work).

It is difficult to get specifics from the companies about how they handle the data, as none of them have made it public. Therefore, in selecting the subjects, we made direct requests to people at the companies with whom we have business relationships. Thus, there is a bias in terms of the type of industry. However, since this study is exploratory, we nevertheless employed this approach.

Table 1. Interviewee affiliations

Company	Industry
A	Manufacturing (construction materials)
B	Manufacturing (nursing care equipment)
C	Scientific research
D	Manufacturing (measuring instruments)
E	Telecommunications
F	Manufacturing (medical devices)
G	Manufacturing (drugs and medicines)
H	Manufacturing (medical devices)
I	Manufacturing (drugs and medicines)
J	Manufacturing (metals)
K	Manufacturing (food)
L	Manufacturing (medical devices)
M	Wholesale (medical devices)
N	Manufacturing (medical devices, drugs, and medicines)
O	Construction
P	Manufacturing (medical devices)

3.2 Interview Methods

This study utilized the semi-structured interview method. The study period lasted from August 2022 to February 2023, wherein each interview ranged from 60 to 120 min in duration (per company). After receiving verbal consent from the interviewees, we recorded these sessions using an IC recorder, then transcribed their statements.

3.3 Analysis Method

While reviewing the interview transcripts, we focused on the essence of each speaker's experience and narrative, then extracted parts of speech where they identified differences between industry and academia and/or any conflicts caused by those differences. Next, we performed a coding procedure on the extracted utterances to generate categories of related codes, which we reapplied to the company interviews for analysis. To ensure the validity of our interpretations, we returned to the data in the process of analysis and documentation to repeatedly examine the generated codes, category structure, and relationships between categories. Finally, we organized the categorized issues into "benefits" and "institutions."

3.4 Definition

We focused on the type of "data" defined for the purposes of this study as follows:

Data handled in the course of research for industry–academia collaboration activities, including data collected and generated as a result of the research and data provided by universities or companies for their own or joint industry–academia research activities.

In this context, handled data included experimental data, clinical data, observation and measurement data, simulation data, and clinical trial data, with attributes including numbers, images, waveforms, sounds, and text. The "industry–academia collaborative activities" for which these data were handled included joint research, contract research (including clinical research and clinical trials), and academic guidance.

4 Results

Our thematic analysis of the interview transcripts produced a total of 15 codes pertaining to issues with data handling in industry–academia collaboration activities. We organized these codes to generate seven categories, which could more broadly be positioned as "profitable factors" (four categories) and "institutional and rule factors" (three categories) (Table 2). The latter of these included differences in both the recognition of laws and regulations (e.g., the Personal Information Protection Law) and data storage rules and formats. Because these factors can be considered common issues at each organization, we decided not to include them in our analysis, which was more focused on issues that emerged due to differences in organizational objectives. Here, we discuss the interview results with a focus on profit factors that manifest differences in the character of organizations. Hereafter, we denote categories with brackets (i.e., []) and codes with quotations (i.e., "").

As shown in Table 2, profitable factors covered a total of four categories, including [Attribution], [Publication], [Cost], and [Information management]. These categories further included eight codes: "1. Commitment to data attribution," "2. Attribution of intermediate products," "3. Timing of data publication," "4. Availability of data publication," "5. How to value data," "6. How to treat the payment for the data," "7. Compensation for use of clinical trial data," and "8. Concerns about university information management." The following subsections provide categorical descriptions for each code.

Table 2. Created codes and categories

Codes	Categories	Factors
1. "Commitment to data attribution" 2. "Attribution of intermediate products"	Attribution	Profitable factors
3. "Timing of data publication" 4. "Availability of data publication"	Publication	
5. "How to value data" 6. "How to treat the payment for the data" 7. "Compensation for use of clinical trial data"	Cost (expense)	
8. "Concerns about university information management"	Information management	
9. "Different interpretations of personal information for data" 10. "Different interpretations of the scope of secondary use" 11. "Restrictions on the use of data due to lack of informed consent" 12. "Difficulty obtaining patient consent for data utilization" 13. "Request for anonymized processing by the hospital"	Personal information Protection law	Institutional and rule factors
14. "The need for data preservation"	Preservation	
15. "Data format varies depending on the institution from which it is obtained"	Data format	

4.1 Attribution

First, we combined the codes "1. Commitment to data attribution" and "2. Attribution of intermediate products" under the [Attribution] category.

(1) Code 1: "Commitment to data attribution."

Since data are inanimate objects, the correct legal interpretation is "right of use" rather than "right of ownership," but the term "attribution" is often used in industry–academia collaboration agreements. Indeed, the interviews produced statements indicating that industry and academia held particular views on "attribution." For example, one interviewee described a case in which a contract was concluded to attribute all deliverables to the university at their insistence. Thus, the data were not immediately available for use when needed at a later date, which hindered commercialization (Company H, a medical device manufacturer).

The corporate side is also concerned about the attribution of data rights. For example, the legal department at Company K, a food manufacturer, believed that the results of any contract research conducted by the university at the request of the company should belong to the company because it bore the research costs. Similarly, Company M, which incurred heavy cost burdens for a large number of clinical trials and research, naturally believed that the rights to the data belonged to the company, and thus concluded all contracts as such. At Company D, a measuring instrument manufacturer, the intellectual property department had concerns about the attribution of rights to research results as a matter of corporate policy, but the individual researchers did not have strong opinions on the matter.

- *All research results belonged to the university. Later, the data were needed as evidence for licensing applications, but it was not immediately available, making it a challenge to commercialize the project. (Company H)*
- *Sometimes it is agreed with the university that the data belong to the company that bears the cost. The legal department thought it would be strange if our company did not retain the clinical trial data, especially since the cost burden was so high, so we had a dispute with the university, but in the end the data belonged to our company. (Company K)*
- *Company management is cautious about attributing data and intellectual property. As a researcher, I am not particular about this, but I think it is unavoidable from the perspective of corporate management. (Company D)*

While some companies were particular about data attribution, many companies did not stipulate the issue of data handling in their contracts and could operate without any such disputes between field researchers. We also heard stories in which care was taken to avoid conflicts over data handling. Company N, a medical device manufacturer, which believed that it was important for both parties to maintain equal positions during joint research, was careful to avoid bias in contributions when generating data. In another approach, Company G, a pharmaceutical manufacturer, tried to avoid conflicts by determining whether researchers would assert their rights before starting any research.

(2) Code 2: "Attribution of intermediate products."

AI development research has rapidly expanded in recent years, with increasing popularity in industry–academia collaborations. Data handling issues have also arisen in this context. In one case, Company E, a telecommunication company, clarified that the rights to patient data (raw data) used to train AI models belonged to the donor university, thus prompting concerns over future issues regarding the attribution of intermediate products resulting from the model generation process.

Right now, we do not have the rights because the rights to the intermediate products belong to the university, but we think it depends on the case [of] whether the rights are needed or not. How far the company should have the rights is an issue for the future. (Company D)

4.2 Publication

Companies that seek profits by using research results as intellectual property and know-how may face major problems when universities intend to publish those results, particularly in terms of their intellectual assets and business strategies. For this reason, companies may wish to restrict universities from publishing the outcomes of industry–academia collaborations. Given the potential for this issue, we combined the codes "3. Timing of data publication" and "4. Availability of data publication" under the [Publication] category.

(1) Code 3: "Timing of data publication."

Structural information on compounds is extremely important for pharmaceutical companies. In fact, the timing of release affects their business strategies. For this reason, Company G, a pharmaceutical manufacturer, continuously tried to ensure that the timing of data release was driven by the company. While companies want to keep the structure of a compound as secret as possible, university faculty can use the same information to facilitate acceptance for scientific journal publication, which causes interparty conflict. We heard a similar story during the interview at Company N, a pharmaceutical and medical device manufacturer, which was coordinating with university researchers on the contents and timing so that the publication of their results would not become a business risk. However, neither company stopped papers from being published.

In other cases, companies were largely proactive about issues concerning the publication of results, although slight timing delays could occur due to intellectual property applications.

- *Pharmaceutical companies do not want to disclose the structural formula of the most important compound in the drug discovery process until the very end, so they ask researchers to delay the timing of their publication to accommodate the company's needs. (Company G)*
- *In most cases, the timing and content of publication are discussed with the researcher, as it is necessary to consider the balance between business risk and publication. However, the publication itself will not be stopped. (Company N)*

(2) Code 4: "Availability of data publication."

At Company I, a pharmaceutical manufacturer, there was a clear distinction between open and closed data. In preliminary meetings with researchers for joint research, both the contents and open/closed direction of the expected results were therefore communicated to university faculty for their approval. Even when generated data were supposed to remain private, both parties coordinated their interests in their release (e.g., passing on other compounds so that university researchers could publish their papers). However, the company had experienced issues in which the university refused to make the results publicly available. In one case, the interviewee pointed out the inflexibility of the university's contract administration staff, as they were unable to conclude a contract to open the results due to an injunction therefrom, even though they had agreed with the researcher to open all results in published papers.

We have a clear distinction between data that we want to keep closed and data that we want to keep open, so we talk to the doctor in advance, including [discussions on] the possible results. Some studies are designed to open the results, but the university may refuse to release the results. As a company, we knew that the research was not the kind that would generate intellectual property, but they stubbornly refused to let the faculty members freely publish the results because they might generate something that could be made into intellectual property. Even if we, as a company, think it is good to be open, we cannot be open if the university's administrative department is against it. (Company I)

4.3 Cost (Expense)

We combined the codes "5. How to value data," "6. How to treat the payment for the data," and "7. Compensation for use of clinical trial data" under the [Cost] category. In Japan, the general lack of experience with data transaction agreements means that there is no common understanding when determining the exact conditions. This leads to a range of interparty issues, both in calculating the value of data and choosing a transaction method.

(1) Code 5: "How to value data."

Company H, a medical device manufacturer, occasionally received offers from universities involving data provisions that exceeded their expectations. In such cases, the company believed that it was critical to check whether the costs and considerations were truly commensurate, thus avoiding violations of the Fair Trade Commission's Competition Code. As a standard practice, the company judged these considerations based on the academic teaching fee offered by each university; they comprehensively considered three aspects, including the amount of time and effort the researchers spent on the expected data, whether the doctor was a competent person, and the actual value and rarity of the data.

We tell our researchers to calculate the price based on how much [the] doctor's time and effort is involved. The basic concept of consideration is based on the amount of academic teaching fee indicated by the university, and we check comprehensively how much labor is involved, whether the doctor is prominent or not, and how much the data are worth. For example, he points out that it is questionable to pay millions of yen for an observational study where the doctor's hands are not involved at all and the data are simply taken from monitors. (Company H)

(2) Code 6: "How to treat the payment for the data".

Company H, a medical device manufacturer, experienced a gap in recognition with the university regarding the interpretation of data rights while negotiating the nature of compensation thereof. While the university argued that the data annotated by the physician constituted a copyrighted work, the company believed that mere data could not be considered as such under copyright law. Therefore, the compensation for the data was not a royalty payment for the use of copyright, but rather an expense (research expense) for the work of annotating the data with correct or incorrect judgments. Similarly, Companies O, a general constructor, and P, a medical device manufacturer, did not pay compensation for data they received from universities, but instead incurred a joint research expense. In another case, Company I, a pharmaceutical manufacturer, pointed out that the university did not have rules and systems in place to receive compensation for data.

We once asked a physician to make a judgment on the correctness of data output from our diagnostic equipment, and, at that time, there was a disagreement with the hospital regarding the interpretation of the rights of the data. The hospital administration argued that the data were copyrighted by the physician, but our legal department pointed out that the data were not intellectual property. It was pointed out that it was not correct to treat the payment for that data in the same way as an intellectual property license, and we discussed this internally. Since the company could not consider the data as a copyrighted work, we finally agreed to pay a research fee for the work to determine whether the data were correct or incorrect, and to allow our company to use the results of the research. (Company H)

(3) Code 7: "Compensation for the use of clinical trial data."

In addition to the costs of clinical trials and research, universities may ask companies to pay for the use of clinical trial data. One reason for this is the uniqueness of the medical field, where the practical application of research results is regulated by the Pharmaceutical Affairs Law. If planning to transfer technology in this field, it is first necessary to obtain a clinical proof of concept, which entails considerable cost and effort. This labor is carried out by the relevant university's Academic Research Organization (ARO), which makes significant contributions. However, university patent income is returned only to the inventors who contribute to the creation of inventions, and not to the AROs that contribute to technology transfers. However, several universities have created new compensation rules for both the use of company data and allocations to ARO organizations so that they will also receive compensation. On the other hand, Company L, a medical device manufacturer that was required to compensate for clinical trial data, expressed concern about the rule. They said that it caused a great deal of internal debate because companies have no basis for paying fees for the use of data that does not fall under copyright. Although the company eventually agreed to pay on the grounds of the university's rules, they felt that they had not received a satisfactory explanation.

A few years ago, we had a great deal of trouble with a university regarding its "Rules for Licensing the Use of Clinical Trial Results from Physician-Initiated Clinical Trials." Despite the fact that the data were obtained through a national project, the university demanded compensation for the use of the data on the grounds of its own regulations. There was an argument within the company as to why we should pay for the use of data that were neither patented nor copyrighted. If it is intellectual property, we can imagine the approximate sales from the intellectual property, and we can calculate the amount to be paid based on that. However, for data, it is difficult to calculate the cost because the company honestly does not know how much the data are worth at this point in time. The biggest challenge is that university regulations are made ahead of time without such a sense of market value, and the company is forced to pay with or without notice. (Company L)

4.4 Information management

Finally, we positioned the code "8. Concerns about university information management" under the [Information management] category.

(1) Code 8: "Concerns about university information management."

As mentioned for the [Publication] category, the leakage of technical and business information can lead to significant profit losses for the company as a whole. Companies H and L, both medical device manufacturers, pointed out concerns over the laxity of data (information) management at universities during their collaborations.

We have a procedure manual, we provide education, and we conduct an internal audit once a year. So, I think we are doing a pretty good job of managing personal information, but I don't think the university is going that far. I am not sure to what extent the university actually manages personal information and provides education, but I have a feeling that it probably does not go that far. (Company L)

5 Discussion

Based on our interview results, it is clear that both "how data are generated" and "the way data are generated" significantly impact data-handling procedures in the context of industry–academia joint research. As shown in Table 3, we categorized issues surrounding data management into three types depending on the data generation process.

Of those presented above, Type A pertains to issues affiliated with the [Publication] and [Information management] categories. In this context, our interviews revealed that companies and universities took different positions on data publication. Specifically, the former valued timing in terms of patent and business strategies, while the latter desired quick publication to promote the performance of research papers. Here, it is important to mention that only companies in the medical industry (e.g., Companies G, I, N, and H) expressed concerns related to [Publication] and [Information management]. One reason

Table 3. Data types and issues

Type	Definition and code assignment
Type A	The data are jointly produced by a university and company, often through collaborative research
	Issues: "3. Timing of data publication," "4. Availability of data publication," and "8. Concerns about university information management."
Type B	Data produced by the university are provided to the company upon the company's request. The research is mostly funded and clinical
	Issue: "1. Commitment to data attribution."
Type C	Existing data in universities are provided to companies, often for use in AI research and development
	Issues: "5. How to value data," "6. How to treat the payment for the data," "7. Compensation for use of clinical trial data," and "2. Attribution of intermediate products."

for this appears to be the importance of patents in the pharmaceutical industry, wherein a single patent right is much more likely to play an extremely important role. In this regard, patents directly related to products are basically substance patents, which pertain to the structural data of actual compounds; it is obvious that this type of data must be handled with great care. For pharmaceuticals, patent strategies require enormous development costs, time, and effort, making information management (e.g., data disclosure) a major issue. During the interviews, we did not hear cases in which any other industries adopted the same level of caution, indicating that the healthcare sector uses a unique data management process.

In Type B, the major issue was "commitment to attribution." In this context, the university produces data at the request of the company. Clinical research and trials also fall under this category. Since this type of effort is so-called "contracted work," there is a clear distinction between "the party bearing the costs" and "the party generating the data." Conflicts can easily arise when each side claims its own legitimacy in the right to take the initiative in data. In many cases, this type of data also has a clear purpose (e.g., being used by a company for various types of approval applications). In fact, Companies H and M, which appeared in the narrative of [Attribution], outsourced their data for pharmaceutical applications, while Company K outsourced its data to acquire information for applications related to food with specific functions. The main reasons for insisting on attribution seemed to be that companies desire to use the data freely and to properly manage and store the data in-house in order to fulfill the legal obligations associated with the application.

In contrast, Company O was not particular about attribution even for data used for regulatory applications. It has concluded an agreement that the data belongs to the university on the condition that the company has the necessary "right to use," and has been able to operate without problems. This suggests that it is not very meaningful to be concerned about the attribution of data that can simultaneously be used by multiple parties, as any related problems between industry and academia can be solved by setting appropriate use rights, as done by Company O.

In Type C, the main issue is [Consideration]. In this context, existing university data are provided to the company rather than generating new data. Therefore, it is necessary to evaluate the value of the data and calculate the price at the time the data transaction occurs. The difficulty of calculating the value of data due to unclear cost-effectiveness has already been pointed out. We also found that companies considered it difficult to calculate the value of data for the final product at the point of transaction.

One possible way to avoid the difficulty of calculating the value of data when acquiring it from universities is to adopt Type A over Type C. Although it is unclear whether companies intended this as a "workaround," we indeed found that data were often provided via Type A. If the data are provided as a resource for the university side when conducting joint research, this case can also be established as Type A; however, care is needed when calculating joint expenses. If a company desires valuable data that is difficult to obtain on its own, then Type C is expected to be priced commensurate with its value; again, care is needed when calculating joint expenses. However, if the data are incorporated into a joint research project, then their value may not be reflected in the joint expenses. Moreover, it is important to consider the cost of the labor (cost), especially in cases where the university customizes the data to meet the needs of the other party. Further, if Type A is adopted, then it is necessary to amend the conventional joint research agreement with a clause for a "data provision agreement." In addition to equivalent value, it is important to both set an appropriate data use period and stipulate the handling of any derived data. In the case of data that involve personal information (e.g., patient data), ethical considerations are also required (e.g., how to handle opt-outs in the case of commercialization). Overall, these factors show that new rules should be drafted to smooth the data-handling process between industry and academia. In addition, as noted above, we did not analyze institutional rule factors in this study, so future research should consider the impact of institutional rule aspects like GDPR.

6 Conclusion

This study identified and organized issues that emerged due to interinstitutional differences when handling data in industry–academia collaborations. Considering that the data dealt with in this paper were generated and provided by industry-academia collaboration activities, we can outline the results in three main points. First, issues on data can be classified into three types according to how they are created and handled between parties. Second, the medical industry uses substantially different data handling practices when compared to other industries. Third, given the expansion of data distribution opportunities, an increasing number of cases involving industry–academia collaborative research cannot be handled under the conventional contract pattern, suggesting the need for a new contract format.

In the future, it will be necessary to establish new contract templates that stipulate data use according to the actual nature of the data. This should be accompanied by a contract structure that address newly arising issues. Both provisions should be explored through continued research.

This study has several limitations. First, this study was restricted to 16 target firms, which limits the generalizability of the results. Second, there is a bias in the companies interviewed, i.e., many of them are in the medical industry, so the results do not accurately reflect the current state of industry-academia collaboration in Japan. Third, since this study deals with issues in Japan, different conclusions may be reached in countries with different institutions and practices. Finally, this study was conducted solely from the companies' perspective, and the opinions of university researchers and managers were not analyzed. In the future, we would like to conduct a broader analysis to address these points.

Acknowledgments. The research was supported by ROIS NII Open Collaborative Research 2022-22S0401, and JSPS Grants-in-Aid for Scientific Research, Grant Number JP22K01733.

References

Bakhshi, H., Bravo-Biosca, A., Mateos-Garcia, J.: The analytical firm: estimating the effect of data and online analytics on firm performance. In: Nesta Working Paper 14/05 (2014)

Brynjolfsson, E., McElheran, K.: Data in action: data-driven decision making and predictive analytics in U.S. manufacturing. In: Rotman School of Management Working Paper, No. 3422397 (2019)

Enders, T., Wolff, C., Kienzle, L.: Opening pandora's box? guiding organizations through selective open data revealing. In: PACIS 2021 Proceedings. 207 (2021). https://aisel.aisnet.org/pacis2021/207

Government of Japan: Science, Technology, and Innovation Basic Plan https://www8.cao.go.jp/cstp/english/sti_basic_plan.pdf. Accessed February 2023

Hitachi, Data lifecycle management. https://www.hitachi.com/rd/glossary/d/data_lifecycle_management.html. Accessed February 2023

IBM, Phases of data lifecycle management. https://www.ibm.com/topics/data-lifecycle-management. Accessed February 2023

Ministry of Internal Affairs and Communications, Information and Communications in Japan 2020. https://www.soumu.go.jp/johotsusintokei/whitepaper/ja/r02/pdf/n3200000.pdf. (in Japanese). Accessed February 2023

National Research Council: Sharing Research Data The National Academies Press: Washington. DC, USA (1985)

Northern Illinois University, Data Management. https://ori.hhs.gov/education/products/n_illinois_u/datamanagement/dmmain.html. Accessed February 2023

O'Dwyer, M., Filieri, R., O'Malley, L.:Establishing successful university–industry collaborations: barriers and enablers deconstructed. J. Technol. Transfer. (2022). https://doi.org/10.1007/s10961-022-09932-2

Päällysaho, S., et al.: Key aspects of open data in finish RDI cooperation between higher education and businesses. Data Intell. **3**(1), 176–188 (2021)

Perkmann, M., Schildt, H.: Open data partnerships between firms and universities: the role of boundary organizations. Res. Policy **44**(5), 1133–1143 (2015)

Roman, M., Liu, J., Nyberg, T.: Advancing the open science movement through sustainable business model development. Ind. High. Educ. **32**(4), 226–234 (2018)

Security Culture and Security Education, Training and Awareness (SETA) Influencing Information Security Management

Haneen Heyasat(✉), Sameera Mubarak, and Nina Evans

STEM, University of South Australia, Adelaide, Australia
Haneen.heyasat@mymail.unisa.edu.au, {sameera.mubarak, nina.evans}@unisa.edu.au

Abstract. Information security management (ISM) ensures the protection of organisations' data assets. Studying actual security events becomes more critical for ISM preparation. The Capital Market constitutes a wealth of data sources which react to various security incidents. ISM is an essential part of this industry due to high technology dependency. The previous literature emphasises the need for a holistic approach for ISM; therefore, there is necessary to investigate the current state of the ISM to develop a cybersecurity and ISM culture. Research should further explore the impact of national and organisational culture and its effects on ISM and explore ISM practices and initiatives that organisations implement to develop a security culture. This paper explores the factors in order to improve how employees' culture and IS awareness affect ISM implementation. A qualitative approach using the case study method was applied to understand the problem. Twenty-two semi-structured interviews were conducted in the Middle Eastern Capital Market. The thematic data analysis revealed that Middle Eastern culture is a dominant factor influencing ISM and the security culture and awareness significantly impact ISM. This suggests that organisations should focus on security culture and, even more, on IS awareness to improve ISM. This research identifies several challenges in current security practices in the Middle Eastern Capital Market industry, including the lack of attention to cultural effects, generic SETA programs that do not consider specific industry needs, and a lack of connection between culture and awareness programs.

Keywords: Information Security Management · Security Culture · Security Education · Security Awareness · Capital Market Industry

1 Introduction

Cybercrime is increasing and it takes longer to resolve attacks, with the result that security is becoming more costly for organisations. Effective information security management (ISM) is becoming an urgent need. This study addresses the weaknesses in security culture and awareness that can weaken and affect ISM within the Capital Market industry in the Middle East.

K. Daimi and A. Al Sadoon (Eds.): ICR 2023, LNNS 721, pp. 332–343, 2023.
https://doi.org/10.1007/978-3-031-35308-6_28

The Capital Market is an important industry that helps create the global market's liquidity. The Capital Market, the main industry for this research, is defined as 'A market where securities are bought and sold' [13]. In more detail, it is a '... market where buyers and sellers engage in the trade of financial securities, and these are undertaken by participants such as individuals and in institutions' [11].

The Middle Eastern region is an area of interest to IS cyberattacks because of its geostrategic location, with its land connecting Asia, Africa and Europe, the size of global investments and political disputes [4]. The Capital Market in the Middle East presents numerous unique challenges and opportunities that need effective ISM preparations [15]. Two regions in the Middle East have been chosen to be research case studies – the Near East region and the Arabian Gulf region.

Human behaviour is largely determined by culture, affecting interactions in the work environment. To improve information security (IS) it is important to understand the people's security culture and awareness as they play a significant role in creating risks and preventing security breaches. The relationship between security culture and awareness has received preliminary support; however, its interplay with organisational culture is yet to be empirically investigated [24]. Therefore, this study explored the relationship of security culture with security education, training and awareness (SETA) with ISM in the Middle Eastern Capital Market by answering the research question: How does security culture and awareness influence ISM in the Capital Market?

This research is unique for focusing on ISM in the Capital Market industry which is increasingly dependent on the internet and information systems. This research will provide practical recommendations for leaders and IT managers in the Capital Market to improve their business performance through proactive IS measures to mitigate security breach damages and address gaps in their security culture and awareness.

2 Related Work

Studies on IS culture and awareness have largely been carried out in developed Western countries. Middle Eastern countries are significantly different from developed Western countries in terms of culture, social attitudes, and government regulations. These differences lead to a different understanding of the importance of security [6]. There is a significant lack of security awareness among users in the Middle East. Security awareness in the Middle East, compared to Europe or the USA, has resulted in less effort being made to raise awareness among users. More significant is that IT decision-makers in the Middle East are often unaware of the cybercrime problem, believing that the Middle East is immune to attacks [12].

2.1 Information Security Culture

Human culture is mainly influenced by the national culture that directly affects human behaviour [23]. Studies conducted mostly in Western and Asian cultures indicate that Western organisational cultures are more individualist, while Asian cultures are more collective [14]. Cultural differences between different countries may sometimes necessitate additional investigations to understand how national culture may influence IS culture

[24]. The Middle East is a rich cultural region, and some research indicates a need for different security training according to the national culture [2].

Organisational culture is another part of the security culture, whether employees are aware of it or not [14]. A strong IS culture exists when individuals are aware of security risks and preventative measures. They assume responsibility and take the required steps to improve the security of their information systems [24]. Recent research supports the idea that organisations need to develop an IS culture to protect their information assets [7] and create an IS culture by identifying key security behaviours and aligning security awareness activities with internal and external campaigns [2, 7, 9].

IS awareness and learning also has a strong relationship with national culture [22, 24]. Organisations effectively manage their time and resources by focusing on what is needed to enhance employee IS awareness [24]. IS awareness content development plans and programs should consider national cultural factors and the area where one grew up on the impact of employees' IS awareness level [16]. IS culture plays an important mediating relationship between organisational culture and IS awareness [24]. This suggests that organisations should focus on security culture rather than organisational culture to improve IS awareness and save time and resources. Security culture should be part of organisational culture, as information is best protected when individuals understand, internalise and adhere to IS standards and best practices [20, 24].

2.2 Information Security Education, Training and Awareness (SETA)

With the continuous increase in attacks that target both individuals and businesses, awareness and ongoing education are needed to protect them [18]. One critical aspect of ISM is employee IS awareness [3] because attackers are more concerned with human behaviour and thus target the systems through employees as their low-security awareness level will increase the likelihood of success for the attackers [10].

Robust cyber laws alone are not enough to protect against cyber threats. Essential components have become building public awareness and educating users about cyber risks and safety [10]. It is essential to spread awareness that IT experts are not responsible for information safety alone. The most crucial step could be to provide awareness regarding protecting data and steps to mitigate attacks [3].

Security awareness is necessary but not sufficient and enough; it is only the first step. Users need to accumulate knowledge and build skills in security [21]. The problem with current awareness programs is that awareness activities are resource heavy and the effects are not that significant and often do not lead to measurable outcomes, which leads to annoyed employees. These problems happen because awareness programs have different shortcomings. These shortcomings mainly include 1) lack of methods to create engaging and appropriate materials for enhancing IS awareness programs [5], and 2) several behavioural factors which are not considered in developing IS awareness [16].

Awareness is typically focused on two aspects – understanding and compliance [10], an understanding of relevant organisational IS policies and the level of engagement between the individual and the principles of IS in their organisations. There are various methods and factors for IS awareness content development that employees need to know [16].

For IS awareness content development methods to be successful, the content of the programs cannot be developed based only on what the technical experts want to teach or based just on technical requirements or best practices; rather it is critical to understand the relevant security beliefs of the employees. To go beyond the traditional awareness programs offered by many organisations in the form of annual computer-based training, organisations need to put considerable investment into compliance or implementing transformative changes to develop IS culture. Awareness programs that include behavioural objectives are more likely to be effective in changing employees' behaviour and commitment to IS [7]. However, there is limited knowledge about methods for enhancing IS awareness and integrated insights into factors affecting employees' awareness levels [16]. Thus, increasing knowledge about effective programs has become a top priority both in research and practice.

2.3 Cyberattacks Targeting the Middle East

Social engineering phishing emails as a successful breach strategy gaining popularity in Capital Market in the Middle East. The KSA has recently experienced a series of cyber-attacks as the wealthiest country globally due to its economic and political position [19]. Oman is another Middle Eastern country that is increasingly experiencing cyberattacks. It was exposed to more than 880 million cyberattacks on government networks in 2017. Recent attacks in the financial sector attacks in Oman have shown the vulnerability of critical national infrastructure systems [4].

3 Methodology

3.1 Approach

This paper explores the effect of security culture and awareness of ISM, which require an in-depth investigation to answer the research question. Hence an exploratory qualitative approach was selected to gain in-depth research understanding and allow more rich input that will contribute to a better outcome. A literature review was first conducted to determine the latest developments in the research interest. A case study method was employed to gain first-hand knowledge from industry participants [25].

3.2 Participants

A total of twenty-two participants from four Capital Market organisations was included in this study. To ensure data quality, participants were selected through specific selection criteria, which required them to have an IT background and be working in the Middle Eastern Capital Market. Participants represented various levels and roles in their organisations evenly distributed between management and non-management positions (Table 1).

Table 1. Participant's Details.

	Managerial position participant	Non-managerial position participant
Org1	IT direct manager; Chief technical officer	System engineer; Infrastructure & operations engineer; Database administrator
Org2	Head: Networks & security section; IT manager; IT security supervisor; Head: Members & operations department	IS specialist; Information & operating officer
Org3	IS manager; Chief IS officer	IS specialist; DBA; System engineer
Org4	Head: Networks & IT security section; Deputy IT manager; Head: Application section	IT system analyst; Director of IT & information officer; Research & development director

3.3 Data Collection and Analysis

The data was collected from the Middle Eastern region through semi-structured interviews that employed open-ended questions, giving the participants the chance to discuss their opinions freely. The questions aimed to investigate how culture and, security education, training and awareness (SETA) programs influence ISM in the Capital Market. Five main questions gave a chance for participants to discuss the security awareness and education programs they have to protect their assets. The questions were about to ask the participants if they have any IS awareness or education programs and the details for these programs. How Middle Eastern culture, values trust and help, affects the security level and practices, and can undermine the role of security awareness and education. Participants were asked to describe the activities they undertake to manage IS. The participants reported based on their current organisational experiences, supported with appropriate real-life examples.

The interviews lasted about 90 min on average. These interviews were audio-recorded and were transcribed into text using Otter software. Then the interview transcripts were coded and themed using the NVivo 12 tool. Finally, thematic data analysis was performed by interrelating the codes and aggregating those themes based on Braun and Clarke guidelines [8].

4 Findings

This section presents the findings obtained in this study. The findings were presented collectively based on the participants' reflections on what was happening in their organisations. The findings demonstrated that the security culture and awareness have a significant impact on ISM in the Middle Eastern Capital Market. It showed that pure technology and spending money on security products without paying enough attention to security culture and awareness would not keep the Capital Markets fully secure. The findings conclude that security awareness is vital at all levels of organisations. Organisations can achieve that by training all different levels of employees, which is no less important than focusing on other security practices.

The subset of participants was provided different answers were based on their different levels within the selected institutions, which reflected their job focus, role and responsibility; (1) Top managers who provided a long-term perspective on organisational objectives, strategies and problem-solving, (2) Senior IT managers, team leaders or administrators who provided information about daily operations and their role as decision-makers, (3) Other IT staff, who explained the functional processes. Exploring the opinions of these different levels of employees is essential to identify issues from a broader perspective and understand different institutions' organisational thinking, experience and decision-making.

4.1 Security Culture

The Middle Eastern region is unique globally as a region full of culture and religious beliefs. These beliefs affect the security level and play a significant role in IS in the Middle East. The findings show that the Middle Eastern culture is a dominant factor influencing ISM in their organisations. However, the culture can undermine the effective role of security awareness and education.

In Middle Eastern culture, participants explained that people's dealing with others were largely based on trust even if sometimes it was unwarranted. They liked to offer help, even if it put the person providing the help in danger. While that kind of friendship culture worked well, sometimes it compromised IS. The most challenging consequence was that the employees were unable easily to change their behaviour and compliance. Middle Eastern employees are generally against changing their compliance with the rules. Learning by mistake rather than knowledge is a new challenge that is connected with the Middle Eastern culture. This Middle East proverb means that no one will learn from another person's experience, they have to do it themselves.

The findings revealed that the Middle Eastern culture is one of the biggest challenges for implementing and managing IS. The Capital Market organisations had to find a way to change the employees' and the organisational culture to have a better security level while they believed that it was hard to change in this context. The participants described the situation in the Middle East-related to the culture: 'We love legacy culture even if it is wrong' [Org2P3], and 'We love legacy rules and regulation' [Org4P1].

One specific cultural challenge in the Middle East is that people do not like sharing their experiences. It was clear from the participants' responses that it was not acceptable to share any information about a security threat or incident from their organisations' experience with their peer organisations, and they were not willing to pass on information about their attacks. All this resistance was because the organisations felt that sharing information could have a negative impact on their reputation.

The findings show that the Middle Eastern culture is not easygoing and does not easily accept change. So, participants were struggling with change management and any change would take a long time to happen. In addition, employees did not welcome cultural issues for security as they were forced to follow certain security measures. Some religious beliefs also guided the people in the Middle East, the belief that God will protect them all the time once they do their job. 'We do whatever we can do, and we will leave the rest to destiny' [Org1P5].

4.2 Security Awareness, Education and Training

The Middle East appears to be generous when it comes to spending money on technology. However, the findings show that they have trouble distributing their budget as it is all consumed on the technical side neglecting the other aspects such as awareness, education and training which indicates a shortage in IS and cause some ISM problems.

(1) Lack of security awareness:

The research findings confirm that security awareness is one of the most critical factors influencing ISM. The level of security awareness in the Middle Eastern Capital Market is unsatisfactory. The participants mentioned difficulties in implementing security solutions because of the lack of awareness in their organisations from different sides – both managers and employees.

(2) Lack of education and training:

It is worth noting that the Middle East has up to now suffered from the lack of high-quality security training. At the same time, if employees received high-quality training, the problem was in the distribution mechanism according to the eligibility of the employees to attend these courses and how to take advantage of them.

(3) Lack of education and training program management:

The Capital Market leaders and business managers do not consider security as a priority. They are not paying enough attention to the quality of the program's content. In addition, they do not have follow-up course-related actions, which create an implementation difficulty. There were no proper management and planning for their SETA programs; for example, email-based awareness training was used rather than interactive sessions. In addition, these Middle Eastern organisations did not include their top management in the security training, which created gaps in their structures. A further weakness of the awareness courses management was they did not have a periodic updates plan.

(4) Weak SETA program content:

Education programs are still weak and need improvement and refinement; nevertheless, it is practised. This research found that the content and activities of SETA programs offer a general security awareness program and IT concept training, which is not specific and detailed to their organisations. These programs lack ways to encourage the trainees to be proactive in implementing IS procedures. When the Capital Market managers have a detailed security program, they do not provide any details of training based on the employee levels, hence keeping all the employees together in the same training and ignoring their background and their different levels of security, which causes a perception of the uselessness of these programs. The second dimension of this weakness is that the programs do not have content related to the top management as decision-makers, which could change the security situation in the organisation. Another weakness was that most of the training content is theoretical. The training is missing the practical part and the real-life examples of the content, making it harder to apply what they learned practically.

(5) Implementing and evaluating SETA programs:

The evaluation of education programs happens in various ways. However, the findings show that the Capital Market organisations still could not see the benefits of their education programs, and even if they could see some benefits, the need to improve was still acknowledged.

One of the main points discussed in relation to their education programs is that it is imperative to pay attention to regular awareness updates. Otherwise, as they experienced, the employees' level of awareness would steadily decrease with the passage of time. The findings recorded that the level of awareness of the employees is at its peak after the completion of the training workshops, which causes a high level of security in the organisation and errors related to IS are reduced. This level gradually begins to decrease after a relatively short period of time and thus the problems start again.

The non-affordable delivering mechanism for non-IT specialists is another challenge of the Capital Market. Unsuitable customisation for non-IT specialists and the highly specialised delivering mechanism for non-IT employees.

5 Discussion

Protecting information assets in the Capital Market and preventing and managing security breaches and incidents are becoming more important than ever. Security culture and SETA represent essential issues in ISM in organisations [1]. Extant literature reveals that the human factor aspect is one of the emerging research areas in IS. Security culture and SETA are part of this main factor. Thus, this research explores the security culture and SETA effect in ISM used to reduce internal threats and how Capital Market organisations perceive them and create a new security culture that works in parallel with SETA.

However, the study's findings exposed two concepts of IS in the Capital Market industry. Firstly, the current culture of the employees in the Capital Market organisations does not promote IS. Secondly, the awareness of the employees towards IS is poor due to a lack of adequate security training and skills. The study findings show a relationship between the culture and the SETA concept. Accordingly, IS involves training employees, enhancing their knowledge and security skills and promoting a culture that helps secure information. This, in turn, will help achieve the business goals and objectives. Figure 1 below gives more explanation in the sense that culture has a stronger influence than the awareness level in ISM and it has a strong influence in SETA itself.

The cultural environment is a multi-disciplinary factor that includes the culture of the country in which the organisation is located (national culture), and the management culture in the organisation and the organisational culture itself. In the context of this research, the Middle East with its distinct cultures, is strongly influenced by religious values, and these strongly influence the Middle Eastern Capital Market regarding implementing IS.

The influence of Middle Eastern culture is strong, as culture dominates people's awareness and education. The Middle Eastern culture is characterised by its great reliance on mutual trust between all parties in the institution and the policy of tribalism and friendship that justifies abuses in laws and regulations. For example, one challenge is that friends will share passwords even when they are security specialist. In other words, they depend on trust and give some employees broad privileges related to their culture.

Various weaknesses of SETA programs were identified. One weakness is that leaders should pay attention to making SETA programs compulsory for everyone or some

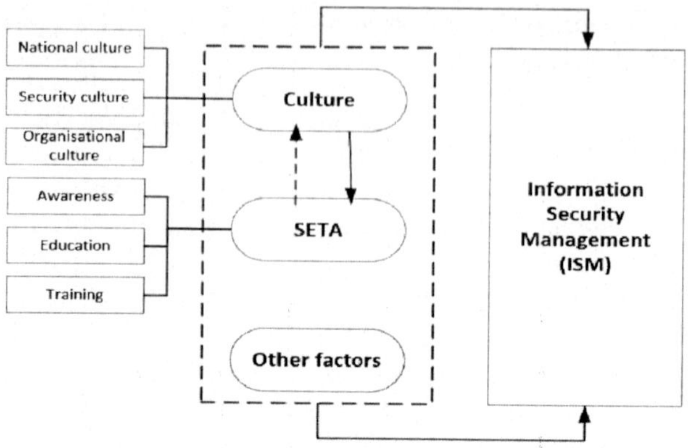

Fig. 1. Security Culture and SETA Influence

employees will miss the security rules and regulations for the Capital Market. As the SETA program is optional for some employees, they will never think about having that kind of education.

The lack of sustainable awareness effects after the course is related to human nature. The level of security will be high once the employees finish the security course, but after around two weeks, the level will go down, and after one month the level will go down more. The Capital Market should be provided a quarterly alert from their organisations regarding security threats would be helpful and keep them on the right track. These alerts should not be the basis of the awareness program as it is now, but it could be with supportive steps.

In conclusion, SETA programs were consistently recognised as being a need for Capital Market organisations. They need to build robust security awareness programs. This program must establish a common understanding that everyone plays an essential role in keeping the organisation secure. Training is an important piece of an institution's overall information security strategy. The overall discussion about SETA programs highlighted that all participants wanted some training for the users but faced time, budget and manpower constraints while also not including the institution's general staff. Even fewer participants could get any training in this area for management.

The findings of this study match literature demonstrating that the organisations are missing good quality training but in addition, the research case shows that the Capital Market has another problem which is misallocating the right training to the right person.

The Capital Market institutions have to prepare a plan with a long-term vision for their educational and training sessions. They have to pay attention to the criteria they are using to choose the right employees for the related training and there should be an evaluation process for the employees after each training. The Capital Market has to be mindful when offering appropriate security awareness content that suits individuals and their culture. All the Capital Market employees must know that cybersecurity is everyone's business, so it is crucial to understand how to protect the data they access at work and how they keep themselves protected against common cyber attacks.

Some literature [6, 24] mentioned that demographic characteristics such as age (higher awareness is positively associated with age) are affecting the awareness level. The findings found that is not the case in the Middle East. Culture is the main factor that could influence awareness. The other factor that the literature [4] focused on is the experience (the more experienced staff become, the less damage from attacks will occur in the organisation).

Although the literature highlighted that SETA would improve the users' understanding of security concepts and improve security behaviour [21], this research also highlighted that culture plays a significant role in security behaviour, and without collaboration between the culture and the SETA the security behaviour will never improve in the needed way.

The main contribution of this study is the advancement of the theoretical and practical basis for IS in proposing a model for developing, assessing and modelling how the security culture and SETA can influence ISM. Furthermore, it improves the understanding of risks in the security incident stages in relation to these factors. The research contributes to the current knowledge of information security by demonstrating the importance and critical role of the cultural factor in managing IS in the Middle Eastern Capital Market. It also contributes by showing that the culture can damage the role of education and awareness.

The previous studies proved that SETA programs are very beneficial. They could help with increasing the individuals' awareness levels [4], motivating employees to pay attention to cyber threats and Facilitating implementing security controls making effective security policy [17, 21].

This study investigates the effect of security culture and awareness only in four Capital Market organisations in the Middle East. Future studies can overcome this limitation by examining more organisations in and out of the Middle East and comparing the effect of the culture. Although this study strives to address a focused topic of convergence of these areas, comprehensive coverage by future studies is still required.

6 Conclusion

The research demonstrates that investing heavily in technical controls yet paying less attention or not being invested enough in employee training and awareness will open the door for attackers to manipulate the organisation's human element. Therefore, the Capital Market has to pay more attention to the lack of knowledge in understanding the main security concept and improving the general IS concept. The findings show that both security culture (organisational culture and country culture) and security awareness are essential factors influencing ISM in the Middle Eastern Capital Market industry.

Middle Eastern culture is the dominant factor in this research context, eliminating the role of security education and awareness in some cases. It is more influential than security awareness in influencing ISM. Culture has a huge effect and it is a major factor cause of security breaches. This research adds to the body of knowledge that the human factor in the Middle East is influenced mainly by culture. This research points to the need for SETA programs for decision-makers in the Capital Market. Security knowledge at the top management level helps Capital Market leaders know the threats that influence their assets and identify their impact to determine what they need to do to prevent attacks by selecting appropriate countermeasures.

The study suggests that the Capital Market should focus on security culture and apply the same degree of focus to the SETA to improve ISM. Focusing on culture, saving time and resources. SETA programs are essential to protect organisational information resources. This study of Capital Market industry security practices exposed three key insufficiencies. First, they ignore the cultural effect on the ISM process. Second, the SETA programmes are generic without considering the special features of the Capital Market context without any customisations for their needs. Third, there is no connection between the culture and the awareness programs. To achieve the desired benefits, all these factors must be considered.

This qualitative research study emphasises the quality of the collected data rather than the quantity of the data. Nevertheless, this research still has some limitations to how far these empirical findings can be generalised. The main limitation of this study was not getting full access to the Capital Market institutions due to the sensitivity of this industry. Despite having access to 5 Capital Market institutions in the Middle East, this study would have been stronger with more Middle Eastern Capital Market institutions involved. The fact that the study represents only 5 Middle Eastern Capital Market institutions limits the relevance of the findings to Capital Markets in different areas.

References

1. Abebe, G., Lessa, L.: Human factors influence in information systems security: towards a conceptual framework. Paper presented at the African International Conference on Industrial Engineering and Operations Management, Harare, Zimbabwe
2. Aboul Enein, S.: Cybersecurity challenges in the Middle East (2017). https://www.gcsp.ch/publications/cybersecurity-challenges-middle-east
3. Ahmed, N.N., Nanath, K.: Exploring cybersecurity ecosystem in the Middle East: towards an SME recommender system. J. Cyber Secur. Mob. **10**(3), 511–536 (2021)
4. Al-Harethi, A.A.M., Al-Amoodi, A.H.A.: Organisational factors affecting information security management practices in private sector organisations. Int. J. Psychol. Cogn. Sci. **5**(1), 9–23 (2019)
5. Al Mughairi, B.M., Al Hajri, H.H., Karim, A.M., Hossain, M.I.: An innovative cyber security based approach for national infrastructure resiliency for Sultanate of Oman. Int. J. Acad. Res. Bus. Soc. Sci. **9**(3), 1180–1195 (2019)
6. Alotaibi, F., Furnell, S., Stengel, I., Papadaki, M.: A survey of cyber-security awareness in Saudi Arabia. Paper presented at the in ICITST 2016: International Conference for Internet Technology and Secured Transactions (2016)
7. Alshaikh, M.: Developing cybersecurity culture to influence employee behavior: a practice perspective. Comput. Secur. **98**, 1–10 (2020)
8. Braun, V., Clarke, V.: One size fits all? What counts as quality practice in (Reflexive) thematic analysis? Qual. Res. Psychol. **18**(3), 328–352 (2021). https://doi.org/10.1080/14780887.2020.1769238
9. Da Veiga, A., Astakhova, L.V., Botha, A., Herselman, M.: Defining organisational information security culture - perspectives from academia and industry. Comput. Secur. **92**, 1–50 (2020)
10. Dharmawansa, A.D., Madhuwanthi, R.: Evaluating the information security awareness (ISA) of employees in the banking sector: a case study. Paper presented at the in KDU IRC 2020:

Kotelawala Defence University International Research Conference, Kuliyapitiya, Sri Lanka (2020)
11. El-Guindy, M.N.: Middle East cyber security threat report 2014. Cybersec. Energy Utilities **25**, 1–7 (2013)
12. Hayes, A.: Capital markets, Investopedia, viewed 30 June 2021. https://www.investopedia.com/terms/c/capitalmarkets.asp
13. Hughes-Lartey, K., Li, M., Botchey, F.E., Qin, Z.: Human factor, a critical weak point in the information security of an organisation's internet of things. Heliyon **7**(3), 1–13 (2021)
14. Jamall, A., Ghazali, M.: Banking and capital markets, PwC (PricewaterhouseCoopers) Middle East, viewed 12 June 2021 (2020). https://www.pwc.com/m1/en/industries/banking-capital-markets.html
15. Khando, K., Gao, S., Islam, S.M., Salman, A.: Enhancing employees information security awareness in private and public organisations: a systematic literature review. Comput. Secur. **106**, 1–22 (2021)
16. Ključnikov, A., Mura, L., Sklenár, D.: Information security management in SMEs: factors of success. Entrepreneurship Sustain. Issues **6**(4), 2081–2094 (2019)
17. Kuchibhotla, H.N., Murray, P., McFarland, R.: Addressing the financial services cybersecurity threat (2017). https://thecybersecurityplace.com/addressing-financial-services-cybersecurity-threat/
18. Mahfuth, A., Yussof, S., Baker, A.A., Ali, N.A.: A systematic literature review: information security culture. Paper presented at the in ICRIIS 2017: International Conference on Research and Innovation in Information Systems (2017)
19. Alqurashi, R.K., AlZain, M.A., Soh, B., Masud, M., Al-Amri, J.: Cyber attacks and impacts: a case study in Saudi Arabia. Int. J. Adv. Trends Comput. Sci. Eng. **9**(1), 217–224 (2020)
20. Renaud, K., Flowerday, S., Dupuis, M.: Moving from employee compliance to employee success in the cyber security domain. Comput. Fraud Secur. **2021**(4), 16–19 (2021)
21. Soomro, Z.A., Shah, M.H., Ahmed, J.: Information security management needs more holistic approach: a literature review. Int. J. Inf. Manage. **36**(2), 215–225 (2016)
22. Topa, I., Karyda, M.: From theory to practice: guidelines for enhancing information security management. Inf. Comput. Secur. **27**(3), 326–342 (2019)
23. Uchendu, B., Nurse, J.R., Bada, M., Furnell, S.: Developing a cyber security culture: current practices and future needs. Comput. Secur. **109**, 1–38 (2021)
24. Wiley, A., McCormac, A., Calic, D.: More than the individual: examining the relationship between culture and information security awareness. Comput. Secur. **88**, 1–8 (2020). https://doi.org/10.1016/j.cose.2019.101640
25. Yin, R.K.: Case Study Research and Applications: Design and Methods, 6th edn. SAGE, Thousand Oaks, CA (2018)

Building a Knowledge Model of Cayo Santiago Rhesus Macaques: Engaging Undergraduate Students in Developing Graphical User Interfaces for NSF Funded Research Project

Martin Q. Zhao[1(✉)], Ethan R. Widener[1], George Francis[2], and Qian Wang[2]

[1] Department of Computer Science, Mercer University, Macon, USA
zhao_mq@mercer.edu, ethan.ransom.widener@live.mercer.edu

[2] Department of Biomedical Sciences, Texas A&M University School of Dentistry, Dallas, USA
gfrancis@exchange.tamu.edu, qian.wang@tamu.edu

Abstract. In this paper, we introduce an NSF funded project that aims to develop a database that integrates genetic, environmental and age-related information to study their effects on health conditions of a rhesus monkey colony at Cayo Santiago, Puerto Rico, which has been founded since 1938. In this project, we will combine the osteology data with the rich genealogy and demographic information into a searchable and computer-interoperable knowledge model accessible through user-friendly interfaces. Backed by the integrated database, this system will provide researchers and the public information from the Cayo Santiago rhesus colony and the derived skeletal collection, a powerful non-human model for datamining to study human disease. Undergraduate and graduate students from diverse communities have been incorporated into research and development activities. Related materials are used as case studies in relevant classes at Mercer University to help train these undergraduate students into problem solvers.

Keywords: Problem-based learning · Computer science education · Data management for analytics · Information integration · Graphical user interface

1 Introduction

An interdisciplinary team led by Qian Wang of Texas A&M University, funded by NSF, is developing a database that integrates genetic, environmental and age-related information to study their effects on health conditions of a rhesus monkey colony at Cayo Santiago, Puerto Rico. Founded in 1938, the Cayo Santiago colony is the source of a rare skeletal collection with associated details about each individual's sex, age, and pedigree (up to twelve generations) [3, 6, 15, 19]. This skeletal collection, housed at the Caribbean Primate Research Center, has been highly useful in anthropological and biomedical studies (i.e., [2, 5, 7, 14, 16–18]).

In this project, bone dimensions, bone density, body mass, tooth eruption, and observable disease conditions of the rhesus monkey will be incorporated into the database with

K. Daimi and A. Al Sadoon (Eds.): ICR 2023, LNNS 721, pp. 344–353, 2023.
https://doi.org/10.1007/978-3-031-35308-6_29

details on each individual's sex, birth and death dates, parentage information, and social rank (when available). Once the integrated database is available to researchers and the public, information from the Cayo Santiago rhesus colony and the derived skeletal collection will provide a powerful non-human model for datamining to study human disease, family history, development, individual experiences, and aging. The team brings together expertise in anthropology, biology, biomedical sciences, and computer sciences. Database development incorporates undergraduate and graduate students from collaborating institutions, providing unique learning opportunities. For building the Cayo Santiago rhesus health database, we will combine the osteology data with the rich genealogy and demographic information into a searchable and computer-interoperable Knowledge Model.

"Using the program opportunity in the project to train undergraduate students at Mercer University", one of the Broad Impacts in the original proposal to NSF, has been planned since the project began. Courses relevant to the database and user interfaces development and data analytics are taught at the Computer Science Department at Mercer University through its Computer Science, Information Science and Technology, and Data Science programs. Martin Q. Zhao (M.Q.Z.) has been using projects based on real world problems in his Software Engineering, Programming, Database Systems, and Data Science Applications courses. This paper will focus on how students have been involved in the design and implementation of the proposed database system, especially the front-end application codenamed as CSViewer, now in v1.0.

2 Database and Application System Design

A conceptual design for the CS rhesus database and the graphical user interfaces (GUI), which support data management and analytics needs, has been discussed in [11]. This section will focus on system design aspects for the database and especially graphical user interfaces provided in the CSViewer frontend application. Implementation of the current version (v1.0) and redesign/enhancement effort for v1.1 will be discussed in the subsequent sections.

A. ***Database Design***

As shown in Fig. 1, a relational data model [11] has been proposed for the integrative database to manage subject genealogy information of the rhesus families maintained by the CPRC, plus health data (to be) obtained in this project (including scans, measurements, and observation data). A relational design similar to a human health database [4] is used, which shows great extensibility. More tables need to be added to keep track of valid users, access control, user activities, etc. in a later stage.

B. ***Data Collection and Preparation***

Various datasets have been collected from historical records at CPRC and bone measure activities conducted by George Francis for this project. Measuring and picture taking are still ongoing after being delayed by the pandemics and maintenance of CPRC facilities.

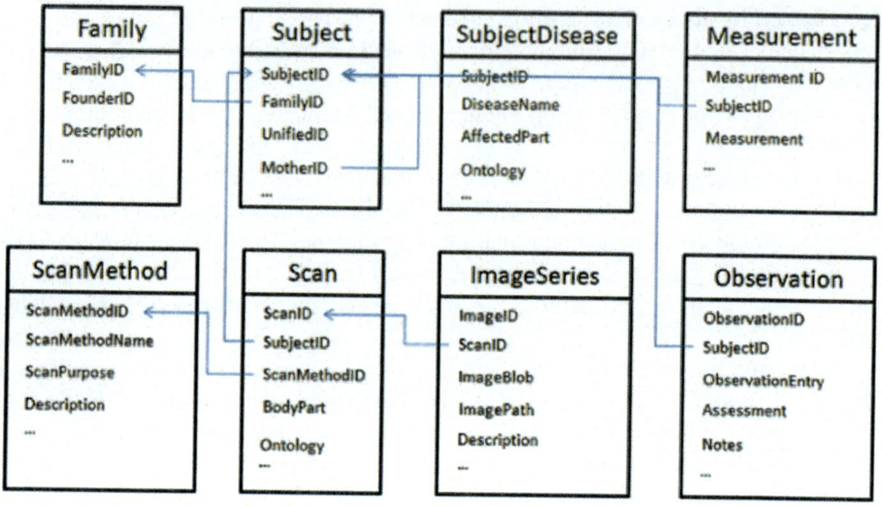

Fig. 1. Conceptual data model for the Cayo Santiago Rhesus Health Database.

Data quality analysis have been conducted for all incoming datasets received for this project, including

1) Census data from 2020 and 2013: The two datasets were merged to generate a complete animal dataset with 10949 distinct animals. Another dataset is available for 77 founding mothers with only the year they were born.
2) Catalog data for skeletons curated at CPRC: This dataset has more than 4800 entries, including 2292 entries from the CS population.
3) Bone measure data: Data collection using cataloged CS specimens has been conducted since 2020. The raw data including dimensions of skull, upper and lower limbs, suture and joint conditions, as well as bone density for 1509 CS specimens (by the end of 2021) are used in the initial building of the database and application system.
4) A small collection of bone pictures has been included in the initial database for testing purposes. Full-scale imagery data collection is currently conducted at CPRC.

C. ***Software Architecture***

The proposed Knowledge Model consists of a comprehensive database managing existing and new collected data from the CS population. The CSViewer application is the frontend that provides friendly user interfaces for analysts to access the data and perform data analytics tasks. A standard layered architecture is adopted (as shown in Fig. 2), which consists of multiple layers of abstraction coalescing to facilitate the transfer and display of data from the database. For version 1.0, the CSViewer system is based on local files with more stable data structures (such as matrilineal and patrilineal family trees) extracted from the censor and catalog datasets. Design of the middle layer uses the metaphor of Business Managers to help make the design flexible such that functions for processing different kinds of data (family, measure, image, etc.) can be supported separately to be suitable for an incremental development approach. The managers (that are key objects in functional partitions in the middle layer) are responsible for accessing data using the relevant data accessor objects (DAOs), and create value objects (VOs, such as animal or measure objects) that map to the relational data entries. Information to be displayed to the user will be prepared by the corresponding manager in the form of a page bean and feed to the GUI component that consumes it. Some design details regarding "managers" will be given in Section III Part B, with descriptions on how Ethan Widener and his teammates in M.Q.Z.'s Software Engineering class contributed to the development of CSViewer v0.1.

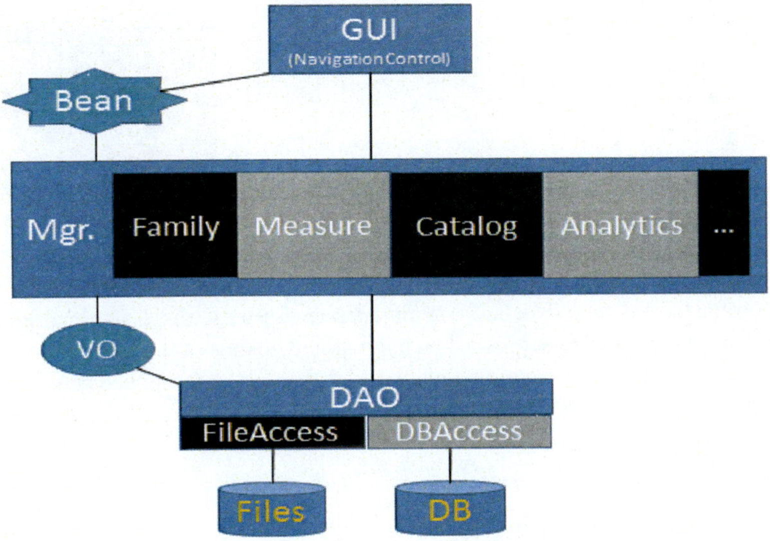

Fig. 2. Layered architecture with Data accessibility, Business Managers, and GUI.

With such a template, each layer is responsible for a distinct set of operations and is in contact with the layers directly above and below it, ensuring a stable chain of command for efficient and clear communication of data from the back end to the front end of the system.

D. ***Graphical User Interfaces***

The graphical user interface displayed upon launch of the application is the user's means of interacting with and navigating the program. The CSViewer window (Fig. 3) features a myriad of menus to support various visualization and analytical tasks. The main results of the current task are displayed in the main content panel (matrilineal family trees as in the screenshot). Views for multiple tasks can be displayed as tabbed pane structures for easy navigation.

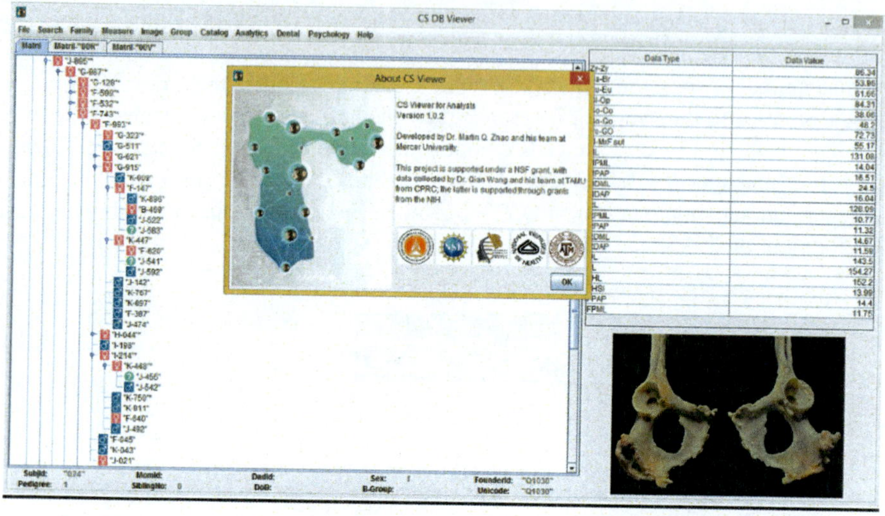

Fig. 3. Screenshot of the Main Window of CSViewer v1.0. (with the About Box laid over)

Below the tabbed pane structure, a summary pane is used to display animal summary information on the selected subject when interacting with one of the tabbed pane views. Any additional relevant information is displayed to the right of the tabbed pane structure. This information can include measure data in table format, and/or images relating to the subject and measure data.

E. *Data Structures*

As mentioned above, this version (v1.0) reads data from local files. Animal records are already sorted in a sequential order based on mother or father bloodlines. Internally, the managers use collection classes in the standard Java collections framework (JCF) to store data, and prepare bean objects to feed to various content panes using Java Swing classes, such as JTree and JTable. The JTree view and related data model, a Java-specific implementation of an n-tree data structure, plays an important role in rendering family trees. In this project, the founders of each matrilineal line serve as top-level nodes, while their offspring are displayed as expandable child nodes. Direct children of founders can further be expanded to show their children, and so on to provide a complete and navigable view of the dataset and the relationships between each specimen. The Patrilineal trees are constructed from each animal's father identity and can be traced back to the earliest male subject (with DNA screening) of a respective tree. The construction process also uses the animal information as available in the matrilineal tree input file to reduce redundancy. Map types as available in JCF are also used to track cross-referencing patterns between animals and their catalog entries, and through which linking to measure/image data when they exist.

3 Software Engineering Education

Martin Q. Zhao has been teaching various software and database courses at Mercer University in the undergraduate Computer Science (CSC) and Information Science and Technology (IST) programs, and recently also teaching for the graduate Software and System Engineering (SSE) program.

A. ***Teaching Pedagogies and Student Engagement***
We believe that software and database development topics can be best learned by applying design principles and programming techniques in practice; and ideally, in real-world projects. The case studies and project topics used in M.Q.Z.'s classes evolved from workshops [12] extended from popular textbooks [1], to externally funded research and development projects [8–10, 13].

Courses involved and teaching/learning activities:

1) Database implementation and essential queries have been assigned to student teams in several database and software engineering classes since the NSF grant was awarded in 2019.
2) The recent CSViewer release was refactored and extended from the codebase finished by a team in the latest Software Engineering I (CSC 480). The student project was based on CSV files listing animal entries sorted by father/mother in chronicle order that are prepared by M.Q.Z. and a layered software architectural template introduced in class.
3) Analytical result visualization (using the JFreeChart API [21]) and related selection features are then added to form version 1.0. As a member of the CSC 480 team, Ethan Widener continues to contribute to source control and redesign for v1.1 (to be detailed in the next section), while taking research and internship courses.

   Implementation, testing, and continuation among classes:

4) Providing DB and GUI design and codebase to student teams with specific tasks seems to be more effective. Incremental development process and source and document control can help establish a foundation securing continued feature building across many classes during subsequent academic terms. Students can contribute through class assignments, volunteer and paid commitments in multiple (software engineering, database systems, research and internship) courses.

B. ***Student Contributions in Building the CSViewer App***
Certain details about contributions made by the student team in a Software Engineering class in Fall of 2022 will be presented here. Their work helped with the integration of partially working modules into CSViewer (version 0):

1) Merged separate tree views for matrilineal and patrilineal lineage, using a single CSFamilyTreePanel class as provided by M.Q.Z.
2) Laid out four major content panes in the CSViewer main window, as described in Section I Part D.
3) Implemented the "measure partition" in the middle layer, which includes
   a. A MeasureHash class using the DAO object to access measure data in a CSV file, and

b. Generating "measure bean" objects with attributes holding values that can be used by the JTable in the MeasureTablePanel.
4) Established cross-references among the CSFamilyTreePanel, the subject summary pane (beneath the main content pane), and the MeasureTablePanel.

The students were trained with several workshops demonstrating topics like layered architectural design, GUI and JDBC programming. A team of five helped with this project, including Ethan A. Widener, who continues to work in this project with additional research and internship courses.

What impressed EAW the most is to work closely with a "client" on a complex system with evolving needs. Instead of being given with a clearly defined problem and a fixed set of steps to write a program, students need to communicate with the client to analyze what exactly is needed, and translate that model into a product. In addition, using third APIs (such as JFreeChart [21] and Tablesaw [20]) significantly extended the capability of the software solution, and exposed students to component-based design and development.

C. *Enhancements Leading to CSViewer v1.0*

The integrated system (Version 0 of CSViewer) was then refactored by M.Q.Z. to give it a consistent look. Additional features have been added to make the app to take the shape that can be a useful tool for researchers managing and analyzing the valuable data collected from the CS colony.

1) A menu structure has been added, with a tabbed panel to hold major contents.
2) A ChartPanel (opened in the Analytics menu) is added to display analytical results.
3) Professional graphics design elements are used, as app logo and on the About box, etc.
4) An easy to deploy set of deliverables are zipped and sent out for user testing.

Significant features of CSViewer v1.0 will be summarized in the next section.

4 Results and Redesign

A. *Results of the Current Design*

By the time of writing this paper, CSViewer is now in v1.0.3, and just started user testing. Essential functions in this version can be accessed through its menu structure, which include:

1) Matrilineal and patrilineal family trees starting from 77 founders or first male ancestors with DNA tracing data. The trees are expandable, and a search function can automatically expand and show the path leading to a chosen animal in either a matrilineal or patrilineal family tree.
2) Cross-reference between animal family information (in the tree panel and the summary pane beneath it) and bone measure data (in table pane on the right) is established. Animal summary and available measure data can be displayed when a tree node is selected.

3) For selected measure data (using the Search menu), scatter plots of measure vs. animal's estimated age at death (EAAD) can be displayed through the Analytics menu (Fig. 4). Analytic plots are generated using JFreeChart API [21] and support
   a. Tooltips when moused over and popup menus for left mouse click;
   b. Short menu with built-in functions for right mouse click. These functions include Save chart as an image (PNG) file, Copy it to a Word file or send to print, as well as Zoom in and Zoom out.
   c. Planned redesign using Tablesaw API [20] (to be discussed next) will make selection and chart generation more streamlined.
4) While large-scale picture taking is still ongoing, linkage between the family tree and corner image pane is established. An available image (though limited in amount so far) can be displayed when the corresponding tree node is selected.
5) A small number of group transfer entries and images taken from earlier studies are included in this current version for proof of concept and are planned into the next release (as v1.0.4).

B. ***New Design with Tablesaw***

While enhancements are still being added to the current version (v1.0), a redesign is carried out to streamline data analytic support. One important goal is to use the Tablesaw API (which was initiated in 2017 and is still in version 0) to provide a generic DataFrame-like construct that is widely used in data analytics. This addition will make the CSViewer application not just a visualization tool, but also a real toolkit for Analysts, supporting endless analytical and modeling tasks upon this comprehensive CS rhesus monkey data collection. The Tablesaw API allows software developers to organize data into tables and manipulate those tables in ways that core Java does not support. Given the vast amount of data involved in this project, as well as the myriad of categories the data falls under which often intersect and need to be cross-referenced with one another, an underlying

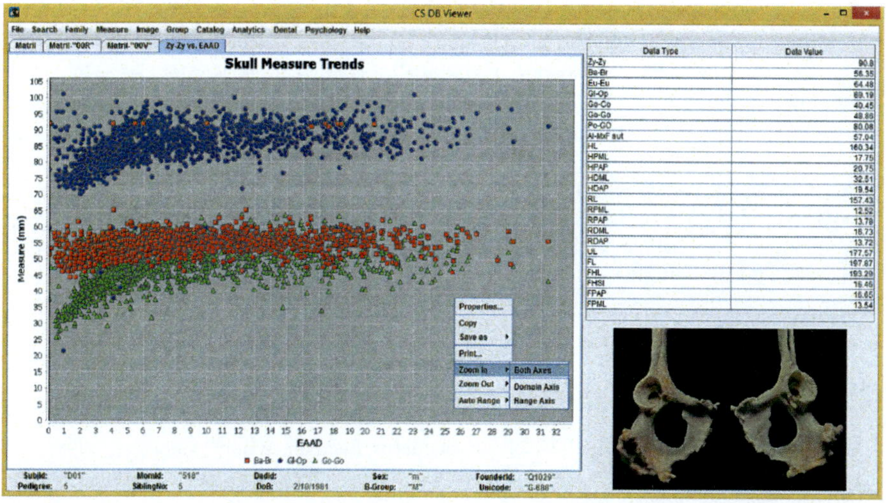

Fig. 4. Screenshot of a chart tab for analytical results, with features like copy, save, and print.

table structure is preferred. Tablesaw API will allow the data to be placed into large tables that can then be cut down into relevant subsets without additional overhead.

The new design will be included in version 1.1, which aims to utilize Tablesaw and related new development (such as the XChart API [22]) to help make the system more modular and extensible. It will pave the way for additional features in future iterations and fulfill the goal of a Knowledge Model for hypothesis-based investigations.

5 Conclusions and Future Work

An initial version of the CSViewer for Analysts (v1.0) has been developed and sent for user testing. This user-friendly application helps make it easy to access and analyze data from the Cayo Santiago rhesus colony, one of the most useful primate sources in biomedical and anthropological research. Essential visualization features are now available for family trees based on historical records and recent census data, as well as dimension measures collected from the derived skeletons. Design and development topics of this real world application have been used in related courses (including programming, database, software engineering, and data science) offered by the Computer Science Department at Mercer University. Undergraduate students in those courses have been involved through lectures, hands-on exercises, and contributing to building parts of the system. Teams of students worked to analyze the needs of the client, design a solution using third party APIs, and translate their models into working software.

With more existing datasets (such as dental data) and new data being collected (such as imagery and pathological data), we will continue to build both the backend database system and add more features to CSViewer. Efforts will be made to make cross-referencing data from different sources consistent and to provide more data analysis and modeling support to establish a unique Knowledge Model for hypothesis-based investigations.

Acknowledgments. The CPRC Skeletal Collection has been supported by National Institutes of Health NIH contracts NIH 5P40OD012217. This project is supported by NSF grants to M.Q.Z. and Q.W. (#1926402, #1926601). Melween I. Martinez Rodriguez (Current CPRC Director), Bonn V. Liong Aure, Terry B. Kensler, Elizabeth Maldonado, Giselle Caraballo Cruz, and other CPRC staff members for their support and help. Andres Boullosa, Adrian Faircloth, Jesus Rijo, and Zaina Khutliwala worked on the team together with E.R.W. that contributed to CSViewer 1.0. Rajwol Chapagain helped in system testing and preparing user instructions. Robert Allen, Jesse Sowell and the students at the Mercer University's Computer Science Department provided their supports and contributions. Special thanks go to Pegasus Vertex, Inc. in Houston, TX for providing graphics design used in the user interfaces.

References

1. Horstmann, C.: Object-Oriented Design and Patterns, 2nd edn. Wiley, Hoboken (2005)
2. Guatelli-Steinberg, D., et al.: Male Cayo Santiago rhesus macaques (Macaca mulatta) tend to have greater molar wear than females at comparable ages: exploring two possible reasons why. Am. J. Biol. Anthropol. **178**, 437–447 (2022). https://doi.org/10.1002/ajpa.24519

3. Sade, D., Chepko-Sade, B., Schneider, J., Roberts, S., Richtsmeier, J.: Basic Demographic Observations on Free-Ranging Rhesus Monkeys. Human Relations Area Files Press, New Haven (1985)
4. Seo, D., Lee, S., Lee, S., Jung, H., Sung, W.K.: Construction of Korean spine database with degenerative spinal diseases for realizing e-spine, KSII. In: The 8th Asian Pacific International Conference on Information Science and Technology (APIC-IST), Jeju, Republic of Korea (2013)
5. Li, H., et al.: The odontogenic abscess in Rhesus macaques (Macaca mulatta) from Cayo Santiago. Am. J. Phys. Anthropol. **167**, 441–457 (2018)
6. Kessler, M., Rawlins, R.: A 75-year pictorial history of the Cayo Santiago rhesus monkey colony. Am. J. Primatol. **78**, 6–43 (2016)
7. Kessler, M., et al.: Long-term effects of castration on the skeleton of male rhesus monkeys (Macaca mulatta). Am. J. Primatol. **78**, 152–166 (2016)
8. Zhao, M.: Knowledge representation and reasoning for impact/threat assessment in cyber situation awareness systems – Technical report. ARFL/RI, Rome, NY (2010)
9. Zhao, M.: Knowledge models for SA applications and user interface development for the SITA system, Final report. ARFL/RI, Rome, NY (2011)
10. Zhao, M., Kensler, T., Guatelli-Steinberg, D., Kohn, L., Francis, G., Wang, Q.: Reproduction of Cayo Santiago Rhesus Colony based on the patrilineal family trees: the missing patterns. Poster presentation at AABA '23, Reno, NV (2023)
11. Zhao, M.Q., Maldonado, E., Kensler, T.B., Kohn, L.A.P., Guatelli-Steinberg, D., Wang, Q.: Conceptual design and prototyping for a primate health history knowledge model. In: Arabnia, H.R., Deligiannidis, L., Shouno, H., Tinetti, F.G., Tran, Q.-N. (eds.) Advances in Computer Vision and Computational Biology. TCSCI, pp. 509–520. Springer, Cham (2021). https://doi.org/10.1007/978-3-030-71051-4_40
12. Zhao, M., White, L.: Engaging Software Engineering Students Using a Series of OOAD Workshops. Proceeding of ASEE, Chicago (2006)
13. Zhao, M., Allen, R.: Training problem-solvers by using real world problems as case studies. Poster paper accepted by ICR '23, Madrid, Spain (2023)
14. Wang, Q. (ed.): Bones, Genetics, and Behavior of Rhesus Macaques: Macaca mulatta of Cayo Santiago and Beyond. Springer, New York (2012). https://doi.org/10.1007/978-1-4614-1046-1
15. Wang, Q.: Dental maturity and the ontogeny of sex-based differences in the dentofacial complex of rhesus macaques from Cayo Santiago. In: Wang, Q. (ed.) Bones, Genetics, and Behavior of Rhesus Macaques. Developments in Primatology: Progress and Prospects, pp. 177–194. Springer, New York (2012). https://doi.org/10.1007/978-1-4614-1046-1_8
16. Wang, Q., Dechow, P.: Divided zygomatic bone in primates with implications of skull morphology and biomechanics. Anat. Rec. **299**, 1801–1829 (2016)
17. Wang, Q., Kessler, M., Kensler, T., Dechow, P.: The mandibles of castrated male rhesus macaques (Macaca mulatta): the effects of orchidectomy on bone and teeth. Am. J. Phys. Anthropol. **159**, 31–51 (2016)
18. Wang, Q., Turnquist, J., Kessler, M.: Free-ranging Cayo Santiago rhesus monkeys (Macaca mulatta): III. Dental eruption Patterns and dental pathology. Am. J. Primatol. **78**, 127–142 (2016)
19. Rawlins, R., Kessler, M. (eds.): The Cayo Santiago Macaques: History, Behavior and Biology. State University of New York Press, Albany (1986)
20. Tablesaw: A Platform for Data Science in Java, https://github.com/jtablesaw/tablesaw. Retrieved 16 Feb 2023
21. The JFreeChart Project. https://www.jfree.org/jfreechart/. Retrieved 16 Feb 2023
22. The XChart API. https://knowm.org/open-source/xchart/. Retrieved 28 Feb 2023

Emotional Intelligence of Teachers in Higher Education: Stress Coping Strategies, Social Self-efficacy, and Decision-Making Styles

Mahshid Lonbani[1](✉), Shintaro Morimoto[2], Joane Jonathan[1], Pradeep Khanal[3], and Sanjeev Sharma[4]

[1] Kent Institute Australia, Sydney, Australia
lonbanimahshid@gmail.com, joane.jonathan@kent.edu.au
[2] Study Group Australia, Darlinghurst, Australia
[3] Expert Education and Visa Services, Sydney, Australia
pradeep.khanal@experteducation.com.au
[4] Queensland International Business Academy (QIBA), Brisbane, Australia
Sam@qiba.edu.au

Abstract. This article discusses the significance of emotional intelligence (EI) in the professional development of teachers and the function that it plays in that development. The purpose of this paper is to explain the relationship between EI and three important factors named Stress Coping Strategies, Social Self-efficacy, and Decision-Making Styles among higher education teachers and its impact on teaching quality. It proposes a conceptual model for improving teaching equality by improving workplace social interactions, decision-making and reducing teacher attrition rates. This article also examines some prior research studies on emotional intelligence and the three above mentioned variables that contribute to the formation of the conceptual framework. Domain knowledge in this area can improve teaching quality by reducing teacher attrition rates through better stress coping, better decision-making in the classroom, and improved morale from better social self-efficacy. This study also provides justification for considering EI as an assessable component during the teacher recruitment process.

Keywords: Emotional Intelligence · Teacher Performance · Coping Strategies · Social Self-Efficacy · Decision-Making Styles

1 Introduction

Interest in Emotional Intelligence (EI) has gained significant attraction since its popularisation in 1995 by Daniel Goleman's publication on EI [1]. Research studies have revealed the critical role of emotions in decision-making, work performance, stress coping, career progression and more [2–5]. In the higher education sector, EI research bears particular significance to both students and teachers as they operate in a high-stress and high social interaction environment. In the US alone in 2014, teacher attrition resulted in an estimated cost of $2.2billion annually [6]. This figure does not include

K. Daimi and A. Al Sadoon (Eds.): ICR 2023, LNNS 721, pp. 354–366, 2023.
https://doi.org/10.1007/978-3-031-35308-6_30

the costs borne by students from high teacher turnover rates. With evidence suggesting the important role of EI in aiding teachers cope better with stress, further knowledge in this domain is critical to improving the quality of education by reducing teacher attrition rates. The academic community is segregated into three different schools of thoughts stemming from the popularisation of EI since Goleman. The original Goleman model, now known as the mixed EI model, includes constructs that measure both EI ability and traits. EI ability measures the capacity of an individual whilst EI traits measure the actual behaviour of an individual. The criticism of Goleman's model was that an individual's ability does not necessarily translate to traits. This has led to the emergence of an EI ability model and an EI trait model. Whilst there are many different instruments used to measure ability model, mixed model or trait model, the following are the most notable for each type: Mayer-Salovey-Caruso Emotional Intelligence Test (MSCEIT) [7], Emotional Competence Inventory (ECI) [8], and Emotional quotient inventory (EQ-i) [9], respectively. Although there are many studies available to examine the effect of EI on teacher's behaviour in higher education, there is lack of study proposing the way each EI subscale interacts with each components of stress coping strategies, social self-efficacy and decision-making styles.

The following research questions and hypotheses have been set in this study:

1. Does EI ability have a significant positive direct relationship with stress coping strategies?
   - Null (H10): EI ability has no significant positive direct relationship with stress coping strategies
   - Alternate (H1a): EI ability has a significant positive direct relationship with stress coping strategies
2. Does EI ability have a significant positive direct relationship with social self-efficacy?
   - Null (H20): EI ability has no significant positive direct relationship with Social Self-Efficacy
   - Alternative (H2a): EI ability has a significant positive direct relationship with Social Self-Efficacy
3. Does EI ability have a significant positive direct relationship with decision-making style?
   - Null (H30): EI ability has no significant positive direct relationship with decision making style
   - Alternative (H3a): EI ability has a significant positive direct relationship with decision making style

The aim of this study is to explore the impacts of EI amongst higher education teachers in terms of their behaviour management based on the above three mentioned factors subscales. In the other word, the aim is to investigate the impact of EI on stress coping strategies, social self-efficacy, and decision-making style. This paper is organised as follows, Sect. 2 presents a literature review in the area of EI and related subject areas relevant to the three behavioral components influenced by EI. Following which, the approach to developing a framework (Sect. 3) will be detailed along with the proposed conceptual framework (Sect. 4). The last two sections (Sects. 5 and 6) present discussion together with some conclusion remarks of this paper.

2 Literature Review

2.1 EI Theoretical Concepts and EI Research

The academic community approaches EI through three different models. Whilst terminologies can vary, all EI models revolve around perceiving, understanding, managing and utilising emotions. The ability model places emphasis on measuring skills and competencies. Among all ability model scales Mayer-Salovey-Caruso developed the most notable one, MSCEIT 2.0 [7]. The trait model, is another model which emphasises on measuring actual behaviour. Researchers who support the trait model argue that knowledge and ability of EI constructs do not necessarily translate to actual behaviour, hence measuring traits independently will provide more meaningful results. The most notable trait model instrument is the Bar-On Emotional Quotient Inventory (Bar-On EQ-i 2.0) [10]. Goleman's EI mixed model measures constructs with a combination of ability and trait approaches [8]. None of the models can be considered to be superior to the other as they all offer valid uses. Most researchers choose the type of model based on research requirements. Much of the existing literature explores EI effects on positive outcomes such as job performance, job satisfaction, mental health, and organisational commitment. The consensus is that EI has significant positive relationship on job performance [2], job satisfaction, work attitude, leadership, and organisational commitment [3, 4, 11–13]. EI was also negatively correlated with 'poor' outcomes such as emotional exhaustion, stress, and burnout [5, 14]. This is significant to the current study as the teaching profession is known to be a high-stress environment with high burnout. Research studies reveal that learning EI is possible through training and hence should be taught as a skill or competence rather than intelligence [10, 14–17]. Through EI training and measuring participant's EI pre, post, and a follow-up of six to twelve months later, the lasting effects of EI training were confirmed [10, 14–17]. These studies support the idea that EI is a learnable form of skill or competence rather than inherent intelligence. To investigate EI impact on teacher behaviours in detail, the following three components were chosen: Stress Coping Strategies; Social Self-Efficacy; Decision-Making Styles. The first two factors were chosen due to the high-stress, high interpersonal interaction environment of the teaching profession. Decision-Making Style was included in the study given that emotion is a critical component of the decision-making process.

2.2 Stress Coping Strategies

EI has been shown to be an important concept in both theory and practice. It has the ability to assist individuals to better cope with stressful situations and suffer less stress, contributing to a healthy and stable workforce [18]. Fteiha and Awwad [19] carried out a study with the objective of determining the nature of the relationship that exists between EI and the ways in which university participants cope with stress. Participants' EI was evaluated using Goleman's theory of EI. In order to determine the nature of the relationship, a Stress Coping Style Inventory that was adapted to the UAE setting was also used in this study. According to the findings of the research, all of the correlation coefficients that were calculated for the various subdomains of the EI scale and the stress coping styles of active emotional coping and active issue coping were positive. The correlation coefficients between the different domains of the EI scale and the stress coping such as passive emotional and issue coping were negative. This study found there is a significant relationship between the level of EI and the strategies employed to deal with the effects of stress.

The capacity of teachers to exercise emotional control will assist them in coping with the stressful job elements that they are exposed to throughout the course of their workday (discipline problems, arguments with parents, excessive numbers of students in class, etc.). It is possible for teachers to experience negative emotions as a result of the factors listed above; however, if they are able to control these feelings in an appropriate manner, it will be possible for them to decrease their levels of occupational stress without reaching levels of burnout that are problematic [20]. In another relevant research conducted by Nogaj [21], the relationship between emotional intelligence and stress-coping strategies was investigated using a tool known as Popular Questionnaire of Emotional Intelligence (PQEI). According to the findings, it was shown that there was a substantial positive relationship between EI and the utilisation of task-oriented coping methods. The findings indicated that the participants' level of EI was directly correlated to the frequency with which they utilise stress-coping strategies that are efficient and effective; more specifically, these participants concentrated more on the task at hand and less on their feelings. In order to examine and analyse different methods of dealing with stress two suitable stress coping strategy scales were identified, namely The Ways of Coping Questionnaire (WCQ) [22] and COPE Inventory [23]. Whilst WCQ is useful to measure coping methods of teachers, the COPE Inventory covers more coping methods [23]. According to Chaudhry and Khan [24] who adopted a four-factor model (The COPE Brief) the overall Self Report Measure of Emotional Intelligence (SRMEI) score was positively correlated with Problem-Focused Coping and Positive Coping. EI was also negatively correlated to Active Avoidance Coping and Religious/Denial Coping. The advantage of using a self-report scale is that no special qualification is required to administer the questionnaire. This study did not investigate which SRMEI construct influences COPE Brief. Using a four-factor model diminishes the detail and insight to specific coping methods but simplifies the conceptualization of 14 coping methods. This experiment was conducted in Urdu (Hindustani language) where the cultural effects on EI and coping methods are unknown. There is also the risk of bias from translation.

2.3 Social Self-efficacy

Due to the critical nature of EI among teachers, educational institutions have begun to place a greater emphasis on developing this trait. In fact, EI is a form of social intelligence that encompasses the ability to control one's own emotions as well as those of others, the ability to choose between different emotions, and the capacity to use one's emotions to direct the course of one's life. Therefore, having this ability is really necessary in order to make the performance of teachers highly effective. Not only will having this skill enable instructors to communicate effectively with their students, but also with one another in the profession [25]. According to the findings of a study carried out by Wapao [26], emotional intelligence had a great effect on the level of self-efficacy, which in turn could influence the level of occupational stress. In another research study, Kosti-Bobanovi [27] considered a sample of Croatian teachers to evaluate the relationship between EI and self-efficacy in the context of teaching novice and experienced teachers of foreign languages. A positive correlation was found between EI and self-efficacy levels among teachers, which was the primary finding of the study. In line with previous studies, Wang and Wang [28] investigated the relationship between EI, self-efficacy, and burnout among teachers of foreign languages. It should not come as much of a surprise that EI is related to self-efficacy because teachers who could better understand their own emotions as well as those of their students and quickly transform unproductive emotions into productive ones would consider classroom instruction to be less difficult. The significant correlation between EI and self-efficacy was highlighted based on the results obtained from this research study. Recent studies show higher EI is positively associated with a higher level of self-efficacy [29, 30]. Morales-Rodríguez and Pérez-Mármol [31] investigated the relationship between the levels of self-efficacy and anxiety, as well as coping strategies and EI, that are found in university participants in Spain. The dependent variable in this study was identified to be self-efficacy and the independent variables included age, state anxiety, trait anxiety, coping techniques, and EI as measured by the Trait-Meta Mood Scale (TMMS) 24 subscales of emotional attention, clarity, and repair. A direct relationship was discovered between self-efficacy and EI characteristics of repair mood and emotional clarity. It demonstrated the impact of participation in EI training programmes and participants' overall self-efficacy in dealing with stress. In another research study, Debes [32] investigated the relationship between EI and self-efficacy in the context of school principals. This study aimed to establish whether school principals cultivate their emotional intelligence, it also examined the effect of EI on principals' levels of self-efficacy improvement. EI was considered as a predictive capacity on self-efficacy since the data demonstrated that three aspects of the school principals' EI (relationship managements, self regulation, and optimism) exhibited significant correlation with sense of self efficacy. Drawing from current studies, four social self-efficacy scales are identified. Three of the scales, Perceived Social Self-Efficacy Scale (PSSE) [33], The Social Self-Efficacy subscale of the Self-Efficacy Scale [34], and the Social Confidence subscale of the Skills Confidence Inventory [35] depended on the perception of the individual which could produce bias. The Workplace Social Self-Efficacy Scale (WSSE) [36] is based on behaviour which accurately reflects actual outcomes. Developed in the context of workplaces, WSSE is compatible for examining teachers. WSSE uses a 4-factor structure enabling examination of social behaviour in greater detail. Traș [37] explored the relationship between EQ-i and Perceived Social Self-Efficacy. Personal Awareness, Interpersonal Relations, and General Mood were positively correlated with Social Self-Efficacy. The limitation of using the Smith-Betz scale is that social self-efficacy can change depending on the context. This is where WSSE excels beyond the other scales. WSSE considers different contexts such as Social Gatherings, Performing in Public Contexts, Conflict Management, and Seeking and Offering Help. Another limitation to the EQ-i scale is that there are barriers to use.

They need to be purchased and formal qualifications are required for administering the test.

2.4 Decision-Making Style

According to Puertas Molero et al. [38], EI is a capacity that should be developed in teachers given its ability to enhance emotional self-regulation, making them stronger in terms of decision-making in daily situations in teaching environments, as well as being a key factor for the success of education. Research conducted by Zaki et al. [39] investigated the impact of EI training on the decision-making styles. A highly significant correlation was found between EI and the manner in which participants make decisions. The result of this study is comparable to that of El Othman et al. [40], who found that EI has a significant positive effect on intuitive decision-making style and a negative effect on avoidant and dependent decision-making styles. Ademi et al. [41] similarly highlighted the role of EI in decision making styles. According to this study and the results obtained, the scores of decision making can be significantly influenced by EI, meaning that the more emotionally intelligent a person is, the more skilled they would be in making decisions.

To evaluate decision-making styles, three scales were identified. The Melbourne Decision Making Questionnaire, designed for extremely stressful situations, the General Decision-Making Style (GDMS) [42] and the Decision Style Scale (DDS) [43] which is based on GDMS where deemed appropriate. The authors of DSS determined that the GDMS had problematic statistical intercorrelations between dimensions and poor internal consistencies. Consequently, the researchers reduced the number of factors to two: Rational and Intuitive. This produced a more reliable scale. Khan et al. [44] utilised the overall score of Wong & Law Emotional Intelligence scale (WLEIS) to predict decision-making styles. The researchers found that the overall score of WLEIS positively correlated with the intuitive and rational style with a stronger relationship in the latter. The limitation of this study is that it did not explore the effects of the four WLEIS subscales against GDMS. In summary, there are advantages and disadvantages to the above-mentioned studies. Some scales must be purchased and require formal qualification to administer. A self-report questionnaire typically does not have these requirements. The use of WSSE allows examining social self-efficacy under different contexts in contrast to other social self-efficacy scales which are unidimensional. It was also found that some studies only used the overall score of scales to examine relationships rather than investigating the subscales. This provides a research gap wherein the focus of this study is to cross-examine the subscale interactions between different scales. This will shed light on what aspects of EI that may affect the different behavioural components of teachers.

3 Approach to Developing a Framework

To address the gap in the literature examining EI impact on teacher behaviour and addressing the limitations of current studies, a new framework is proposed. Of the three EI models, it was determined that the ability model was best suited for this study as it interprets how EI ability translates to teacher behaviour. In this study, the Wong & Law's Emotional Intelligence Scale (WLEIS) [45] elements was chosen to propose a conceptual framework. The theoretical foundation of WLEIS is built on four constructs: 1) Appraisal and expression of emotion in oneself or Self-Emotion Appraisal (SEA) – This refers to an individual's ability to understand his/her own emotions and be able to express emotions naturally. 2) Appraisal and recognition of emotion in others or Others' Emotional Appraisal (OEA) – This refers to an individual's ability to perceive and understand the emotions of the people around them. 3) Regulation of emotion in oneself. (RoE) – This refers to an individual's ability to regulate his/her own emotions, enabling a more rapid recovery from psychological distress. 4) Use of emotion to facilitate performance. (UoE) – This refers to an individual's ability to make use of his/her own emotions by directing them toward constructive activities and personal performance. In order to develop the framework, the expected interactions between the EI constructs and the three-factor model of Brief COPE Stress Coping Strategies are examined. Chaudhry and Khan [24] demonstrated a significant positive relationship between EI and Problem-Focused Coping, and Positive Coping while having a negative relationship with Active Avoidance Coping and Religion/Denial Coping. Based on this, it is expected that EI will positively correlate to Problem-Focused Strategies. It is also expected that EI will be negatively correlated with Dysfunctional Coping Strategies. It is unclear whether EI will be positively correlated with Emotion-focused strategies as Positive reframing should be positively correlated while Turning to Religion should be negatively correlated. Despite this, it is expected that SEA and RoE will be overall positively correlated with Emotion-Focused Strategies due to the other items contained under this factor. Humour is a form of emotional regulation and SEA can be argued as a requirement for RoE to occur. When examining the relationship between EI and Social Self-Efficacy, it is expected that there will be a significant positive correlation between most constructs as social interactions require interpersonal emotional understanding. Using Bar-On EQ-i and the Social Self-Efficacy Scale of Smith-Betz, Traș [37] found that Personal Awareness, Interpersonal Relations, and General Mood were significant predictors of Social Self-Efficacy among university students. Personal awareness can be thought to be similar to SEA, and interpersonal relations can be thought to be similar to OEA. Therefore, it is expected that some positive correlations exist between SEA, OEA, and social self-efficacy constructs used in WSSE. The perceived social self-efficacy scale, however, does not have sub-constructs the way that WSSE does. Therefore, it is unknown which WSSE constructs will positively correlate to SEA and OEA. SEA and OEA will be positively correlated with Social Gathering. This is likely to be the construct that most closely matches the perceived social self-efficacy scale. For Performing in Public Contexts, it is predicted that SEA and RoE will have significant positive correlations as it requires an individual to appraise their own emotions before being able to regulate their own emotions. Performing well in public contexts should also require a degree of UoE and thus it is also expected to have a significant positive correlation. Conflict resolution requires emotional understanding of the parties involved and the ability to control emotions. Conflict Management between two or more individuals may only require OEA and RoE, but conflict management between the self and others would then also require SEA. Hence, it is expected that SEA, OEA, and RoE will be positively correlated to Conflict Management. Seeking and Offering Help can also be argued that the identification of emotional distress in the self (SEA) or others (OEA) is required before seeking or offering help. Therefore, SEA and OEA should positively correlate to Seeking and Offering Help. Khan et al. [44] found that EI positively predicted rational and intuitive decision-making styles with stronger significance in rational decision making. For both Intuitive and Rational Style, it is expected that RoE will have significant positive correlations as good decision-making requires calmness and controlled emotions, as uncontrollable emotions can cloud an individual's judgement.

4 Proposed Conceptual Framework

The proposed framework aimed at a model, where all four constructs discussed in the previous section are utilised concurrently to examine the relationship between EI subscales against the three behavioural components (stress coping strategies, social self-efficacy, decision-making style). Based on logic and existing literature, the likely interactions in the model are established as presented in Fig. 1. It is anticipated that SEA and RoE, two components of WLEIS, will have a positive influence on the utilisation of emotion-focused strategies, which may refer to factors such as positive reframing, acceptance, humour, turning to religion, and employing emotional support. It is important for teachers to feel that they have more to contribute than simply teaching to the students in their classroom. When they commit to being active participants in the decision-making process, they have the opportunity to play a more significant part in the overall success of the educational environment. Therefore, the ability to make sound decisions and choices is crucial for them. Based on our proposed framework, intuitive and rational decision making styles employed by teachers are expected to be influenced by emotional intelligence, more especially RoE. It is anticipated that the influence of RoE on emotion-focused strategies is positive; however, the effect of RoE on factors such as self-blame, self-distraction, and other components of dysfunctional coping strategies is negative. Emotional intelligence can have a positive effect not only on one's own emotions but also on the emotions of others. Problem-focused strategies, which aim to reduce the source of stress or increase the resources available to confront it, are another factor that will be positively affected by emotional intelligence. SEA and OEA also positively correlate with Active coping, planning, and use of instrumental support among teachers, their effect is similarly positive on teacher's social gathering activities. Teachers with high EI are expected to have a better performance dealing with others as the social self-efficacy can also be positively influenced by EI.

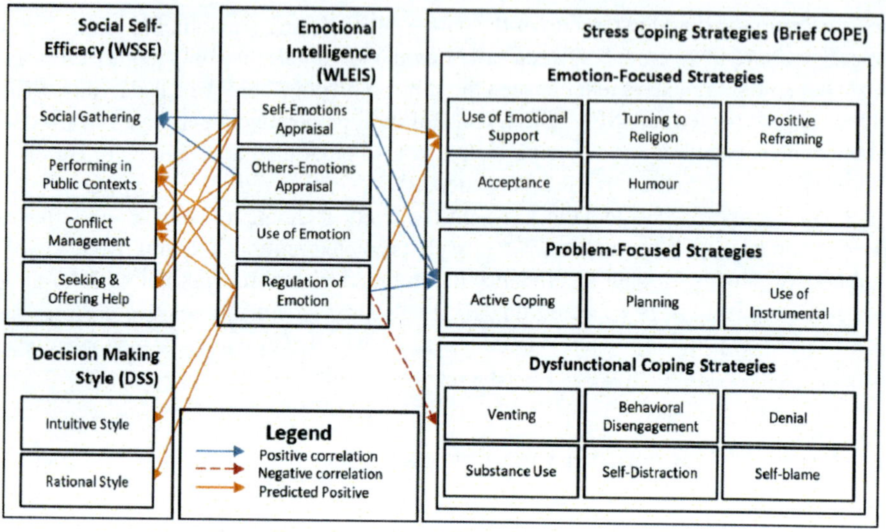

Fig. 1. Proposed conceptual framework of this study

5 Discussion

This study set out to improve the body of knowledge in the domain of the effects of EI on teachers' performance concerning stress coping strategies, decision making styles, and social self-efficacy. There are a variety of ways in which stressful situations manifest for teachers, and they will always make an effort to establish coping techniques whenever they are confronted with one. Better ways for dealing with stress can be developed with the assistance of emotional intelligence, which refers to the capacity to direct one's feelings in a constructive direction. Emotional intelligence has the potential to have a significant impact on three types of coping techniques: emotion-focused strategies, problem-focused strategies, and dysfunctional coping strategies. According to the model that we have proposed, it is anticipated that teachers who have a higher level of emotional intelligence will be less affected by stress. This is because emotionally intelligent teachers have a greater degree of control over how they perceive stress, and as a result, they obtain a greater number of coping strategies. According to our model, there is a possibility that a positive correlation exists between a person's emotional intelligence and their social abilities. The teacher's positive assessments of both their own and their students' emotions have a positive impact on the social gathering. Teachers who have a high level of emotional intelligence are likely to have a superior performance in public settings; they are able to readily seek and offer assistance as well as manage conflict in an efficient manner. EI has a beneficial effect on the quality of decisions made by teachers about students' educational pursuits. It is reasonable to anticipate that a teacher's approach to decision-making may be positively influenced by EI.

This study identified opportunities for new areas of further investigation in relation to teachers' fundamental role of EI in specific subcategories of the three variables mentioned above. This study had some limitations that need to be considered in future studies.

Our proposed conceptual framework and the relationship between components of each parameter are only based on previous literature and research studies. These interactions of the model are proposed to be put to test in future studies by doing data analysis. On the other hand, one of the components of our proposed framework is WLEIS The limitation of WLEIS is that the scale was developed using test subjects in Hong Kong and China. It is unknown if EI varies across different cultures. This limitation can be addressed in future research studies by extending the test to subjects in other countries and contexts, examining the WLEIS in a different cultural setting.

6 Conclusion

Emotional intelligence is one of the influential factors that can have a great impact on teachers' behaviour. Stress coping strategies, social self-efficacy, and decision making styles are among the parameters that can be influenced by EI among higher education teachers. The conceptual model proposed different interactions between EI constructs and three behavioural components. The effect of EI on constructive and destructive stress coping styles has been discussed, and based on that, it is expected that EI can negatively influence dysfunctional coping strategies. On the other hand, emotion-focused and problem-focused strategies can be positively influenced by EI. Therefore, teachers with higher EI can have better behaviours regarding different activities such as the use of emotional support, planning, active coping, etc. Teachers' social self-efficacy is also very important to be examined against EI since it helps them to perform specific interactional tasks, and also develop and maintain positive interpersonal relationships with students. Based on the proposed models, it could be concluded that El can play a significant role in teachers' behaviour regarding social interaction with students, such as social gathering, conflict management, seeking and offering help, etc. Finally, decision-making styles can be considered as a crucial parameter that can affect teachers' performance. Based on the proposed model, it is expected that teachers with higher emotional regulation abilities can make better intuitive and rational decisions in their working environment. A significant number of scholars considered emotional intelligence to be an essential indication in the academic domains of professional education. Teachers that are emotionally intelligent demonstrate care for their students, cultivate an emotional climate in the classroom that fosters an environment conducive to student learning, and assist other educators in becoming more effective in their efforts to assure academic success. It has been found that a teacher's emotional intelligence influences their level of comfort, self-efficacy, and job satisfaction, as well as improving their social relationships with their students. It is worth mentioning that, emotional intelligence has a direct impact on the process of teaching and learning. Therefore, emotional intelligence can be a very useful indicator for the hiring process as well as for determining the credentials required for a job. The enhancement of EI should be given crucial importance by higher educations in order to improve the candidate screening process, and institutes should also implement proper recruitment methods in order to ensure effective teaching and outstanding performance. The implication of this study is that EI could be considered as an assessable component during the recruitment process to hire teachers who are more effective at coping with stress, decision-making, and being socially malleable with colleagues.

References

1. Goleman, D.: Emotional Intelligence: Why it can Matter More than IQ. Bantam Books, New York (1995)
2. Shamsuddin, N., Rahman, A.R.: The Relationship between Emotional Intelligence and Job Performance of Call Centre Agents. Science Digest, pp. 75–81 (2014)
3. Yahyazadeh-Jeloudar, S., Lotfi-Goodarzi, F.: Teachers' emotional intelligence and its relationship with job satisfaction. Adv. Educ. **1**(1), 4–9 (2012)
4. Yin, H., Lee, J.C., Zhang, Z., Jin, Y.-l.: Exploring the relationship among teachers' emotional intelligence, emotional labor strategies and teaching satisfaction. Teach. Teach. Educ. 137–145 (2013)
5. Nizielski, S., Hallum, S., Schütz, A., Lopes, P.N.: A note on emotion appraisal and burnout: the mediating role of antecedent-focused coping strategies. J. Occup. Health Psychol. 363–369 (2013)
6. Haynes, M., Maddock, A., Goldrick, L.: ON THE PATH TO EQUITY: Improving the Effectiveness of Beginning Teachers. Alliance for Excellent Education, Washington (2014)
7. Mayer, J.D., Salovey, P., Caruso, D.R., Sitarenios, G.: Measuring Emotional Intelligence With the MSCEIT V2.0. Emotion, pp. 97–105 (2003)
8. Boyatzis, R.E., Goleman, D., Rhee, K.: Clustering competence in emotional intelligence: Insights from the Emotional Competence Inventory (ECI). In: Bar-On, R., Parker, J.D. (eds.) Handbook of Emotional Intelligence, pp. 343–362. Jossey-Bass, San Francisco (2000)
9. Bar-On, R.: Emotional Quotient Inventory: A Measure of Emotional Intelligence: Technical Manual. MHS. Multi-Health System Inc, Toronto (2004)
10. Zijlmans, L.J., Embregts, P.J., Gerits, L., Bosman, A.M., Derksen, J.J.: The effectiveness of staff training focused on increasing emotional intelligence and improving interaction between support staff and clients. J. Intell. Disabil. Res. 599–612 (2015)
11. Schutte, N.S., Loi, N.M.: Connections between emotional intelligence and workplace flourishing. Person. Individ. Differ. 134–139 (2014)
12. Anari, N.N.: Teachers: emotional intelligence, job satisfaction, and organizational commitment. J. Workplace Learn. 256–269 (2012)
13. Tang, H.-W.V., Yin, M.-S., Nelson, D.B.: The relationship between emotional intelligence and leadership practices - a cross-cultural study of academic leads in Taiwan and in the USA. J. Manag. Psychol. 899–926 (2010)
14. Abe, K., et al.: Expressing one's feelings and listening to others increases emotional intelligence: a pilot study of Asian medical students. BMC Med. Educ. 1–9 (2013)
15. Zijlmans, L.J., Embregts, P.J., Gerits, L., Bosman, A.M., Derksen, J.J.: Training emotional intelligence related to treatment skills of staff working with clients with intellectual disabilities and challenging behaviour. J. Intell. Disabil. Res. 219–230 (2011)
16. Nelis, D., Quoidbach, J., Mikolajczak, M., Hansenne, M.: Increasing emotional intelligence: (how) is it possible? Person. Individ. Differ. 36–41 (2009)
17. Schutte, N.S., Malouff, J.M., Thorsteinsson, E.B.: Increasing emotional intelligence through training: current status and future directions. Int. J. Emotion. Educ. 56–72 (2013)
18. Por, J., Barriball, L., Fitzpatrick, J., Roberts, J.: Emotional intelligence: its relationship to stress, coping, well-being and professional performance in nursing students. Nurse Educ. Today **31**(8), 855–860 (2011)
19. Fteiha, M., Awwad, N.: Emotional intelligence and its relationship with stress coping style. Health Psychol. Open **7**(2), 2055102920970416 (2020)
20. Martínez-Monteagudo, M.C., Inglés, C.J., Granados, L., Aparisi, D., García-Fernández, J.M.: Trait emotional intelligence profiles, burnout, anxiety, depression, and stress in secondary education teachers. Person. Individ. Differ. **142**, 53–61 (2019)

21. Nogaj, A.A.: Emotional intelligence and strategies for coping with stress among music school students in the context of visual art and general education students. J. Res. Music Educ. **68**(1), 78–96 (2020)
22. Austin, V., Shah, S., Muncer, S.: Teacher stress and coping strategies used to reduce stress. Occup. Therapy Int. 63–80 (2005)
23. Carver, C.S., Scheier, M.F., Weintraub, J.K.: Assessing coping strategies: a theoretically based approach. J. Person. Soc. Psychol. 267–283 (1989)
24. Chaudhry, A.G., Khan, S.E.: Relationship between emotional intelligence and coping strategies among university teachers of Khyber Pakhtunkhwa. Pakistan J. Sci. 81–84 (2015)
25. Subalakshmi, S., Sunderaraj, R., Manikandan, M.: Impact of emotional intelligence on stress: with special reference to government school teachers. J. Entrepreneurship Manag. **8**(1), 7–21 (2019)
26. Wapaño, M.R.R.: Emotional intelligence, self-efficacy and occupational stress of academic personnel. Int. J. Res. Innov. Soc. Sci. (IJRISS), **V**(V), 264–275 (2021)
27. Kostić-Bobanović, M.: Perceived emotional intelligence and self-efficacy among novice and experienced foreign language teachers. Econ. Res.-Ekonomska istraživanja **33**(1), 1200–1213 (2020)
28. Wang, Y., Wang, Y.: The interrelationship between emotional intelligence, self-efficacy, and burnout among foreign language teachers: a meta-analytic review. Front. Psychol. **13**, 913638 (2022). https://doi.org/10.3389/fpsyg.2022.913638
29. Wu, Y., Lian, K., Hong, P., Liu, S., Lin, R.M., Lian, R.: Teachers' emotional intelligence and self-efficacy: mediating role of teaching performance. Soc. Behav. Personal. Int. J. **47**(3), 1–10 (2019)
30. Ruiz-Fernández, M.D., Alcaraz-Córdoba, A., López-Rodríguez, M.M., Fernández-Sola, C., Granero-Molina, J., Hernández-Padilla, J.M.: The effect of home visit simulation on emotional intelligence, self-efficacy, empowerment, and stress in nursing students. A single group pre-post intervention study. Nurse Educ. Today **117**, 105487 (2022)
31. Morales-Rodríguez, F.M., Pérez-Mármol, J.M.: The role of anxiety, coping strategies, and emotional intelligence on general perceived self-efficacy in university students. Front. Psychol. **10**, 1689 (2019)
32. Debes, G.: The predictive power of emotional intelligence on self efficacy: a case of school principals. Int. Online J. Educ. Teach. **8**(1), 148–167 (2021)
33. Smith, H.M., Betz, N.E.: Development and validation of a scale of perceived social self-efficacy. J. Career Assess. 283–301 (2000)
34. Sherer, M., Maddux, J.E.: The self-efficacy scale: construction and validation. Psychol. Rep. 663–671 (1982)
35. Harmon, L.W., Borgen, F.H., Berreth, J.M., King, J.C.: The skills confidence inventory: a measure of self-efficacy. J. Career Assess. 457–477 (1996)
36. Fan, J., et al.: Workplace social self-efficacy: concept, measure, and initial validity evidence. J. Career Assess. 91–110 (2013)
37. Traş, Z.: Analysis of social self efficacy and emotional intelligence in university students. Soc. Sci. Educ. Res. Rev. 107–113 (2016)
38. Puertas Molero, P., Zurita Ortega, F., Ubago Jiménez, J.L., González Valero, G.: Influence of emotional intelligence and burnout syndrome on teachers well-being: a systematic review. Soc. Sci. **8**(6), 185 (2019)
39. Zaki, H.N., Abd-Elrhaman, E.S.A., Ghoneimy, A.G.H.: The effect of emotional intelligence program on decision making style. Am. J. Nurs. **6**(6), 524–532 (2018)
40. El Othman, R., El Othman, R., Hallit, R., Obeid, S., Hallit, S.: Personality traits, emotional intelligence and decision-making styles in Lebanese universities medical students. BMC Psychol. **8**(1), 1–14 (2020)

41. Ademi, M., Afendouli, P., Louka, P.: The correlation between perceived stress, emotional intelligence and decision making: a multiple linear regression analysis. Dialog. Clin. Neurosci. Mental Health **5**(4), 149–160 (2022)
42. Scott, S.G., Bruce, R.A.: Decision-making style: the development and assessment of a new measure. Educ. Psychol. Meas. 818–831 (1995)
43. Hamilton, K., Shih, S.-I., Mohammed, S.: The development and validation of the rational and intuitive decision styles scale. J. Person. Assess. 523–535 (2016)
44. Khan, E.A., Riaz, M.N., Batool, N., Riaz, M.A.: Emotional intelligence as a predictor of decision making styles among university students. J. Appl. Environ. Biol. Sci. 93–99 (2016)
45. Law, K.S., Wong, C.-S., Song, L.J.: The construct and criterion validity of emotional intelligence and its potential utility for management studies. J. Appl. Psychol. 483–496 (2004)

Internet of Things

Industrial Air Quality Visual Sensor Analytics

Eleftheria Katsiri(✉)

Department of Electrical and Computer Engineering, Democritus University of Thrace, Xanthi 67100, Greece
ekatsiri@gmail.com

Abstract. Rapid advancements in affordable, miniaturised air pollution sensor technologies and embedded systems are enabling a new wave of reliable air quality sensing devices. Due to their ability to measure air pollution ad hoc and in great spatio-temporal resolution such devices enable advanced processing and analytics.

Our team has been engaged in the development of reliable air quality sensing devices using low-cost sensors, custom sensor boards, embedded software and cloud services. Our devices use pre-calibrated optical Particulate Matter (PM) sensors, measuring concentrations in ug/m^3 of *PM1.0*, *PM2.5* and *PM10*, *NDIR*, CO_2 sensors and electrochemical *CO* sensors, as well as differential pressure sensors, while all devices monitor also humidity and temperature. The data is sampled at a few seconds interval and it is transferred to a cloud-based platform where is stored and visualised in real-time, raising alerts. A delay tolerant middleware stores data locally, temporarily for up to 12 h.

The devices have good accuracy, response time and sensitivity in indoor pollution levels, however, they suffer from low signal strength of the WiFi receiver as a result of which they often become disconnected for long period of times. A sensor data analytics platform was therefore developed using python. We introduce two new algorithms for auditing the sampling process and detecting and removing outliers specific to air quality data. Furthermore we introduce a new methodology for detecting patterns based on visual analytics.

We have conducted a pilot application in a state-of-the art industrial space that is sensitive to infection caused by particulate matter such as dust. Fifteen PM devices were installed in three different production areas with varying air quality sensitivity. Indicative results from two of the devices from the first production area show that mining sensor time-series with the above analytics produces useful insights on the level of pollution and industrial activity while confirming the stable performance of our devices.

Keywords: low-cost sensors · air quality monitoring · internet of things · wireless sensor networks · delay tolerant networking · middleware · analytics · python · pattern detection · outliers · visual analytics

K. Daimi and A. Al Sadoon (Eds.): ICR 2023, LNNS 721, pp. 369–380, 2023.
https://doi.org/10.1007/978-3-031-35308-6_31

1 Introduction

In recent years the development of low-cost sensor technology [1–8] has been a critical factor that changed the pollution detection paradigm [9,10]. The combination of great spatio-temporal resolution and real-time monitoring makes it possible to answer new questions about the underlying causes of poor air quality, ensure more accurate modelling and prediction at local scales [11] improve the ability to identify the links between air quality and human health [12,13], or environmental degradation [14], identify potential air pollution "hot spots", enhance the ability to quantify the impacts of pollutant mitigation techniques and promote savings through *on-demand ventilation* [15].

Three types of reliable air quality measurement devices, *Particulate Matter (PM), Differential Pressure (DP), Air quality Outdoor Gases (AQG)* were developed for monitoring air quality in indoor micro-climates [35]. Although their performance is stable, they have increased maintenance requirements due to harsh industrial environments where heavy equipment and large, walled areas, cause signal deflection and extenuation to which the devices are sensitive due to lack of powerful antennas and real-time clocks.

Furthermore, the embedded middleware which collects data from the sensors and communicates it to the cloud is vulnerable to network outages of more than 12 h, after which, data that is temporarily stored is lost. Furthermore, unavailability of the cloud timeseries database e.g., due to disk space fullness may cause more data to be lost. Although data retention rates can help, this is not realistic as historic data needs to be collected and analysed.

Most of the works reported in the literature have deployed low-cost-sensor devices outdoors, mostly in urban settings where there is significant pollution [16–26]. Issues and challenges like privacy problem, user behavior, and data visualization were studied in [27–29].

2 Methods

This paper focuses in the case of a modern dairy in in Greece that produces milk and yoghurt. Outdoor sources of pollution include a) a flour mill located south of the dairy and b) Saharan dust and c) microorganisms,whose correlation with air quality is proven in the literature [30–32] [33]. The levels of particulate matter concentration in the production areas are and monitored periodically to prove compliance with European workplace legislation. Eighteen sensing devices (15 PM and 3 DP ones) were deployed at two productions areas that are highly sensitive to contaminants; Three PM devices were deployed outdoors and twelve indoors measuring particulate matter concentrations at *points of interest*, i.e., locations identified as critical for health and safety. As a result, a very large volume of additional continuous measurements were collected [34]. Each sensing device is associated with a Grafana [36] dashboard that provides visual analytics. InfluxDB, a time-series database [37], stores the data tuples formatted by the LineProtocol.

2.1 Analytic Functions

Sensor data quality [38] generally requires for sensor data to be available in real-time, not to contain outliers, not to suffer from bias and not to contain missing values. Bias has to do with drift, stuck-at-zero values or constants - indicating a fault of the sensor - noise or uncertainty. Methods in sensor data quality deal with *detection of faults* [39] and *quantification of uncertainty* [40,41] i.e. the presence of inaccurate values [42,43] due to hardware failure, network disruption, software faults or noise.

White noise. A time series can be *white noise* [50,51] if the samples are independent and uniformly distributed with a mean of zero. This means that the standard deviation is the same for each sample and that there is no correlation between each sample and all the others. Time series data are expected to contain some white noise component on top of the signal generated by the underlying process.

$$y(t) = signal(t) + noise(t) \tag{1}$$

In order to quantify the strength and type of relationship between observations and their lags, *auto-correlation plots* were used.

Random walk. A *random walk* is a time-series where the next value in the sequence is a modification of the previous value in the sequence. This dependence provides some consistency from step-to-step rather than the large jumps that a series of independent, random numbers provides.

$$y(t) = B0 + B1 * X(t-1) + e(t) \tag{2}$$

Time-series re-sampling. Each raw timeseries, after being converted to a Pandas data-frame, was re-sampled in order to aggregate it over the time windows of interest. First, the index of the data-frame was set to the "time" column.

```
df.set_index('TIME', inplace=True)
```

Then data sampled are grouped by the desirable interval. e.g., to create a weekly group:

```
weekly_group = df.resample('7D')
```

Last, the aggregate (agg) function of the pandas library is called with parameters a list of functions to summarise the data.

```
weekly_df = weekly_group.agg({'COLUMN_A': ['min', 'max'],
                              'COLUMN_B': ['mean', 'median', std]})
```

2.2 Overall Methodology

In this paper all a) visual analytics, b) descriptive statistics and c) time-series analytics were developed in order to:

- describe the elements of the data-set qualitatively

- explore the temporal structure of the data-set
- understand the distribution of observations
- explore the change of the distribution over intervals

The scope of our analysis approach is two-fold and it encompasses both *production area analytics*, i.e. analysis of multiple time-series generated by devices that are collocated in a production area and *point-of-interest avalytics*, i.e. analysis of a single time-series generated by a single device at a specific point of interest. At point-of-interest level, analytic functions were applied at:

- the entire raw data of each device, ranging from 1/1/2020 to 31/12/2020 and 1/3/2020 to 31/3/2021, respectively
- data grouped per month, day of the week, hour-of-day, shift, weekday/weekend

while at room level the functions were applied at tuples of time-series generated by collocated devices at the same interval.

First the time series are downloaded from InfluxDB and converted to csv. Next, the sampling middleware is audited and one-sample peaks are isolated and removed. Next, the *mean, median, standard deviation, min* and *max* values are calculated and *density, histogram, delay and line plots* are generated in order to check for white noise [44] and random walk [45] and to detect patterns between variables.

3 Air Quality Sensor Data Analysis Algorithms

The ***sampling process auditing algorithm*** first counts number of data points per intervals of different granularity in order to determine data loss. Missing values are ignored as they do not make any difference to the analysis. Next the sampling rate is checked by counting the number of sample pairs that differ by the period of the original time series. This process shows whether any delays e.g. from software timers or communication delays exist. Last the data-sets are tested for NaN values.

The ***outlier detection and removal algorithm*** comprises three steps: First the timeseries were visualised using boxplots (*Interquartile (IQR)* method) to detect any extreme data points. Next, the *z-score* [48,49] is calculated (Eq. 3)

$$z_i = (x_i - \mu)/\sigma \tag{3}$$

where x_i is the sensor observation, μ is the average value and σ is the standard deviation. Next, the number of samples whose value differed more than x times the standard deviation of the time-series where $x > 3$ is plotted. Based on this result, a cut-off value is decided in order to create a set of outliers amounting to less than 0.001% of the data-set. Next, the same process is repeated for annual day-of-the-week averages and a second set of outliers is generated. After the overlapping outliers of the above two sets are removed, the remaining outliers are filtered by comparing them to their predecessor: those that differ more than 20% are removed.

Regarding the ***data-sets:*** *Device 2*, consists of 400,656 samples taken over 66 d while *Device 7*, consists of 2 291 991 samples taken over 292 d.

$$PM1.0(ug/m^3), PM10(ug/m^3), PM2.5(ug/m^3), RH(\%), T(C)$$

$PM*$ variables represent the mass of suspended particles in the atmosphere with a diameter of $< 1um, < 2.5um$ and $< 10um$, respectively. They express how many micrograms of particles we have per cubic meter of indoor air. $RH(\%)$ represents the percentage of relative humidity in the atmosphere and T(C) the temperature in degrees Celsius at the point-of-interest. "time" is the data-point timestamp representing the time at the device end when the microprocessor logged the measurement.

4 Results

Point of interest analysis was carried out on two different data-sets following the methodology in the previous sections. Each of which came from a different sensing device; The first data-set, *Device 2*, consists of 400,656 samples taken over 66 d. The second data-set, *Device 7*, consists of 2 291 991 samples taken over 292 d. None of the data-sets contains any NaN values, however both contain missing values. In Device 2, data ranges from March 2020 to January 2021. May 2020, February 2020, October 2020 and January 2021 have few samples while in Device 7 data ranges from March 2020 to March 2021 and is distributed as follows: October, September, April and July 2020 contribute to the total number of samples with more than 10% each. The months of February, January, November 2020 and June, March 2021 participate in the total number of samples with percentages ranging from 5.5% to 8.76%. Finally, there is May 2020 which is a small percentage of the total samples, 0.162% (5336 samples).

The distribution of data points over the days of the week is similar for both data-sets: in Device 2, most probably because of the missing values, Saturday, Sunday and Monday have similar smaller percentages of samples in comparison with the rest of the week, whereas in Device 7 it is Mondays and Fridays that have a slightly smaller percentage of data points.

The distribution of data points per shift (6:00–14:00, 14:00–22:00, 22:00–6:00) is uniform as there is a relatively even distribution of samples in each of the shifts (33% in each).

The distribution of data points over each day of the data set, shows that for Device 7 some data was missed the first week of July and sometimes the first and last day of each monthly data-set. The number of samples collected each day is stable and close to 140000 samples per day.

The distribution of consecutive samples grouped in groups of different sizes, shows that most datapoints in Device 2 were collected in groups of 4, while in device 7 in groups of 8. This was due to a sleep() statement in troducing a delay in data collection as well as a difference in configuration between the two devices, setting the size of a buffer to 4 and 8 measurements, for Device 2 and 7, respectively. Both oversights were corrected in future measurements.

The timeseries were resampled with a fixed 5 sec interval before they were further analysed, to eliminate the error.

A histogram of gaps between consecutive data points, confirms the missing data and gives an insight in the size of the gaps. The Device 2 histogram has a bimodal shape as 2 gaps fall in the 1–5 days interval and 2 more in the larger than 2 m (May 2020 to September 2020) and (October 2020 to January 2021) intervals. The Device 7 histogram is uniform, as there exist 4 gaps each of a different size, 1–5 days, 10–15 days, 25–30 days (May 2020) and greater than 1m (December 2020).

So by creating the graphs with the overall mean and the mean per day for all the variables, it is observed that no variable has an overall mean of zero and that the mean per day varies without ever becoming zero. So there is an indication of no white noise in all variables in the data-set. This is confirmed by the auto-correlation graphs for each variable. Similarly the data-sets were checked for the existence of random walk but there was no significant evidence.

Histograms of PM1, PM2.5 and PM10 showed overall normal distributions. Lag plots of PM1, PM2.5 at point of interest level of the entire timeseries data, show weak correlation while PM10 almost no corellation. When applied to monthly timeseries they show a weak positive correlation that suggests that they could be modelled at this scale. As expected T(C) anf RH(%) are strongly positively correlated. More analysis at week and few day intervals is required to identify the optimal scale of modelling. Furthermore the lag plots connecting a car a current value with more than the previous recent one would be very useful. Furthermore, autocorrelation plots show weak autocorrelation.

Since no significant randomness exists in the data, Pearson corellation was applied to the two datasets and the results were plotted with a heat map. Both datasets show strong corellation between PM1.0 and PM 2.5, as well as PM2.5 and PM10. In Device 2, the former is 0.92 and the latter 0.73, while in Device 7 the same variables are 0.59 and 0.55. This is expected as PM2.5 contain PM1.0 and PM10 contain PM2.5. There is no significant correllation of the PM variables with either humidity or temperature.

After applying the outlier detection algorithm, for Device 7 16246 outliers were identified per 3302258 total data points, aka 0.005% of the data-set whereas for Device 2 the number of outliers was 2188 out of 400656 samples amounting to approximately 0.005%. Last but not least, by plotting the mean at the level of the re-sampled time-series, the following observations were made.

4.1 Device 7

The ***annual day-of-the-week average values***of both PM1.0 and PM2.5 are significantly higher on Saturdays while PM10 ones on Tuesday. The maximum annual average standard deviation follows this pattern. T(C) peaks on Wednesdays and RH(%) is lowest on Wednesdays.

Conclusion: We observe the following sequential pattern: the T(C) annual day-of-the-week average timeseries rising gradually during Sunday-Monday-Tuesday-

Wednesday, followed by the RH(%) one rising during Thursday-Friday-Saturday-Sunday, followed by the PM* ones rising through Friday-Saturday-Sunday. This means that PMs follow RH(%) with a lag of one and RH(%) follows T(C) with a lag of 4.

The ***annual daily max & min values*** for PM1.0 occur on Thursday (max), for PM2.5 on Tuesday and for PM10 on Mondays. The annual maximum T(C) occurs on Tuesday while for RH(%) on Friday. **Conclusion:** We observe a similar pattern as above with PM1.0, PM2.5, PM10 preceding RH(%) by one lag.

The ***monthly average values*** for PM1.0, PM2.5 and PM10 peak in May 2020 while the minimum monthly average occurred in March 2020. The maximum monthly average for T(C) is on March 2020 and the minimum in May 2020. From May 2020 to March 2021 the monthly average follows the annual seasonality. Vice versa, the maximum monthly average for RH(%) is in May2020 and the minimum in March 2020. The monthly average standard deviation time-series of PM1.0, PM2.5 and PM10 follows the same pattern as the average while for T(C) and RH(%) it is constant.

Conclusion: As before, we observe a pattern starting with T(C) dropping gradually from March to May 2020, rising again until August, dropping till January 2021 etc. Humidity behaves the other way round and all PMs follow humidity without lag in this case.

The ***monthly max & min values*** of PM1.0 peak in September 2020, the ones of PM2.5 in January 2021 and those of PM10 in April 2020. For T(C) the maximum value is in September 2020 while RH(%) has a minimum in November 2021. **Conclusion:** We observe a similar pattern as above with PM1.0. PM2.5, PM10 following RH(%) without lag.

The ***annual hour-of-the-day averages*** for PM1.0 and PM2.5 peak at 8:00, for PM10 at 18:00, for T(C) the minimum average is at 8:00 and the max at 18:00 while for RH(%) the minimum is at 7:00. **Conclusion:** We observe a similar pattern as above with PM1.0, PM2.5, PM10 following RH(%) without lag and RH(%) preceding T(C) by one lag.

The ***annual hour-of-the-day max & min*** for PM1.0,PM2.5,PM10 and RH(%) (minimum) is around 15:00. RH (%) values are high between 10:00 until midnight and low from midnight to 10:00, ranging from 12 to 90 while T(C) values range from 15C to 33C. **Conclusion:** We observe a similar pattern as above with PM hour-of-the-day maximums follow without lag the behaviour of RH(%)

The ***annual averages per shift*** for PM1.0 and PM2.5 the maximum average value per shift occurs during the morning shift (6:00–14:00) while for PM10 it occurs during the afternoon shift (14:00 - 22:00). For RH(%) and T(C) there is no significant difference. **Conclusion:** We observe a similar pattern as above with PM1.0, PM2.5, PM10 preceding by one lag RH(%).

The ***annual max & min per shift*** for PM1.0,PM2.5, PM10 and RH(%) the maximum average value per shift occurs during the afternoon shift (14:00-20:00).

For RH(%) and T(C)there is no significant difference. **Conclusion:** We observe a similar pattern as above with PM1.0, PM2.5, PM10 following RH(%) without lag.

The ***annual weekend vs annual weekday averages*** For PM1.0,PM2.5, PM10 and RH(%) over the weekend is significantly higher to that over weekdays. For RH(%) the average over weekends is slightly higher to that over weekdays while for T(C) the opposite holds. **Conclusion:** We observe a similar pattern as above with PM1.0, PM2.5, PM10 following RH(%) without lag.

The ***annual weekend vs annual weekday min & max.*** For PM1.0,PM2.5, PM10 and RH(%) the maximum value over the weekdays is significantly higher to that over weekends, while for T(C) the opposite holds. **Conclusion:** We observe a similar pattern as above with PM1.0, PM2.5, PM10 following RH(%) with a lag.

4.2 Device 2

The ***annual day-of-the-week average values*** of PM1.0, PM2.5 and PM10 are significantly higher on Wednesdays, for RH(%) on Thursdays and for T(C) on Tuesdays. **Conclusion:** This indicates a pattern of T(C) increasing gradually during Sunday-Monday-Tuesday followed by a similar increase of PMs during Sunday-to-Wednesday and of RH during Tuesday-Wednesday-Thursday. In this case PMs follow T(C) without a lag while RH(%) follows T(C) with a lag of one.

The ***annual day-of-the-week max & min values*** for PM1.0,PM2.5,PM10 and RH(%) follow T(C) by two lags.

The ***monthly average values*** for PM1.0, PM2.5 and PM10 and RH(%) peak in February 2020 while the minimum occurs in May 2020. T(C) follows the annual seasonality. **Conclusion:** As before, we observe a pattern starting with T(C) rising gradually from February to May 2020, then dropping till January 2021. Humidity is the opposite and PMs follow humidity without lag in this case. As there is no data between May and September we don't know if there is a second peak as is the case with Device 7.

The ***monthly max & min values*** for PM1.0 peak in September 2020, for PM2.5 in January 2021 and for PM10 in April 2020. **Conclusion:** As before, we observe a similar pattern with PM1.0, PM2.5, PM10 and RH(%)following T(C) without lag.

The ***annual hour-of-the-day average values*** for PM1.0, PM2.5 and PM10 peak at 4:00 with a second higher at 18:00. RH(%) follows the same pattern while T(C) precedes RH(%)by two lags. T(C) shows daily seasonality with a peak around 14:00 **Conclusion:** As before, we observe a similar pattern with PM1.0, PM2.5, PM10 following RH(%) without lag and T(C) by two lags. Furthermore there is clear activity during the night and evening.

hour-of-the-day annual max & min. All PM1.0,PM2.5,PM10 and RH(%) follow T(C) by four lags. T(C) ranges from 15C to 33C and RH(%) from 20 to 70.

The ***annual averages per shift*** for all PM1.0, PM2.5, PM10, RH(%) and T(C) peak during the morning shift (6:00–14:00). *The* ***annual max & min per shift*** for PM1.0 the maximum occurs during the afternoon shift, for PM2.5 during the morning shift and for PM10 during the night shift. For T(C) and RH(%) during the afternoon shift.

annual weekend vs annual weekday averages. For all PM1.0, PM2.5, PM10,the maximum annual average of weekdays is higher than weekends. The opposite holds for RH(%) and T(C).

5 Conclusions

An air quality sensor data analytics platform developed using python and kaggle. We introduce two new algorithms for auditing the sampling process and detecting and removing outliers specific to air quality data. Furthermore we introduce a new methodology for detecting patterns based on visual analytics.

We applied these methods during an experiment that took place in a modern dairy in Greece where 12 sensing devices were installed monitoring concentrations of particulate matter, humidity and temperature for one year. Both raw and aggregated timeseries generated by two sensing devices were processed in python with visual analytics such as histograms, line, lag and pie plots, checked for noise and randomness, and finally aggregated annually, monthly, daily, hourly, per shift and weekday. With respect to air quality time series we observed that they do not exhibit white noise, random walk and that they can be modelled in order to detect trends and make predictions. Furthermore our work has unveiled a general behaviour/pattern where particulate matter annual and monthly average time-series behaviour follows closely that of humidity either without lag or with a small lag. Similarly humidity follows temperature by a small lag. In the case of particulate matter maximum values, these seem to follow humidity and often temperature without lag. The above results will be confirmed by further testing e.g., calculating time-series synchronicity. Trend detection and prediction more specifically is the subject of an upcoming paper.

References

1. Mahajan, S., Kumar, P.: Evaluation of low-cost sensors for quantitative personal exposure monitoring. Sustain. Cities Soc., 102076 (2020)
2. Kumar, P., Morawska, L., Martani, C., Biskos, G., Neophytou, M., Di Sabatino, S., et al.: The rise of low-cost sensing for managing air pollution in cities. Environ. Int. **75**, 199–205 (2015)

3. Morawska, L., Thai, P.K., Liu, X., Asumadu-Sakyi, A., Ayoko, G., Bartonova, A., et al.: Applications of low-cost sensing technologies for air quality monitoring and exposure assessment: how far have they gone? Environ. Int. **116**(2018), 286–299 (2018). https://doi.org/10.1016/j.envint.2018.04.018
4. Snyder, E.G., Watkins, T.H., Solomon, P.A., Thoma, E.D., Williams, R.W., Hagler, G.S.W., et al.: Applications of low-cost sensing technologies for air quality monitoring and exposure assessment: how far have they gone? Environ. Sci. Technol. **47**(2013), 11369–11377 (2013)
5. Anjomshoaa, A., Duarte, F., Rennings, D., Matarazzo, T.J., deSouza, P., Ratti, C.: City scanner: Building and scheduling a mobile sensing platform for smart city services. IEEE Internet Things J. **5**, 4567–4579 (2018)
6. DeSouza, P., Anjomshoaa, A., Duarte, F., Kahn, R., Kumar, P., Ratti, C.: Air quality monitoring using mobile low-cost sensors mounted on trash-trucks: methods development and lessons learned. Sustain. Cities Soc. **60**, 102239 (2020)
7. Elen, B., Peters, J., Poppel, M.V., Bleux, N., Theunis, J., Reggente, M., et al.: The aeroflex: a bicycle for mobile air quality measurements. Sensors **13**(2013), 221–240 (2013)
8. Dutta, P., et al.: Common sense: participatory urban sensing using a network of handheld air quality monitors. In: Proceedings of the 7th ACM Conference on Embedded Networked Sensor Systems, Berkeley, CA, USA, 4–6 November ACM: New York, NY, USA, 2009; pp. 349–350 (2009)
9. Krzyzanowski, M., Martin, R.V., Van Dingenen, R., van Donkelaar, A., Thurston, G.D.: Exposure assessment for estimation of the global burden of disease attributable to outdoor air pollution. Environ. Sci. Technol. **46**, 652–660 (2012)
10. WHO- Regional office for Europe, Review of evidence on health aspects of air pollution - REVIHAAP project: final technical report (2013)
11. Hasenfratz, D., Saukh, O., Sturzenegger, S., Thiele, L.: Participatory air pollution monitoring using smartphones. Mobile Sens. **1**, 1–5 (2012)
12. deSouza, P., Kahn, A.R., Limbacher, A.J., Marais, A.E., Duarte, F., Ratti, C.: Combining low-cost, surface-based aerosol monitors with size-resolved satellite data for air quality applications. Atmos. Measur. Tech. **13**(10), 5319–5334 (2020). https://doi.org/10.5194/amt-13-5319-2020
13. Koukouli, M.E., et al.: Sudden changes in nitrogen dioxide emissions over Greece due to lockdown after the outbreak of Covid-19. Atmos. Chem. Phys. **21**(21), 1759–1774 (2020)
14. Postolache, O.A., Pereira, J.M.D., Girao, P.M.B.S.: Smart sensors network for air quality monitoring applications. IEEE Trans. Instrum. Meas. **58**, 3253–3262 (2009)
15. Kumar, P., et al.: Indoor air quality and energy management through real-time sensing in commercial buildings. Energy Build. **111**(145–153), 0378–7788 (2016)
16. Hagan, D.H., Gani, S., Bhandari, S., Patel, K., Habib, G., Apte, J., Hildebrandt Ruiz, L., Kroll, H.J.: Inferring aerosol sources from low-cost air quality sensor measurements: a case study in Delhi, India. Environ. Sci. Technol. Lett. **6**(8), 467–472 (2019)
17. Yazdi, M.N., Arhami, N., Delavarrafiee, M., Ketabchy, M.: Developing air exchange rate models by evaluating vehicle in-cabin air pollutant exposures in a highway and tunnel setting: case study of Tehran. Iran, Environ. Sci. Pollut. Res. Int. **26**(1), 501–513 (2019)
18. Bukowiecki, N., Dommen, J., Prévôt, A.S.H., Richter, R., Weingartner, E., Baltensperger, U.: A mobile pollutant measurement laboratory-Measuring gas phase and aerosol ambient concentrations with high spatial and temporal resolution. Atmos. Environ. **36**, 5569–5579 (2002)

19. Apte, J.S., Messier, K.P., Gani, S., Brauer, M., Kirchstetter, T.W., Lunden, M.M., et al.: High-resolution air pollution mapping with google street view cars: exploiting big data. Environ. Sci. Technol. **51**, 6999–7008 (2017)
20. Capezzuto, L., et al.: A maker friendly mobile and social sensing approach to urban air quality monitoring. In: Proceedings of the 2014 IEEE on SENSORS, Valencia, Spain, pp. 12–16 (2014)
21. Murty, R.N., et al.: Citysense: an urban-scale wireless sensor network and testbed. In: Proceedings of the 2008 IEEE Conference on Technologies for Homeland Security, Waltham, MA, USA, 12–13 May 2008, pp. 583–588 (2008)
22. Kadri, A., Yaacoub, E., Mushtaha, M., Abu-Dayya, A.: Wireless sensor network for real-time air pollution monitoring. In: Proceedings of the 2013 1st International Conference on Communications, Signal Processing, and their applications (ICCSPA), Sharjah, United Arab Emirates, 12–14 February, pp. 1–5 (2013)
23. Jiang, Y., et al.: MAQS: a personalized mobile sensing system for indoor air quality monitoring. In: Proceedings of the 13th International Conference on Ubiquitous Computing, Beijing, China, 17–21 September 2011; ACM: New York, NY, USA, pp. 271–280 (2011)
24. Jelicic, V., Magno, M., Brunelli, D., Paci, G., Benini, L.: Context-adaptive multimodal wireless sensor network for energy-efficient gas monitoring. IEEE Sens. J. **13**, 328–338 (2013)
25. Mansour, S., Nasser, N., Karim, L., Ali, A.: Wireless sensor network-based air quality monitoring system. In: Proceedings of the 2014 International Conference on Computing, Networking and Communications (ICNC), Honolulu, HI, USA, pp. 545–550 (2014)
26. Sun, L., Wong, K.C., Wei, P., Ye, S., Huang, H., Yang, F., Westerdahl, D., Louie, P.K., Luk, C.W., Ning, Z.: Development and application of a next generation air sensor network for the Hong Kong marathon 2015 air quality monitoring. Sensors **16**, 211 (2016)
27. Honicky, R., Brewer, E.A., Paulos, E., White, R.: N-smarts: networked suite of mobile atmospheric real-time sensors. In: Proceedings of the Second ACM SIGCOMM Workshop on Networked Systems for Developing Regions, Seattle, WA, USA, 18 August 2008; ACM: New York, NY, USA, pp. 25–30 (2008)
28. Lane, N.D., Miluzzo, E., Lu, H., Peebles, D., Choudhury, T., Campbell, A.T.: A survey of mobile phone sensing. IEEE Commun. Mag. **48**, 140–150 (2010)
29. Helbig, C., Bauer, H.-S., Rink, K., Wulfmeyer, V., Frank, M., Kolditz, O.: Concept and workflow for 3D visualization of atmospheric data in a virtual reality environment for analytical approaches. Environ. Earth Sci. **72**(10), 3767–3780 (2014). https://doi.org/10.1007/s12665-014-3136-6
30. Setti, L., et al.: Evaluation of the potential relationship between Particulate Matter (PM) pollution and COVID-19 infection spread in Italy:first observational study based on initial epidemic diffusion. BMJ Open; 10 (2020)
31. Wu, X., Nethery, R.C., Sabath, M.B., Braun, D., Dominici, F.: Air pollution and COVID-19 mortality in the United States: Strengths and limitations of an ecological regression analysis. Sci. Adv. **6**(45) (2020)
32. Saadat, S., Rawtani, D., Hussain, C.M.: Environmental perspective of COVID-19. Sci. Total Environ. Aug 1;728 (2020)
33. Le Quéré, C., et al.: Temporary reduction in daily global CO2 emissions during the COVID-19 forced confinement. Nat. Clim. Chang. **10**, 647–653 (2020)
34. Katsiri, E.: Sensor networks with edge intelligence for reliable air quality monitoring in the Covid-19 Era. In: Proceedings of the ICR'22 International Conference on Innovations in Computing Research, pp. 83–396 (2020)

35. Katsiri, E.: Developing reliable air quality monitoring devices with low cost sensors: method and lessons learned. Int. J. Environ. Sci. **6**, 425–444 (2020)
36. Grafana: The open observability platform. https://grafana.com
37. Fadhel, M., Sekerinski, E., Yao, S.: A comparison of time series databases for storing water quality data. Mobile Technol. Appl. Internet Things, IMCL (2019)
38. Buelvas, J., Múnera, D., Tobón, V., D.P., et al.: Data quality in IoT-based air quality monitoring systems: a systematic mapping study. Water Air Soil Pollut. **234**, 248 (2023)
39. Sharifi, R., Langari, R.: Nonlinear sensor fault diagnosis using mixture of probabilistic PCA models. Mech. Syst. Sign. Process. **85**, 638–50 (2017)
40. Wang, R.Y., Strong, D.M.: Beyond accuracy: what data quality means to data consumers. J. Manag. Inform. Syst. **12**(4), 5–33 (1996)
41. Li, Y., Parker, L.E.: Nearest neighbor imputation using spatial-temporal correlations in wireless sensor networks. Inform. Fusion. **15**, 64–79 (2014)
42. Aggarwal, C.C.: An introduction to outlier analysis. Outlier analysis. Springer: New York, pp. 1–40 (2013)
43. Ahmad, N.F., Hoang, D.B., Phung, M.H.: Robust preprocessing for health care monitoring framework. In: 2009 11th International Conference on e-Health Networking, Applications and Services (Healthcom), pp. 169–74 (2009)
44. Anderson, R.L.: Distribution of the serial correlation coefficient. Ann. Math. Stat. **13**(1), 1–13 (1942)
45. Bosman, H.H., Iacca, G., Tejada, A., Wörtche, H.J., Liotta, A.: Spatial anomaly detection in sensor networks using neighborhood information. Inform. Fusion **33**, 41–56 (2017)
46. Moursi, A.S., El-Fishawy, N., Djahel, S., Shouman, M.A.: An IoT enabled system for enhanced air quality monitoring and prediction on the edge. Complex Intell. Syst. **7**(6), 2923–2947 (2021). https://doi.org/10.1007/s40747-021-00476-w
47. InfluxDB line protocol reference. https://docs.influxdata.com/influxdb/v1.8/write_protocols/line_protocol_reference/
48. Glantz, S.A., Slinker, B.K., Neilands, T,B.: Primer of Applied Regression & Analysis of Variance (Third ed.), McGraw Hill (2016)
49. Aho, K.A.: Foundational and Applied Statistics for Biologists (First ed.), Chapman & Hall / CRC Press (2014)
50. Bartlett, M.S.: On the theoretical specification and sampling properties of autocorrelated time-series. Supplement J. Royal Stat. Soc. **8**(1), pp. 27–41 (1946). JSTOR, http://www.jstor.org/stable/2983611
51. Quenouille, M.H.: The joint distribution of serial correlation coefficients. Ann. Math. Stat. **20**(4), 561–571 (1949)

Social Spider Optimization Meta-heuristic for Node Localization Optimization in Wireless Sensor Networks

Zahia Lalama[1](✉), Fouzi Semechedine[2], Nabil Giweli[3], and Samra Boulfekhar[4]

[1] Faculty of Sciences, University of Setif 1, 19000 Setif, Algeria
zahia.lalama@univ-setif.dz

[2] Mechatronics Laboratory-E1764200, Optics and Precision Mechanics Institute, University of Setif 1, 19000 Setif, Algeria
fouzi.semcheddine@univ-setif.dz

[3] Western Sydney University, Sydney, Australia
n.giweli@westernsydney.edu.au

[4] Research Unit, LAMOS, Faculty of Exact Sciences, University of Bejaia, 06000 Bejaia, Algeria
samra.boulfekhar@univ-bejaia.dz

Abstract. Localization is one of the most important system parameters in Wireless Sensor Networks (WSNs). It consists of the determination of the geographical coordinates of nodes forming the network. Traditional localization algorithms suffer from the high error of localization, then they need to be enhanced. This paper proposes a new localization algorithm namely Centroid Localization Algorithm based on Social Spider Optimization Algorithm (CLA-SSO). The proposed algorithm uses the Social Spider Optimization metaheuristic (SSO) to improve the localization of the basic Centroide Localization Algorithm (CLA) which is a range free localization algorithm. In our method, the initial spiders are initialized by the locations obtained by the CLA and optimized using the SSO metaheuristic. Simulation results show that our proposed algorithm outperforms the basic CLA in terms of localization accuracy. These results are obtained by changing some factors such as transmission radius, ratio of anchor nodes and the number of unknown nodes which affect the localization accuracy.

Keywords: Wireless Sensor Networks · Localization Optimization · Meta-heuristics · Social Spider Optimization Meta-heuristic · Centroid Localization Algorithm

1 Introduction

Wireless Sensor Networks (WSNs) are networks which composed of a great number of costly effective sensor nodes. These nodes are randomly or manually deployed in the environment which to be monitored and cooperate for collecting information about it. In WSNs, localization is one of the most important challenges where the locations

K. Daimi and A. Al Sadoon (Eds.): ICR 2023, LNNS 721, pp. 381–391, 2023.
https://doi.org/10.1007/978-3-031-35308-6_32

of sensor nodes are very preferred to be the most possible accurate. In the literature, many algorithms have been proposed to tackle with this challenge. These algorithms are divided into range based and range free algorithms [4].

The range-based schemes use extra hardware capabilities to inter-sensors distances determination, the popular range based techniques use Received Signal Strength Indicator (RSSI), Time of Arrival (ToA), Time Difference of Arrival (TDoA) and Angle of Arrival (AoA) to inter-sensors distances estimation [4, 5]. These algorithms are more accurate, but the requirement of additional hardware makes it expensive. Hence, these methods are generally not preferred.

The range free algorithms use the content of messages circulated in the network between sensor nodes (anchor and non anchor sensor nodes) [5] to estimate the unknown sensor nodes positions. Compared with range-based algorithms, range free schemes achieve low accuracy but provide cost effective localization. The most used range free algorithms [4] are Distance Vector-Hop (DV-Hop) and Centroid localization algorithm (CLA) [1].

The CLA has the advantage that it is simple and uses few parameters; however, it calculates the unknown sensor nodes coordinates with large error. Then, this error need to be optimized.

In recent years, meta-heuristics such as Genetic Algorithms (GA) [12], particle swarm optimization (PSO)[13], Ant Colony Optimization (ACO) [14], BAT optimization algorithm (BAT) [15], Firefly Optimization Algorithm (FFA) [16], Flower Pollination Algorithm (FP) [7], Grey Wolf Optimization algorithm (GWO) [17], Artificial Bees Colony Optimization Algorithm (ABC) [6], Fish Swarm Optimization Algorithm (FSA) [18] and other become among the most methods used to optimize the error of traditional localization algorithms in WSNs as they simple, effective and give good results [19].

Social spider optimization algorithm (SSO) is one of the new metaheuristics, which was developed in 2013. It is inspired from the cooperative behavior of the social spiders to resolve the optimization problems [8]. SSO metaheuristic has been used to resolve many problems in various areas, such as Center-Based Clustering [20], and Cloud detection in satellite images [21]. In this work, the SSO is used to reduce the localization error of the basic CLA.

In the proposed algorithm, called CLA-SSO, which consist of an hybridization of two algorithms CLA and SSO, the CLA is used firstly to find out the positions of unknown sensor nodes, second, the SSO is used to optimize these initial locations and reduce the localization error of the CLA method.

The rest of this paper is organized as follows: In Sect. 2, we present the Social Spider Optimization meta-heuristic (SSO). Our proposed approach for localization is detailed in Sect. 3. In Sect. 4, we present simulation results and performances of the proposed algorithm. Finally, we end our work with a conclusion in Sect. 5.

2 Social Spider Optimization Algorithm Principle

SSO [9] is a novel meta-heuristic inspired from the cooperative behavior of social spiders which live in groups by forming colonies. Members of social spider colony can be classified based on their gender into two groups: Females and Males spiders. Female spiders represent the largest proportion in the spider colony which may reach up 90% of the total number (Ns) of the colony members. Male spiders can in turn be dominant or non-dominant, where the dominant spiders have best fitness than non-dominant spiders.

To resolve an optimization problem, the original SSO algorithm follows many steps as described below:

1. Initialize the N_s spiders of the initial population randomly as follows:

Generate randomly N_f female spiders between 65% and 90% and N_m male spiders using the following equations:

$$N_f = Fix[(0.9 - rand * 0.25)] \tag{1}$$

where: Fix transforms the real number to an integer number and rand a random number within the range [0,1].

The number of male spiders is calculated as follows:

$$N_m = N_s - N_f \tag{2}$$

2. Initialize randomly each female and each male spider as follows:

$$f_{i,j}^{initial} = p_j^{min} + rand(0, 1) * \left(p_j^{max} - p_j^{min}\right) \tag{3}$$

$$m_{k,j}^{initial} = p_j^{min} + rand(0, 1) * \left(p_j^{max} - p_j^{min}\right) \tag{4}$$

3. Calculate the weight of each spider depending on its fitness value by using the following equation.

$$w_i = \frac{fitness(s_i) - worst_s}{best_s - worst_s} \tag{5}$$

where: $fitness(s_i)$ is the fitness value of the spider i, $best_s$ and $worst_s$ represent respectively the best and the worst fitness among the population S. This weight represents the quality of solution obtained by the spider. The spider with the highest weigh is the fittest member.

4. Calculate vibrations received by each spider from different spiders in the colony depending on the weight and the distance of the spider which has transmitted them according to the following equation.

$$v = w_j * e^{-d_{ij}^2} \tag{6}$$

where: w_j is the weight of the spider s_j and d_{ij}^2 is the Euclidian distance between the spider s_i and the spider s_j . In fact, each spider receives three types of vibrations:

a) Vibrations $v_i cb_i$ are received by the spider Si from the closest spider s_j which has more weight $(w_j > w_i)$
b) Vibrations $v_i b_j$ are received by the spider s_i from the fittest spider s_i that has the biggest weight of the whole population (the fittest spider).

c) Vibrations $v_i f_i$ are received by the spider s_i from the nearest female spider s_j.

5. Update the position of each spider colony member depending on its gender by using different cooperative operators as mentioned below:

a) Female cooperative operator: Female spiders present an attraction or repulsion movement over other spiders in the colony as modeled in the following equation:

$$f_i^{k+1} = \begin{cases} f_i^t + \alpha.v_i cb_j(s_c - f_i^t) + \beta v_i b_j(s_b - f_i^t) + \varphi(rand - \frac{1}{2}) if p < PF \\ f_i^t - \alpha.v_i cb_j(s_c - f_i^t) - \beta v_i b_j(s_b - f_i^t) + \varphi(rand - \frac{1}{2}) if p > PF \end{cases} \quad (7)$$

b) Male cooperative operator: Male spiders can be dominant or non dominant, then the male group is divided into dominant male (d) and non dominant male (Nd) spider based on the solution quality of the male member spider where the dominant spiders have best fitness than non-dominant spiders.

$$m_i^{t+1} = \begin{cases} male(d), w_i > median(w) \\ male(Nd), w_i < median(w) \end{cases} \quad (8)$$

where median is the spider situated in the middle of the male population in regard of its weight.

Dominant male spiders are attracted to the nearest female spider of the colony, while the non dominant male spiders have a propensity to stay in the middle of the dominant male spider population. Then, the male spider's position change depends on their weights and can be modeled as follows:

$$m_i^{t+1} = \begin{cases} m_i^t + \alpha.v_i f_j(s_f - m_i^t)\varphi(rand - \frac{1}{2}) if w_j > w_{mn} \\ m_i^t + \alpha(\frac{\sum_{i=1}^m m_i^t w_i}{\sum_{i=1}^m w_i} - m_i^t) if w_j < w_{mn} \end{cases} \quad (9)$$

where: s_f is the position of the closest female to the spider i, w_{mn} is the weight of the median spider and $(\frac{\sum_{i=1}^m m_i^t w_i}{\sum_{i=1}^m w_i})$ is the weighted mean position of male spider in the population.

6. Update the spider population members according to the mutation operator by adopting the roulette wheel technique.

Mating takes place between dominant male spiders and female spiders within a specific range (range of mating) which can be computed using the following equation:

$$r = \frac{\sum_{j=1}^n (p_j^{max} - p_j^{min})}{2.n} \quad (10)$$

where p_j^{max} and p_j^{min} are respectively the maximum and minimum boundaries of the search space, whereas n is the dimension of the search space.

The new spider s_{new} generated from the mating process is compared to the worst spider s_{worst} of the population in regards of its weight. If the new spider is better than the worst spider, this later is replaced by the new one. Otherwise, the colony does not change. In case of replacement, the new spider takes the same gender of the replaced spider.

7. Repeat the steps 2 to 7 until reach a termination criterion.

3 CLA-SSO Details

The objective of localization process by CLA -SSO approach is to estimate the locations of N unknown sensor nodes which are deployed randomly in the 2-dimensional (2D) space using prior information about the position of M anchor sensor nodes. The transmission range of both unknown sensor nodes and anchor nodes is R. Our approach, first estimates the unknown sensor nodes locations by using the traditional Centroid Localization Algorithm. Second, it uses The SSO meta-heuristic to optimize the locations calculated by the CLA.

Centroid localization algorithm (CLA) is proposed by Bulusu et al. [1]. In this algorithm, when the unknown sensor node receives position information from at least three anchor sensor nodes within its transmission range, it localizes itself based on that information. The CLA has the advantage that it is simple and uses few parameters; however, it calculates the unknown sensor nodes coordinates with large error [2, 3].

The location of an unknown sensor node is calculated by the following equation:

$$(x_{est}, y_{est}) = (\frac{\sum_{i=1}^{k} x_a}{k}, \frac{\sum_{i=1}^{k} y_a}{k}) \tag{11}$$

where: (x_{est}, y_{est}) is the estimated position of the unknown node and k is the number of anchor sensor nodes within the transmission range of this unknown sensor node.

The main steps followed by our proposed algorithm to obtain optimal locations are given in the following subsections.

3.1 Initial Positions Estimation by CLA

In our algorithm, the first step of CLA is to estimate distances between every unknown node and anchor nodes within its transmission range. It is important to note that we take into account an additive noise when calculating estimated distances [7, 11]. Then the distance between an unknown node and each anchor node is calculated as follows:

$d_i = d_a + n_a$, where d_a is the actual distance which can be calculated according to the Eq. (12) and n_a is a Gaussian noise.

$$d_a = \sqrt{(x - x_a)^2 + (y - y_a)^2} \tag{12}$$

where: (x, y) are the coordinates of unknown sensor node and (x_a, y_a) are the coordinates of anchor sensor node.

Once estimated distances are calculated, each unknown node checks if there are at least three anchor sensor nodes within its transmission range, if it is the case, that sensor node is considered as localizable node and it can estimate its location by using the Eq. (11). We note that each unknown sensor node uses the three nearest anchor node to estimate its position by CLA.

Nodes succeed to obtain their locations by CLA (nodes have at least three anchor sensor nodes in their transmission radius) are optimized by the SSO as in the following subsection.

3.2 Locations Optimization by SSO

At the beginning of the optimization process, our algorithm generates randomly Ns spiders (Nf female spiders and Nm male spiders) around each position initially calculated by traditional CLA. Then, each unknown sensor node runs the SSO meta-heuristic to find out its optimal location. Our proposed method minimizes the objective function described in the following equation:

$$f(x, y) = \frac{1}{m}(\sum_{a=1}^{k} \sqrt{(x - x_a)^2 + (y - y_a)^2 - d_a^2}) \tag{13}$$

where (x, y) the estimated coordinates of the unknown node, (x_a, y_a) the coordinates of the anchor nodes a = 1;..,k, d_a the estimated distance between anchor nodes, the unknown node and m the number of neighboring anchor nodes to this unknown node.

At the end of each generation of the SSO method, the estimated position of each sensor node is compared to the position obtained in the previous iteration in terms of its fitness. The best location (location which has the min distance to the neighboring anchor nodes) becomes the optimal position of the target sensor node.

Finally, after a maximum number of iterations (*MaxIter*), CLA-SSO finds out the optimal positions of unknown nodes.

The main steps of the proposed algorithm CLA-SSO are described below:

Step1: Deploy Randomly N unknown nodes and M anchor nodes in 2-D space.

Step2:

- Calculate distances between unknown sensor nodes and anchor nodes to determine the set of localizable nodes (nodes haves at least 3 neighboring anchor nodes)

  $UL = (UL_1, UL_2, ..UL_n)$.

- Determine R, *maxIter* and Ns.

Step3: Find out initial positions by CLA.

Step4:

- Define the initial set of optimal positions as the set of initial position found by CLA.
- Generate Ns spiders (N_f female and N_m male spiders) around each initial position.

Step5: Calculate the fitness value of each spider.

Step6: Update the set of optimal positions.

Step7: Calculate weighs.

Step8: Calculate vibrations received by each spider.

Step9: Update spiders positions based on their gender.

Step10: Update the spider population by applying mutation operator.

Step11: Repeat the steps from 5 to 11 until reach the maximum number of iterations.

4 Simulation Results

To evaluate the performance of our proposed algorithm namely CLA-SSO, simulations are done by using the MATLAB platform. Then, the proposed algorithm is compared to the original CLA in terms of localization error and average localization.

In our simulation, we use a square area of 50*50 m^2, and both of unknown sensor nodes and anchor sensor nodes are deployed randomly and have a transmission radius set to 20 m (m).

For the proposed algorithm parameters, we deploy ten (10) spiders around each position found by the CLA, so the size of the spider colony is NL *10, where NL is the number of the sensor nodes localized by CLA.

Among the ten spiders deployed around every location, we use seven (7) female spiders and three (3) male spiders. So, the total number of female spiders in the population is calculated as a multiplication of the total number of nodes localized by CLA and 7 according to the following equation:

$$N_f = N_l * 7 \tag{14}$$

The total number of male spiders in the population is calculated by multiplying the total number of nodes localized by CLA and 3 as shown in the equation:

$$N_m = N_l * 3 \tag{15}$$

To evaluate the performance of the proposed algorithm, 50 unknown sensor nodes and 10 anchor nodes are deployed randomly in the simulation environment, then the localization error of each localized sensor node and the average localization error are calculated according to the following two equations: Eq. (16) and the Eq. (17) respectively.

$$error_i = \sqrt{(x - x_i)^2 + (y - y_{i)}^2} \tag{16}$$

This error represents the distance between the estimated location (x, y) and the real location (x_i, y_i) of each localized sensor node.

$$Averageerror = \frac{1}{NL}\sum\nolimits_{i=1}^{NL}\sqrt{(x - x_i)^2 + (y - y_{i)}^2} \tag{17}$$

where: (x, y), (x_i, y_i) are the real and the estimated coordinates of the unknown node respectively and NL is the number of localized nodes in the network (nodes can be localized by CLA).

Figure 1 represents the localization error of every unknown sensor node for both basic CLA and CLA-SSO algorithm, Results obtained show clearly that our proposed algorithm reduces the localization error of the **original** CLA which also reduces the average of localization error from 5.64123 m in basic CLA to 3.25691 m in CLA-SSO as shown in the Table 1.

Table 1. Average localization error for CLA and CLA-SSO algorithms

Average localization error	CLA	CLA-SSO
	5.64123	3.25691

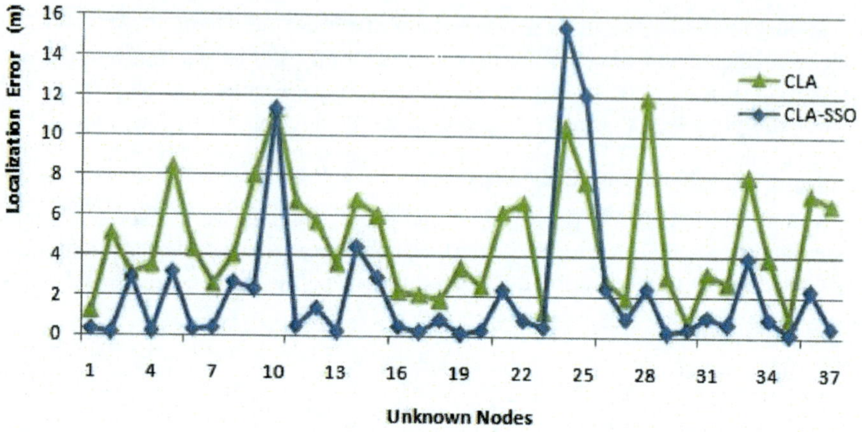

Fig. 1. Localization error for every unknown node for both CLA and CLA-SSO algorithms

To show the results of localization by CLA-SSO algorithm in different configuration, the average localization error is calculated by changing some parameters, first we fix the number of unknown nodes and the transmission range and change the values of the ratio of anchor nodes. Second, we change the number of unknown nodes and fixe the other parameters. Finally, we change the communication range, and we fix the other parameters.

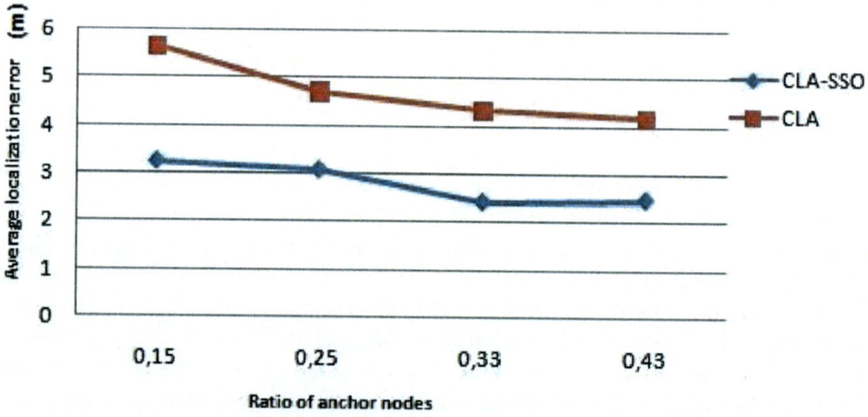

Fig. 2. Average localization error Vs Ratio of anchor nodes for both CLA and CLA- SSO algorithms.

Simulation results shown in Fig. 2 represent the average localization error of two algorithms, CLA and CLA-SSO by varying the ratio of anchor nodes and fixing the other parameters. These results show that the average localization error is reduced in CLA-SSO in comparison to the traditional CLA. We can also see that the average localization error decrease when ratio of the anchor nodes and thus for both CLA and CLA-SSO.

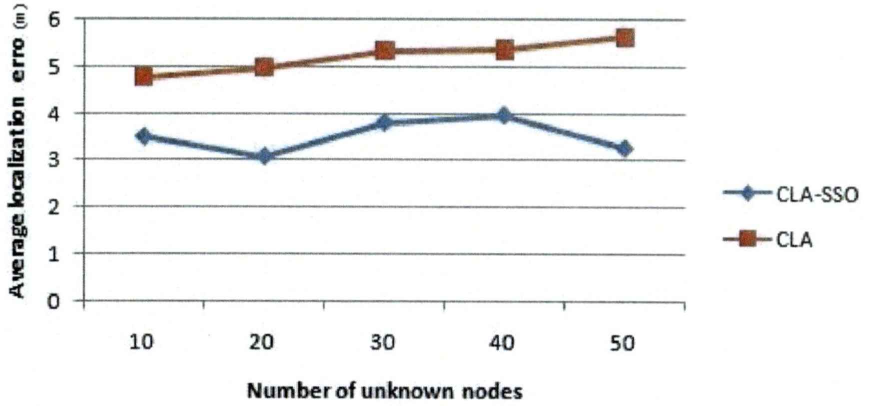

Fig. 3. Average localization error vs number of unknown nodes for both CLA and CLA-SSO algorithms

The average localization error of tow algorithm CLA and CLA-SSO calculated by changing the number of unknown nodes from 10 to 50 is shown in Fig. 3. Results obtained show that the average localization error stays stable for different number of unknown nodes. In addition, the average localization error is minimized in CLA-SSO compared to traditional CLA. From these results, we can demonstrate the effectiveness of the SSO metaheuristic for localization optimization.

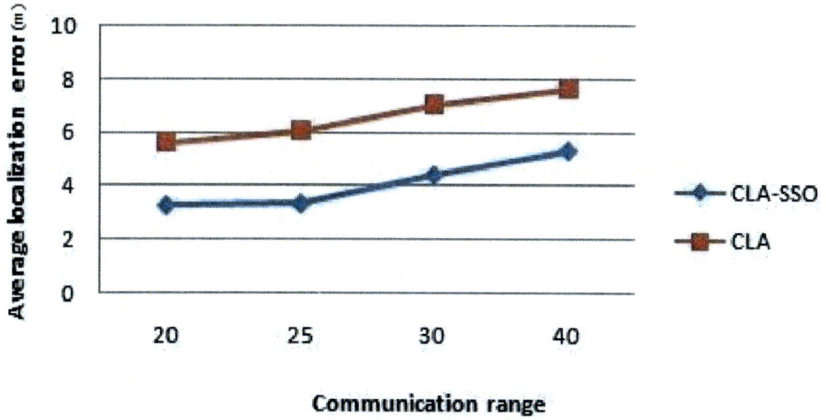

Fig. 4. Average localization error Vs communication range for both CLA and CLA-SSO algorithms.

Figure 4 illustrates the simulation results obtained by varying the communication range and calculating the average localization error of two algorithms, basic CLA and CLA-SSO algorithms. From this figure, the average localization error is increasing when increasing the communication range and it minimized in CLA-SSO compared to basic CLA.

5 Conclusion

The main objective of the work proposed in this paper is to increase the localization accuracy by decreasing the localization error. To reach our aim, we used the sso meta-heuristic to optimize the Exact location is very demanded for many WSNs applications. Traditional localization algorithms such as CLA and other are suitable for the localization problem but the localization error of these methods is high and need to be optimized. In this work, the CLA is enhanced by using the meta-heuristic SSO. In our proposed algorithm, the locations firstly obtained by the CLA are optimized by the SSO meta-heuristic. The simulation results showed that our proposed method significantly reduces the localization error compared to the basic CLA. Then we can conclude that the meta-heuristic optimization algorithms are suitable techniques to improve the localization accuracy of the traditional localization algorithms.

References

1. Bulusu, N., Heidemann, J., Estrin, D.: GPS-less low-cost outdoor localization for very small devices. J. IEEE Pers. Commun. **7**, 28–34 (2007)
2. Tuncer, T.: Intelligent centroid localization based on fuzzy logic and genetic algorithm. J. Comput. Intell. Syst. **10**, 1056–1065 (2017)
3. Gupta, V., Singh, B.: Study of range free centroid based localization algorithm and its improvement using particle swarm optimization for wireless sensor networks under log normal shadowing **12**, 1–7 (2018)
4. Paul, A.K., Sato, T.: Localization in wireless sensor networks: a survey on algorithms, measurement techniques, applications and challenges, journal of sensor and actuator. Networks **6**, 1–23 (2017)
5. Sivakumar, S., Venkatesan, R.: Meta-heuristic approaches for minimizing error in localization of wireless sensor networks. J. Appl. Soft Comput. **36**, 506–518 (2015)
6. Gupta, V.: Centroid based localization utilizing artificial bee colony algorithm. J. Comput. Networks Appl. **6**, 47–54 (2019)
7. Kaur, R., Arora, S.: Nature inspired range based wireless sensor node localization algorithms. J. Interact. Multimedia Artif. Intell. **4**, 7–17 (2017)
8. Gupta, R., Jagannath Nanda, S., Prakash Shukla, U.: Cloud detection in satellite images using multi-objective social spider optimization. J. Appl. Soft Comput. **79**, 203226 (2019)
9. Cuevas, E., Cienfuegos, M., Zaldvar, D., PrezCisneros, M.: A swarm optimization algorithm inspired in the behavior of the social-spider. J. Expert Syst. Appl. **40**, 6374–6384 (2013)
10. Blumenthal, J., Grossmann, R., Golatowski, F., Timmermann, D.: Weighted Centroid localization in Zigbee-based sensor networks. In: The Proceedings of the IEEE International Symposium on Intelligent Signal Processing, pp. 1–6 (2007)
11. Singh, P., Khosla, A., Kumar, A., Khosla, M.: Wireless sensor networks localization and its location optimization using bio inspired localization algorithms: a survey. J. Current Eng. Sci. Res. **4**, 74–80 (2017)
12. Uraiya, K., D. Kumar Gandhi, K.; Genetic algorithm for wireless sensor network with localization based techniques. J. Sci. Res. Publ. **4**, 1–6 (2014)
13. Alhammadi, A., Hashim, F., Fadlee, M., Shami, T.M.: An adaptive localization system using particle swarm optimization in a circular distribution form. J. Technol. **78**, 105–110 (2016)
14. Qin, F., Wei, C., Kezhong, L.: Node localization with a mobile beacon based on ant colony algorithm in wireless sensor networks. In: The Proceeding of Communications and Mobile Computing Conference, pp. 303–307 (2010)

15. Goyal, S., Patterh, M.S.: Modified bat algorithm for localization of wireless sensor network. J. Wirel. Pers. Commun. **86**, 657–670 (2015)
16. Nguyen, T., Pan, J., Chu, S., Roddick, J.F., Dao, T.: Optimization localization in wireless sensor network based on multi-objective fire fly algorithm. J. Network Intell. **1**, 130–138 (2016)
17. Asghar Heidari, A., Pahlavani, P.: An efficient modified grey wolf optimizer with levy flight for optimization tasks. J. Appl. Soft Comput. 115–134 (2017)
18. Sivakumar, S., Venkatesan: Error minimization in localization of wireless sensor networks using fish swarm optimization algorithm. J. Comput. Appl. **159**, 39–45 (2017)
19. Lalama, Z., Boulfekhar, S., Semechedine, F.: Localization optimization in WSNs using meta-heuristics optimization algorithms: a survey J. Wirel. Pers. Commun. **122**, 1197–1220 (2022)
20. Leon, J., Chullo-Llave, B., Enciso-Rodas, L., Luis Soncco-Alvarez, J.: A multi-objective optimization algorithm for center-based clustering. J. Electron. Notes Theoret. Comput. Sci. **349**, 4967 (2020)
21. Gupta, R., Jagannath Nanda, S., Prakash Shukla, U.: Cloud detection in satellite images using multi-objective social spider optimization. J. Appl. Soft Comput. **79**, 203226 (2019)

Privacy-Aware IoT Based Fall Detection with Infrared Sensors and Deep Learning

Farhad Ahamed[1,2](✉), Seyed Shahrestani[1], and Hon Cheung[1]

[1] Western Sydney University, Kingswood, NSW 2747, Australia
{farhad.ahamed,s.shahrestani,h.cheung}@westernsydney.edu.au
[2] Kent Institute Australia, Sydney, NSW 2000, Australia

Abstract. Falls among the elderly are a major worry for both the elderly and their care-takers, as falls frequently result in severe physical injury. Detecting falls using Internet of Things (IoT) devices can give elderly persons and their care-takers peace of mind in case of emergency. However, due to usability and intrusive nature of wearable and vision-based fall detection has limited acceptability and applicability in washroom and privacy sensitive locations as well as older adults with mental health condition. Privacy-aware infrared array sensors have great potential to identify fall in a non-intrusive way preserving privacy of the subject. Using a secondary dataset, we have utilised and tuned time series based deep learning network to identify fall. Experiments indicate that the time-series based deep learning network offers accuracy of 96.4% using 6 infrared sensors. This result provides encouraging evidence that low-cost privacy-aware infrared array sensor-based fall monitoring can enhance safety and well-being of older adults in self-care or aged care environment.

Keywords: Fall Detection · Deep Learning · Privacy · Internet of Things · Machine Learning · Infrared sensors

1 Introduction

Falls have negative consequences for the elderly. Falls among the elderly are a severe health concern that can lead to hip fractures, traumatic brain injuries, and even death. 25% of older individuals age 65 and older fall per year [1]. 20% of these 25% have significant injuries [1]. The typical approach to protecting the safety of the elderly involves continual and watchful supervision of their daily activities by hired nurses and caretakers. The physical health risk associated with falls is one of the key concerns for carers. The residents of residential care facilities are likewise particularly concerned about the potential threat posed by falls. Mobility is essential for elderly persons to keep their independence. Falls can diminish mobility and constitute a serious health risk. Even a fear of falling can result in decreased exercise [6]. It places a significant load on the carer to constantly supervise and accompany the elderly. Consequently, one carer often cares for one or a small number of patients, which ultimately increases the

K. Daimi and A. Al Sadoon (Eds.): ICR 2023, LNNS 721, pp. 392–401, 2023.
https://doi.org/10.1007/978-3-031-35308-6_33

number of staff needed in a nursing home. Hiring such a staff personally at home or collectively in a shelter for elderly folks is quite expensive. In addition, while caretakers are absent, the elderly may fall and get significant injuries, as it is very difficult to oversee everyone and at all times. They require immediate medical attention, but it may be delayed until the carer returns or becomes aware of the mishap. This form of delays presents a big concern regarding absolute dependability. To ensure the safety and security of the elderly, it is necessary to evaluate more cost-effective and dependable choices. An infrared (IR) sensor is an electrical sensor that can detect overall movement. As humans emit infrared radiation predominantly, IR sensors can be used to monitor human mobility. Infrared-based systems are likewise primarily focused on surveillance. IR sensor-generated data are typically utilised to build 3D pictures or blocks containing information about environmental infrared radiation [7].

2 Literature Review

Fall has some features that a human easily identifies. A person can promptly make noise, vibration, and visual analysis of a fall. However, for machines, fall identification is not a very simple task. Wearable sensors like pendant and bracelet are in use for fall detection for older adults. However, wearable sensors has intrusive nature, low security, shorter battery life, and usability issues. There are many challenges when we use ambient devices to detect falls. A fall may happen either during a day or night. Therefore, only image analysis of the fall event may not be adequate to cover monitoring for the whole day. The brightness and darkness level of the image add complexity to fall detection. When the ambient sensors are considered, the fall has a similar movement signature like lying down, exercising, and others. Additionally, the surrounding environment may impact the detection signature. These conditions will have an impact on the identification of a fall. The movement signature and the living place are different for each person and place, implying an additional challenge for fall detection with accuracy. Therefore, fall detection features are dependent upon various dynamic parameters and dynamic environment. A combination of motion and movement

Table 1. A comparison among most of the fall detection methods

Fall detection type	Advantage	Disadvantages
Computer vision, camera-based, image processing, depth camera.	Widely available, wide-coverage, inexpensive	Night or darkness issue, occlusion
Remote sensors (Infrared array, acoustic, Wifi-CSI, PIR sensor, and others)	Inexpensive, privacy-aware, non-intrusive	smaller coverage, high signal interference
Body-worn sensors (mobile devices, smartwatch, implant devices and others)	Broad coverage, reliable, mobile	Intrusive, power lifespan, Need to be carried

signature, audio and vibration signature, object recognition and co-ordination can aid in accurate fall detection. Audio-visual inspection by an assistance robot may help to confirm the fall scenario further. However, this is still being far from the reality of a simple solution specially to cater fall detection when the older adult require non-intrusive and privacy-aware solution. The computer vision-based method is resource expensive and slower compared to the ambient sensory method. Moreover, occultation in video input poses a challenge to distinguish a specific object, like a human, among background objects. Body-worn accelerometers detect impacts and changes in an orientation associated with falls, however, they need continuous power and wearable sensors are intrusive by nature. [1]. Table 1 presents a comparison among most of the fall detection method.

2.1 Privacy Aware Fall Detection

In hospitals and aged-care facilities patient falls are among the major incidents that require urgent attention. Patients with low blood glucose or another medical condition as well as older adults has higher risk of falling. Falls in patients can occur in toilets when no one is around. To identify fall in closed areas, privacy-aware fall-detection is required. In acoustic and ambient sensors-based technique to detect falls, systems may include infrared sensors, microphones or vibration sensors. An acoustic sensor-based system also provides an unobtrusive way of monitoring older adults, just like computer vision based techniques. The hardware, software and infrastructure are relatively inexpensive and straightforward for such systems, in most cases, when compared to computer vision-based methods that require expensive and faster Graphical Processing Units (GPU). A group of researchers proposed a design for a floor vibration-based fall detection system [2]. Their system utilised a particular piezoelectric sensor coupled to the floor surface using spring and mass arrangement. The vibration patterns of a human fall from other activities and falls of other objects are the key differentiators for this fall detection system. Using anthropomorphic dummies, field experiments have been conducted. The system demonstrated a 100% fall detection rate, however, the drawbacks of these approaches are (1) the minimal range of the vibration sensor was set 20 feet only, and (2) floor materials as the vibrations could not be detected on all kinds of floor materials. Some researchers have developed a fall detection method based on an array of acoustic sensors [9]. To recognise a fall, the loudness and height of the sound are used. Two microphones are placed 4 m apart, and they are mounted on the vertical z-axis. Firstly, they remove noise and then use both sensors for fall detection decisions on the signal received energy. They have achieved a 70% recognition rate with no false alarm. A 100% success rate is achieved by adjusting the system but with a penalty of 5 false alarms every hour. Their system can only be used in indoor environments. Ultrasonic sensors are accurate to detect movements and can detect an object from far away. Additionally, it can detect object movement even if the line of sight is not established. The downside of applying an ultrasonic sensor to detect falls is that these sensors are too sensitive and prone to produce too many false alarms [9]. Non-intrusive infrared sensors are also used for fall detection by various researchers. In [6], after feature extraction, various machine learning and statistical models are employed to detect falls and activities of daily life (ADL) incidents. The authors in [7] took similar approach of utilising machine learning using kinect's infrared sensor. The authors in [8] developed a fuzzy inference system consists of infrared and ultrasonic sensors for non-intrusive fall-detection. Additionally, the authors in [3] utilised an infrared sensor array where the sensors connected to distinct locations on the wall and captured three-dimensional infrared image data. The temperature differential feature is then utilised to subtract the image from the background model in order to identify the human body's foreground. The collected features are then classified as fall or non-fall events using the k-Nearest Neighbor (kNN) classification model. This technique distinguished autumn events with an overall accuracy of 93%. The authors in [5] presented a method based on readings from infrared depth sensors. A block of feature selection by Gram-Schmidt orthogonalization and a block of Nonlinear Principal Component Analysis (NPCA) are used to enhance the performance of discriminative statistical classifiers (multi-layer perceptron). The feature selection block defines how the features are ranked. The NPCA block turns the raw data into a nonlinear manifold, hence lowering the data's dimensionality to two. The system had a 93% accuracy rate. The authors in [12] have developed a fall detection system called WiFall that claims to achieve fall detection for a single person with high accuracy [12]. They have demonstrated by the experimental results that WiFall yields 90% detection precision with a false alarm rate of 15% on average using a one-class Support Vector Machine (SVM) classifier in all testing scenarios. The authors in [11] have developed RT-Fall, an indoor fall detection system using commodity Wi-Fi devices [11]. The system uses the phase and amplitude of the fine-grained Channel State Information (CSI) accessible in commodity Wi-Fi devices and attempts to segment and detect the falls automatically in real-time. They claim that their experimental results in four indoor scenarios outperform the state-of-the-art approach WiFall with 14% higher sensitivity and 10% higher specificity on average. In the following section we present our privacy-aware fall detection system.

3 Fall Detection System Using Infrared Sensors

A privacy-aware fall detection system scans the user movements and activities of daily life from a smart environment. The infrared array-based fall detection system is trained with dataset from simulated real-life fall events and generic activities of daily life such as walking, seating, running and others. Figure 1 shows the architecture of the fall detection system (FDS) used in this research using privacy-aware and non-intrusive infrared sensors. The FDS is trained from the movements of the users as shown in Fig. 1. After the training is completed, trained FDS is tested from the sample movements of the users. The machine learning (ML) model of FDS will decide if a fall has occurred as shown in Fig. 1 The sensor data are stored in a plain text file or CSV file format imported to

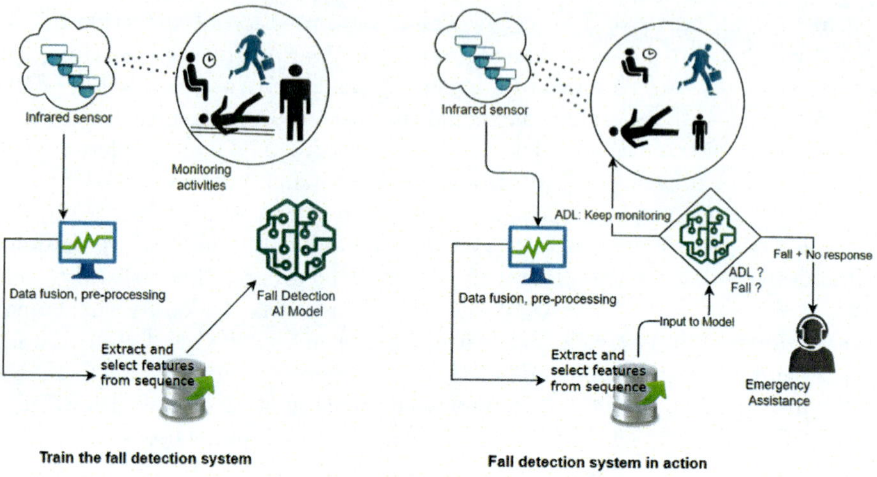

Fig. 1. Fall detection system workflow.

Matlab for analysis, classification and pattern recognition. The high-level steps that are used for the machine learning-based FDS are provided as follows,

1. Import data from Sensors
2. Filtering and cleaning the data
3. Feature extracting, ranking, selecting
4. Train the models of fall detection
5. Validate and test the models for FDS

In step one, raw sensory data files are input to the Matlab tool. In the next step, data is filtered and cleaned to readable for machine learning model. In case of building the model for first time, we need to make sure we have a good proportion of data to represent daily activities, like walking, sitting, lying, and enough fall scenarios on the other side. Preparing dataset is vital to train the model with machine learning algorithms. In the third step, we conducted data analytics to check for any patterns or anomalies for choosing machine learning algorithms and popular classifiers. Due to timeseries nature of multimodal sensor data, we choose popular deep learning network Long Short-term Memory (LSTM). In step four, actual learning is started by the model from the data. Machine learning algorithms are used in this step. The data received from the sensors can be viewed as a time-series graph. Ideally LSTM use time series-based learning to discover patterns in the signals to identify fall and distinguish it from other activities, such as walking, running, climbing stairs, sitting, lying down, picking up objects from the floor, and others. The trained models are also tested against the test dataset. A good rule of thumb of the dataset utilisation is to use the split of 80/20 or 70/30 for a training-test to achieve an optimal intelligent model for FDS. Generally, this depends on the size of the source dataset. If there is plenty of data, we may not need a significant fraction of data for the evaluation. After completing previous steps, the model will be ready for further improvement and actual deployment and measurement of the success rate. The further details of the ML-model and experiment procedures are described in the following sections.

4 Dataset Overview and Analysis

We have utilized a secondary dataset HAR-UP in our experiment [6]. This labeled dataset contains multiple types of sensor readings of various types of fall and ADL of 17 subjects. Each infrared sensor contains over 294000 sensor readings. Apart from other sensors such as video camera and wearable sensors, these six infrared sensors are used to capture the movements of the subjects from specific location and perimeters. Based on the captured data we have plotted eleven types of movements in Fig. 2. The colored line represents sensor activation. It can be observed from the Fig. 2 that, fall related movements have activated (1) different types of infrared sensors, and (2) frequent activation of infrared sensors in a short period of time. The infrared sensors array was activated in a discrete time-sequence manner. These patterns are picked up by the ML algorithms as classifier of the motions: walking, seating, standing and fall models. Due to time-sequence properties, we design a timeseries based deep learning network to recognize the discrete pattern of the fall from the labeled data.

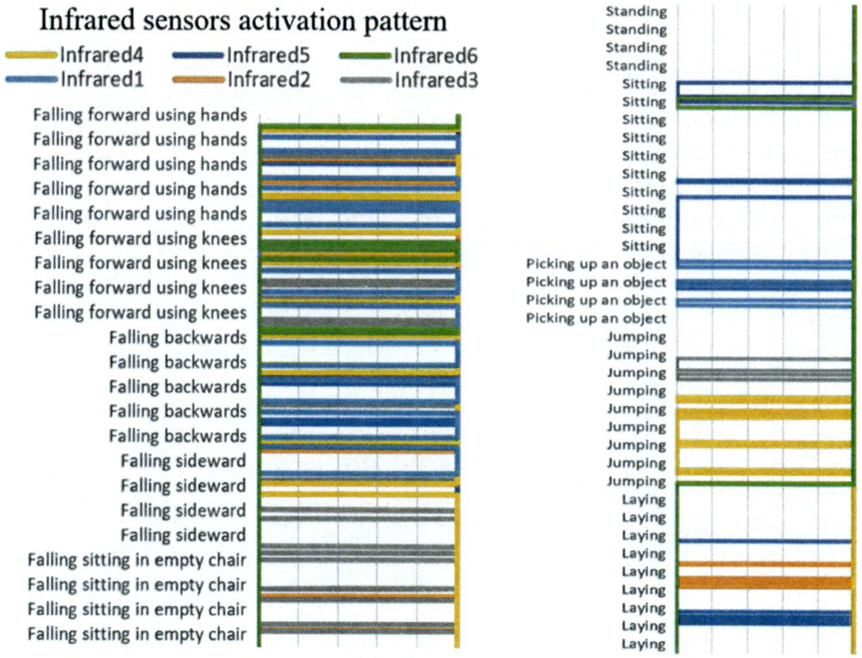

Fig. 2. Infrared sensors activation intensity.

5 Experiment Details

A novel remote sensor-based fall detection method is provided in this section that uses six pairs of infrared sensors, as shown in Fig. 3. Out of these six pairs, the sensors are positioned at 90-degree angles as four pairs by two pairs. Figure 3 shows the layout of the sensors. When a movement occurs inside the sensor coverage area, these sensors will generate events. When anyone moves inside the sensor coverage area, a movement pattern is registered and identified as a fall or ADL event. These movements generally occur in a time domain, walking, sitting, running, jumping, falling, standing and other events. Moreover, the movement pattern is also expected to be identified by the machine learning process. Due to the time-varying and pattern matching properties of the movement data, LSTM based model should be considered. Therefore, in this experiment, LSTM based model will be used to distinguish a fall from ADL events. The publicly available UP-Fall dataset contains infrared sensor information for fall and ADL events. The infrared sensor provides binary data. If anyone is blocking the line of sight, the sensor will trigger the value '1'; otherwise, it will trigger the value '0'. The six infrared sensors produce six binary values whenever a participant moves through the line of sights. These six lines of sights in a time sequence fashion can provide insights into the movement sequence of the participants. Therefore, a Bi-LSTM network-based model with six input layers should estimate the type of movements of participants. To distinguish between a fall and ADL activities, an ML model is presented in Fig. 3 The model has six input layers due to the data stream from six infrared sensors. The layers are connected with the Bi-LSTM layer, which contains 100 hidden units. The Bi-LSTM is connected with a fully connected layer that has only two output neurons. The fully connected layer is connected with a softmax layer followed by a classification layer of 2 outputs (1) fall or (2) ADL. There are 17 participants in these experiments. However, due to missing values from the sensors of 3 participants, 14 participants' data are considered to train and test the model. Each participant has three trials to generate movements for five types of fall and six types of ADL activities. The dataset is split into train and test portion in the ratio of 70/30. Various hyperparameter range was tested to reach optimal value to train the model is presented in Table 2. Figure 4 illustrates the training progress chart that represents sequential learning over time. In the next section, the trained model is tested with testing data.

Table 2. Hyperparameter values

Hyperparameter	Values
Optimiser	ADAM
Maximum epochs	100
Batch size	32
Learning rate	0.01
Gradient threshold	1

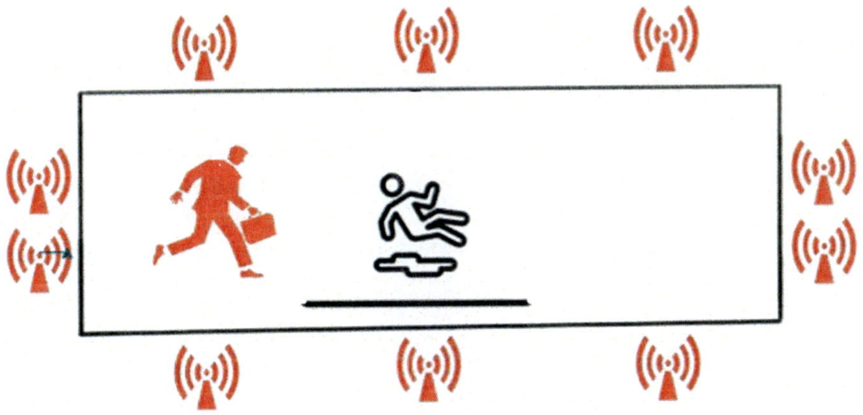

Fig. 3. Positioning of the array of infrared sensors.

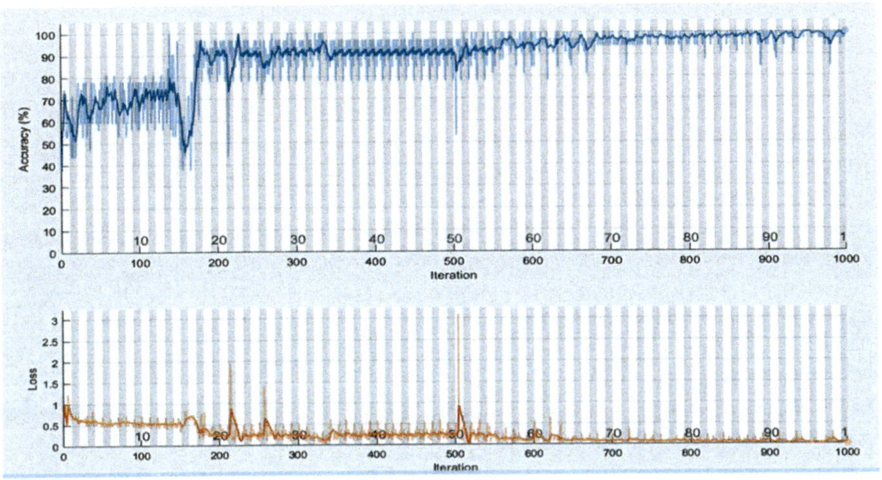

Fig. 4. Training progress of infrared sensor array based FDS

6 Results

A series of experiments were conducted with the set of hyperparamers, finally, we have used the optimised parameters that is presented in Table 2. The training and testing results from the selected hyperparameters are presented in Table 3. Using the LSTM based model from 138 testing samples, the model demonstrates 96.4% accuracy. The training and testing accuracy difference is less than 2% that demonstrate the model is not overtrained. The sensitivity level of the trained model is showing 98.3%.

Table 3. Result of infrared array sensor based FDS

Experiment	Sensitivity	Specificity	Precision	Accuracy	F1 Score
Training	99.3%	97.1%	96.7%	98.1%	98.2%
Testing	98.3%	94.9%	93.7%	96.4%	96.6%

The performance of the LSTM-based FDS is encouraging as the model of this FDS covers five types of fall and six different ADLs. The UP-Fall dataset researchers have tried to build an activity model with 11 classes (5 types of fall and six types of ADL). They have achieved 67% accuracy when only the infrared sensors are considered to classify the falls and ADL. The experiment presented in this work shows a simple remote, and privacy aware FDS that is trained from infrared sensor movement data can achieve better accuracy. Comparing to Doppler sensor based approach in [10] that achieved 89.4% accuracy, IR sensor based technique provided encouraging result. Our deep learning approach also demonstrated better accuracy ($>$ 3.5%) and F1-score ($>$ 3.9%) comparing with [4].

7 Conclusion

The use of a privacy-aware non-intrusive IF sensor to distinguish between different types of falls and activities of daily living is a promising low-cost technology and a tool for long-term continuous monitoring of older adults and post-surgery populations at risk of falls. However, currently, the evidence is limited because these studies have primarily involved simulated laboratory events in young adults. Future studies should focus on validating fall detection in larger units and include data from (a) people at high risk of falling, (b) activities of daily living, (c) both near falls and actual falls, and (d) naturally occurring near falls. To improve coverage, privacy and assurance, infrared sensor-based fall detection with wearable sensors can be included and gradually added to the multimodal FDS. Remote FDS is also presented using infrared array sensors, which shows 96.4% accuracy.

References

1. Ahamed, F., Shahrestani, S., Cheung, H.: Intelligent fall detection with wearable IoT. In: Barolli, L., Hussain, F.K., Ikeda, M. (eds.) CISIS 2019. AISC, vol. 993, pp. 391–401. Springer, Cham (2020). https://doi.org/10.1007/978-3-030-22354-0_35
2. Alwan, M., et al.: A smart and passive floor-vibration based fall detector for elderly. In: 2006 2nd International Conference on Information & Communication Technologies, vol. 1, pp. 1003–1007. IEEE (2006)
3. Chen, W.H., Ma, H.P.: A fall detection system based on infrared array sensors with tracking capability for the elderly at home. In: 2015 17th International Conference on E-health Networking, Application & Services (HealthCom), pp. 428–434. IEEE (2015)
4. He, C., et al.: A non-contact fall detection method for bathroom application based on mems infrared sensors. Micromachines **14**(1), 130 (2023). https://doi.org/10.3390/mi14010130. https://www.mdpi.com/2072-666X/14/1/130
5. Jankowski, S., Szymański, Z., Dziomin, U., Mazurek, P., Wagner, J.: Deep learning classifier for fall detection based on IR distance sensor data. In: Computer Systems for Healthcare and Medicine, pp. 169–192. River Publishers (2022)
6. Martínez-Villaseñor, L., Ponce, H., Brieva, J., Moya-Albor, E., Núñez-Martínez, J., Peñafort-Asturiano, C.: Up-fall detection dataset: a multimodal approach. Sensors **19**(9), 1988 (2019)
7. Mastorakis, G., Makris, D.: Fall detection system using Kinect's infrared sensor. J. Real-Time Image Proc. **9**, 635–646 (2014)
8. Moulik, S., Majumdar, S.: FallSense: an automatic fall detection and alarm generation system in IoT-enabled environment. IEEE Sens. J. **19**(19), 8452–8459 (2018)
9. Popescu, M., Li, Y., Skubic, M., Rantz, M.: An acoustic fall detector system that uses sound height information to reduce the false alarm rate. In: 2008 30th Annual International Conference of the IEEE Engineering in Medicine and Biology Society, pp. 4628–4631. IEEE (2008)
10. Su, B.Y., Ho, K., Rantz, M.J., Skubic, M.: Doppler radar fall activity detection using the wavelet transform. IEEE Trans. Biomed. Eng. **62**(3), 865–875 (2014)
11. Wang, H., Zhang, D., Wang, Y., Ma, J., Wang, Y., Li, S.: RT-Fall: a real-time and contactless fall detection system with commodity WiFi devices. IEEE Trans. Mob. Comput. **16**(2), 511–526 (2016)
12. Wang, Y., Wu, K., Ni, L.M.: WiFall: device-free fall detection by wireless networks. IEEE Trans. Mob. Comput. **16**(2), 581–594 (2016)

Smart Cities/Smart Energy

Heterogeneous Transfer Learning in Structural Health Monitoring for High Rise Structures

Ali Anaissi[1(✉)], Kenneth D'souza[1], Basem Suleiman[1], Mahmoud Bekhit[2], and Widad Alyassine[1]

[1] School of Computer Science, The University of Sydney, Sydney, Australia
{ali.anaissi,kenneth.souza,basem.suleiman, widad.alyassine}@sydney.edu.au

[2] School of Computer Science, Kent Institute, Sydney, Australia
mahmoud.Bekhit@kent.edu.au

Abstract. Structural Health Monitoring aims to utilise sensor data to assess the integrity of structures. Machine learning is opening up the possibility for more accurate and informative metrics to be determined by leveraging the large volumes of data available in modern times. An unfortunate limitation to these advancements is the fact that these models typically only use data from the structure being modeled, and these data sets are typically limited, which in turn limits the predictive power of the models built on these datasets. Transfer learning is a subfield of machine learning that aims to use data from other sources to inform a model on a target task. Current research has been focused on employing this methodology to real-world structures by using simulated structures for source information. This paper analyzes the feasibility of deploying this framework across multiple real-world structures. Data from two experimental scale models were evaluated in a multiclass damage detection problem. Damage in the structures was simulated through the removal of structural components. The dataset consists of the response from accelerometers equipped to the structures while the structures were under the influence of an external force. A convolution neural network (CNN) was used as the target-only model, and a Generative adversarial network (GAN) based CNN network was evaluated as the transfer learning model. The results show that transfer learning improves results in cases where limited data on the damaged target structure is available, however transfer learning is much less effective than traditional methods when there is a sufficient amount of data available.

Keywords: Transfer Learning · Convolution Neural Network · Damage Detection · Sensors · Structural Health Monitoring

1 Introduction

Structural health monitoring (SHM) is a branch of science dedicated to developing systems to monitor buildings' structural health via different sensor technolo-

K. Daimi and A. Al Sadoon (Eds.): ICR 2023, LNNS 721, pp. 405–417, 2023.
https://doi.org/10.1007/978-3-031-35308-6_34

gies. The goal is to extract information from these sensors to make inferences about the current state of health in a structure. This reduces the need for visual inspections by enabling the dynamic real-time monitoring of structures. Machine learning (ML) is advancing this field by making data-driven models possible that can extract information from patterns in data to make these inferences. This approach relies on the presence of a lot of data so that enough scenarios can be observed to mine out the patterns and relations between sensor data and corresponding damage scenarios. The crux of the problem in machine learning approaches to SHM is that data is scarce. This is because an ML-based SHM model is fine-tuned to the idiosyncrasies of a particular building, meaning the data for the model must be acquired from the building being monitored. This makes it difficult to predict states that have not been previously observed, or do not occur frequently enough for a pattern to be discerned from the building's existing data. This highly limits the feasibility of ML-based SHM models in many applications because damage states are relatively infrequent for structures. This data problem can be ameliorated if we can transfer knowledge learned from a similar structure to make inferences on a target structure. This would enable access to a much larger history of data from damaged buildings, to inform model predictions when the data from the building of interest is sparse. This methodology is called transfer learning (TL). Transfer learning is currently applied to structures that are nominally equivalent (population-based SHM) i.e. A set of wind turbines in a wind farm. Inferences become more challenging as structures begin to differ in dimensions and materials. The existing research in transfer learning SHM across heterogeneous structures is limited to knowledge transfer across simulated building models, or from simulated models to an experimental model. The goal of this study is to investigate the feasibility of applying these methodologies across different real-world structures. This feasibility study will be evaluated using two experimental scale models containing slightly different materials and dimensions, but a similar topology. These conditions should enable relevant and informative information to be transferable across the structures. In particular, we will use a 3-story aluminum scale model to inform damage predictions on a 4-story steel highrise scale model.

2 Related Work

The field of structural health monitoring is rapidly developing in response to concurrent advances in machine learning and sensor technologies [16,18]. This warrants the need for a prefatory cost-benefit analysis of the existing sensor technologies available, the associated analytic methodologies, and their scope in terms of application and deliverables. SHM methodologies can be broadly categorized into two groups: global methods that can detect if there is damage present in general and local methods that pinpoint the location and specifics of the damage event [2,17]. Frangopol and Messervey [7] expounded on these classifications by subdividing global methods by sensors applicable. This includes piezometric sensors, deformation sensors, accelerometers, and deflection monitoring. The local methods can also be subdivided to include photogrammetry, displacement sensors, electrochemical monitoring, and fatigue measurements. Over time accelerometers in particular have become increasingly promising due to dropping costs, miniaturization, and broader applicability [15]. Accelerometers can be leveraged for a global vibration-based SHM methodology. These vibration-based methodologies exploit the fact that natural frequencies (modal and resonant) are inherent properties of structures, and are in turn determined by physical properties such as mass and stiffness. Since these properties change with damage, natural frequencies serve as a sensitive indicator of structural damage [1,3]. The goal is to use vibration data to obtain these frequencies from the source building (aluminum scale model) to make inferences about the target building (steel scale model) and use transfer learning as a vehicle to get us there. The foundations for transfer learning were conducted on homogenous structures which are nominally identical. This assumes the same materials and dimensions are present across a group of structures. If this condition holds, then the distribution of parameters across structures must also be equal. This allows a general model to be developed to represent the entire population of structures (PBSHM) [5]. This work was later expanded to heterogeneous structures where the assumptions of mutual parameter space are removed. These developments were materialized through a subcategory of transfer learning called domain adaptation. 'Domain adaptation assumes labeled data are available in a source domain and that this can be used to aid classification in an unlabelled target domain, by mapping the two domains onto a common latent space on which the data distributions coincide' [9,12]. Laura Ierimonti et al. [14] used this approach to develop an SHM model for a monumental structure, based on an analytic finite element model. P. Gardener et al. [8] expanded the scope of the application of heterogeneous transfer learning to populations with inconsistent feature spaces. This was achieved via a method called Kernelised Bayesian transfer learning. Kernelised Bayesian transfer broadly works in two stages. The first stage learns an optimal linear projection matrix that maps the domains onto each other in a shared latent space. The second stage learns a discriminative classifier in this shared latent space using a set of shared parameters.

In [10] P. Gardner et al. applied domain adaptation SHM to a 3-story scale model based on vibration SHM and a set of simulated numeric models. The framework of learning in a shared latent space that was laid out in kernelized Bayesian transfer was later adapted via a class of General Adversarial Network (GAN) models. The state-of-the-art models generate the embedding space using a generator and discriminator. GAN models use a generator to generate instances of data from an underlying distribution, with the objective of having those instances match a target distribution. The discriminator subsequently outputs the probability that data belongs to the target distribution. The generator and discriminator are trained in an adversarial manner using a min-max optimization until convergence when the source and target distributions are identical, and the discriminator outputs a 0.5 probability for all inputs [11]. In the context of the SHM problem, the generator computes the embedding for data from both the target and source building, and the discriminator outputs the probability that the embedding is a representation of data from the target building. The trained generator is used to map data from the two buildings into a shared latent space. To compute damage predictions from the embeddings, a classifier is needed. Convolutional neural networks (CNN) have proven to be very successful for this task. In [20] Puruncajas et al. developed a vibration-response CNN for SHM monitoring of off-shore wind turbines. The time series data from these vibration responses can be noisy, however, and noisy time series data can bias the building response so that it no longer reflects the structural condition of a building. This can ultimately hinder the performance of a CNN classifier or other ML-based classifiers. The data can be effectively denoised by transforming the time series representation into the frequency domain. In [3,4] vibration signals were converted into frequency responses and used in a support vector machine to localize concrete cracks. Y. He et al. [13] developed a CNN classifier for SHM using the Fast Fourier Transform (FFT) to compute the data inputs in the frequency domain. The framework of utilizing a GAN for latent embeddings and a CNN for classification has also been adopted on numerous tests across simulated data. Xu and Noh [21] developed the PHYDAN model which integrates multiple source buildings into a GAN framework by using a different discriminator for each building and a mutual CNN predictor. This model trains the discriminator, generator, and CNN-based classifier simultaneously in a 3-entity optimization problem under the assumption that labeled data only exists for the source buildings. The training and testing of the model are evaluated using a series of simulated models. Such a training scheme has proven very effective for knowledge transfer in SHM. This is because training the generator and discriminator allows for data representations to be generated where the distributions of data under the embeddings are equivalent for all buildings, while training the classifier ensures that the discriminative resolution of the data is not lost through the embeddings. Simultaneous training ensures that an optimal trade-off between embedding space consistency and discriminative resolution can be obtained. This is important because a domain invariant embedding may not hold any predictive information on the structural health of a building, meanwhile, a highly discriminative embedding may not be shared amongst the buildings, making the discriminative resolution of the source data non-transferable to the target building [21]. This paper adopts the methodologies employed in [21] to the case where labeled data on the target domain is available and integrated into the training process. The evaluation is also transferred from simulated models to the case of real-world physical structures to investigate the applicability of this framework across existing structures.

This paper aims to investigate the feasibility and potential benefits of deploying transfer learning-based SHM models to classify damage on high-rise structures. To be a viable solution for ameliorating data sparsity in ML models, transfer learning should be shown to bolster the performance of models trained exclusively on the target building. That is, the knowledge gained from supplementary buildings should produce a model with a performance gain over models which are naive to this information. The idea motivating this method of compar-

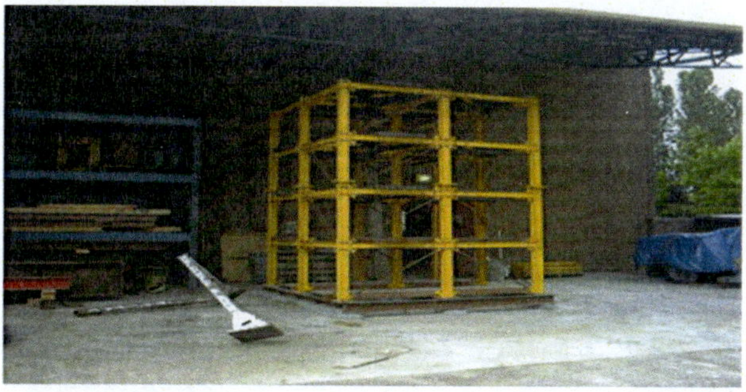

Fig. 1. UBC steel structure (Target structure) Adapted from [6]

ison is the notion that with severely limited data on the target building, there could be a lot of benefit in having supplementary data to gain more information on rare structural states. As the dataset from the target building increases, reliance on supplementary data may not prove to be as beneficial. This can be due to a lack of additional useful information from the source buildings, or due to prediction bias introduced by a partial discrepancy in the data distributions.

3 Method

3.1 Data Collection

The data for this research was collected from two sources. The data for the target building was downloaded off the DEEDS database and contains a zip file of data on a scale model structure, tested at the University of British Columbia [12]. The zip file contains MAT files of data recorded from 15 accelerometers placed throughout the frame, one accelerometer on the shake bed, and a force transducer under the rubber tip of a hammer for impact tests. The data was recorded by researchers at UBC using FBA accelerometers oriented along the strong axis, and EPI sensors along the weak axis. The accelerometers were connected to a 16-channel DasyLab acquisition system to record the accelerometer signals. The data files are divided between ambient data, as well as data under stresses from a shaker table and hammer under different simulated damage scenarios. The data from the hammer tests were sampled at a frequency of 1000 Hz, and the remaining scenarios were sampled at a rate 200 Hz. The structure analyzed is a 4-storey, 2-bay by 2-bay steel scale model. It measures 2.5 m $\times$ 2.5 m in the horizontal plane, and 3.6 m in height. A photograph of the structure is shown in Fig. 1, and a more complete description of the structure and experimental design, as well as access to the data is available at [6].

The other data for the source building is downloaded as a zip file off of the SHM data repository from the website of the Los Alamos National Laboratory Engineering Institute [19]. The source data is on a three-story frame structure. It consists of MAT files of data from 24 piezoelectric single-axis accelerometers (two per joint), as well as data from a force transducer to measure the input force

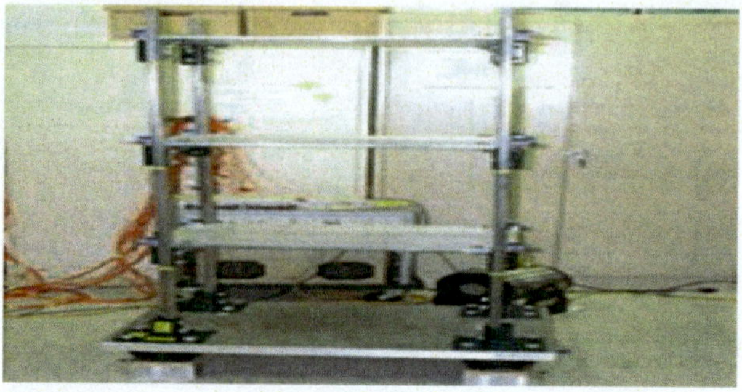

Fig. 2. Los Alamos aluminum structure (Source Building) Adapted from [19]

Table 1. The three distinct cases description

Label	Damage Description
0	Undamaged (baseline)
1	Damaged-removal of a single bracket on the first floor
2	Damaged-removal of a bracket on the first floor and opposite corner of the top floor

from the shaker. The data files are divided between the undamaged structure and various simulated damage scenarios. Each file contains the accelerometer data as a time series of 8192 samples, sampled at a rate of 1600 Hz. The structure is a 3-story scale model, constructed of unistrut columns and aluminum floor plates. The floor plates are mounted to the unistrut columns via brackets secured with two bolts. The structure has a base measuring 0.610 m × 0.762 m and a height of 1.553 m. A photograph of the structure is shown in Fig. 2. For a more complete description of the structure and experimental design, refer to [19].

3.2 Data Preparation

The datasets for both buildings were imported into python data frames. Effective knowledge transfer requires the label space to be equivalent [6]. To ensure this criterion was met, only data from mutual damage cases were retained. The shared label space consists of three distinct cases described in the Table 1.

The sensors used for the analysis were reduced to a mutual subset to ensure that the distributions of the training data were similar. This was done by only using three time-series inputs. The first is the acceleration history for the shakers used to simulate earthquakes on the test structures. The other two inputs consist of single-axis accelerometers oriented in the strong axis of the top and bottom floors of both structures. This choice of sensors creates a more symmetric relation of features in comparison to the case where all sensors are used for each building. Furthermore, this data limitation stresses the importance of using supplementary data for classification, so that the effectiveness of transfer learning can be evaluated.

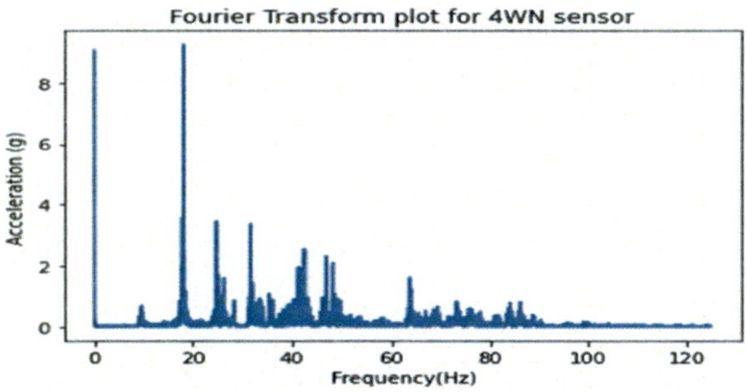

Fig. 3. Fourier transform plot for 4WN sensor

The data on the Los Alamos structure was downsampled from 1600 Hz 200 Hz so that it matched the sampling frequency of the UBC model. Data augmentation was also performed by upsampling the data using a sliding window. At each iteration, the vibration data contained within the window is used as a single instance of the data with its corresponding damage label. The window size was set at 800 data points (4 s). The stride of the sliding window was varied to create datasets of varying sizes so that the effect of training data size on the models could be determined. The window slicing serves a couple of additional functions. Firstly it upsamples the data. This is necessary since the UBC scale model building contains only one experiment from each damage case. More data is therefore required to train and test a model. Secondly, window slicing allows for a constant length input size to be generated. This is necessary since the sample durations for the models are different, and CNN's require a fixed input size for training and evaluation.

The sliced time series were converted to the frequency domain using the FFT algorithm. The Frequency domain data has the effect of denoising the time series input [15]. The frequency domain data of the time-sliced accelerometer measurements were used as the input features for the downstream modeling tasks. The frequency representation makes the underlying trends in time series data more prevalent. Figure 4 shows the frequency domain representations for acceleration responses in the undamaged UBC model at the location of a joint on the top floor of the structure. It is evident that a frequency of 20 Hz is the modal excitation frequency for the structure at the 4 WN sensor location. These modal frequencies are highly correlated to the integrity of a structure and therefore provide rich damage-sensitive features for the downstream models [4]. The frequency spectrums for each test case were stacked into an array and reshaped from a 3×400 array to a 30×40 array. This served as the input representation for the CNN architectures (Fig. 3).

3.3 GAN-CNN Model

We proposed a novel GAN-CNN model consists of an embedding generator, discriminator, and predictor. The layout of the network is shown in Fig. 4. During

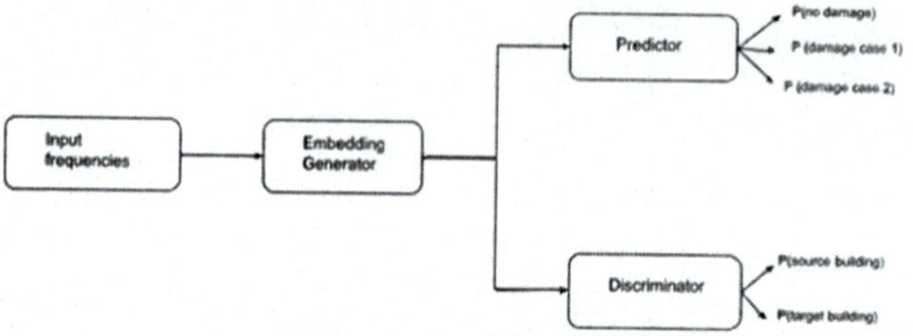

Fig. 4. GAN-CNN Architecture

Table 2. GAN-CNN settings

Network	Function	Parameters
Embedding Generator	conovolution kernel	30 feature maps, 5×5 size, 1×1 stride
	max pool	2×2
	convolution kernel	80 feature maps, 5×5 size, 1×1 stride
	max pool	2×2
	convolutional kernel	120 feature maps, 2×2 size, 1×1 stride
Discriminator	fully connected	$12{,}480 \times 1$
Predictor	conovolution kernel	80 feature maps, 2×2 size, 1×1 stride
	fully connected	6720×60
	fully connected	60×20
	fully connected	20×5
	output	5×3

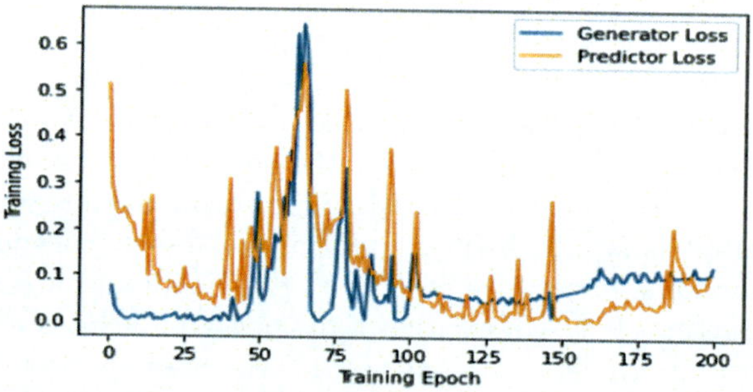

Fig. 5. The convergence of the loss functions for the predictor and generator over 200 epochs.

training, sample frequencies from both structures are fed into the model. The first stage is an embedding generator that uses a CNN to embed the frequency input into a latent space. The embedding is then passed to the discriminator. The discriminator flattens the embedding and uses a fully connected layer to compute the probability that the embedded input belongs to the target structure. The embedding is also passed to the predictor. The predictor uses a CNN to compute the probabilities that the embedding is representative of each damage state. A full description of the parameters of each network is provided in Table 2. The loss function for the discrimator is binary cross entropy loss computed using the probability of the target structure predicted by the discrimator, and the actual structure label. The loss function for the predictor is binary cross entropy loss computed using the predicted damage state probabilities and the actual damage label. Conversely, the loss of the generator is the binary cross entropy loss of the discriminator predictions and the opposite of the actual labels. The loss function of the generator is set this way so that loss is minimized when the discriminator performs poorly. These loss functions are used for backpropgation in the network parameter updates. Training a GAN model is notoriously difficult due to the competing objectives of the generator and discriminator. The addition of the predictor adds further complexity to the geometry of the parameter space. Early trials resulted in the discriminator loss converging to 0 while the generator loss continuously increased, as the gradients vanished, preventing parameter updates in the generator. This was corrected by simplifying the discriminator into a shallow network so that the generator loss and predictor loss could converge at some equilibrium. Figure 5 shows the convergence of the loss functions for the predictor and generator over 200 epochs.

4 Experiments and Results

Our model was evaluated on both the UBC and Los Alamos structures. The structure of the training data and results on the test set are presented in Table 3. Each case used a train:validation:test ratio of 60:20:20, and was trained using 100 epochs. The loss was calculated using binary cross entropy loss. The model parameters at the epoch that minimized this loss on the validation set were retained for the test set evaluation.

As can be seen from Table 3, it is clear that the CNN architecture is able to easily discriminate between the scenarios of damaged and undamaged structures for both buildings. Given enough data, the model can perfectly differentiate the cases, and even in training settings of limited data the performance is still excellent. This demonstrates that there are clear differences in structural responses between damaged and undamaged structures, which makes it evident which binary state is present.

The next experiment is to do a three-class classification task which aims to further split the damage cases into two distinct cases as shown in Table 1. Evaluation is performed on the target structure (UBC structure). Two models are contrasted in this setting. The baseline model is a CNN adapted for 3-class classification, which is trained and tested on the target structure. The transfer learning model is a GAN-CNN model. This model was trained on training data from both the source and target structure, and then evaluated on a test set from the target structure only.

The predictive accuracy of the two models under different data constraints is presented in Table 4. The first test evaluates the classifiers in the presence

Table 3. The structure of the training data and results on the test set

Model	undamaged case		damaged case		accuracy	macro average F1
	window stride	training samples	window stride	training samples		
UBC (Target)	100	140	200	140	1	1
	100	140	800	36	0.92	0.87
	100	140	1200	24	0.91	0.81
Los Alamos (Source)	50	90	50	90	1	1
	100	54	50	90	0.99	0.98
	200	36	50	90	0.98	0.98

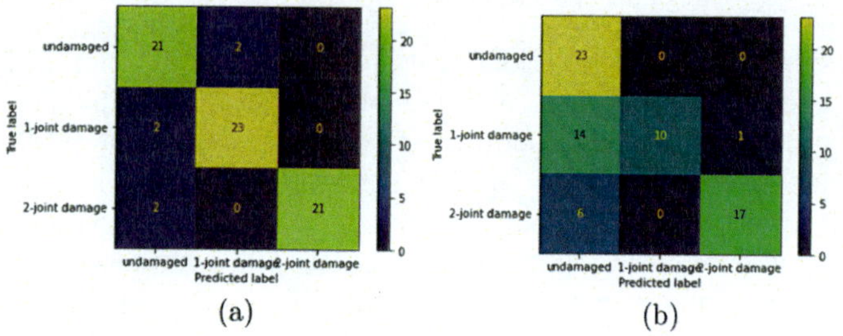

Fig. 6. (a) CNN trained on full data. (b) GAN- CNN trained on full data.

of a sufficient amount of training data. The second test evaluates the classifiers with limited data from the undamaged case. This is an unlikely scenario as undamaged data is the most prevalent scenario. This evaluation was done for completeness however. The final test compares the models when there is limited damage data available on the target structure. As can be seen from Table 4, it is evident that the CNN model outperforms the transfer learning model when sufficient data on the damaged states of the structures is provided. The transfer learning GAN-CNN model outperforms the CNN model in the case of limited damage from case 2.

The Confusion matrix for the CNN and GAN-CNN model predictions when trained on the full dataset is displayed in Figs. 6(a) and 6(b). The CNN model is able to accurately classify the damage state of the target structure as there are only a few cases of misclassified samples. The GAN-CNN model does not perform as well as the CNN model in this setting. This is likely due to the model bias introduced by training across two structures.

The Confusion matrix for the CNN and GAN-CNN model predictions when trained with limited samples of damage case 2 is displayed in Figs. 7(a) and 7(b). We can see that the CNN performs extremely poorly in this case. A noteworthy observation is that the model never predicts that damage case 2 is present. This is likely because the model is too uninformed on this state to make predictions about it. The GAN-CNN model does comparatively better in this scenario since it is informed on this damage state from information gained from the source building. This model does not perform as well as the CNN when there is an abundance of data. A noteworthy observation from Figs. 6(b) and 7(b) is that the

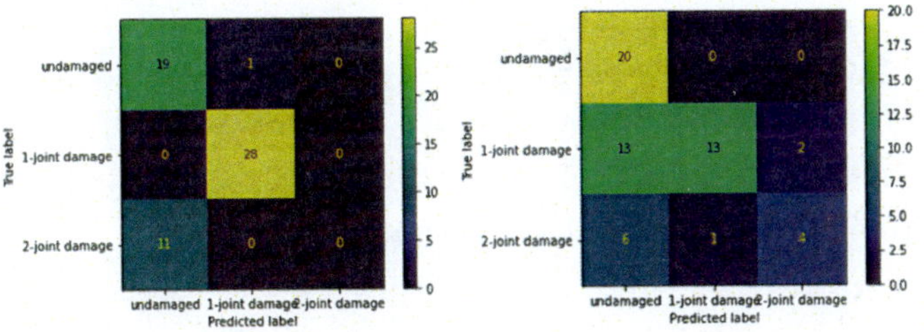

(a) (b)

Fig. 7. (a) CNN trained on limited damage. (b) GAN- CNN trained on limited damage.

Table 4. The predictive accuracy of the two models under different data constraints

Undamaged case		Damage case 1		Damage Case 2		Macro average F1	
window stride	training samples	window stride	training samples	window stride	training samples	CNN	GAN-C NN
200	117	200	117	200	117	0.92	0.70
400	59	200	117	200	117	0.80	0.61
200	117	200	117	400	59	0.48	0.59

GAN-CNN model performs consistently across cases, while the CNN deteriorates quickly when damage data is not available. The GAN-CNN was also able to predict the undamaged state perfectly in all cases.

4.1 Discussion

The results of this work indicate that the transfer learning model has a comparative advantage over the target-only model in cases where damage data on the target structure is limited. However, the target-only model performs significantly better when trained on a sufficient amount of data from the damage cases. This trend is likely the product of a combination of different factors. The transfer learning model improves model predictions when damage cases are rare in the target building because the model can leverage information on damage from a source building. The downside is that a bias is introduced by training on other structures, and some predictive power is still lost in the embedding since this trade-off is necessary to ensure embeddings are distribuitionally equivalent across structures. This experiment also validates the potential for transfer learning by extending the existing literature to a real world comparison, so that the effectiveness of the models outside simulated data can be observed. Transfer learning across existing structures as exemplified in this report opens the door to a much greater range of applications in the future. This paves the way for future research in the field which can expand on the methodology and potentially increase the scope of how dissimilar structures can be while still appreciably benefiting from transfer learning. The overarching implications of this are that the demands for the large quantity of data required in machine learning SHM models can be met, opening the door for applications of SHM at larger scale. This will also define a positive feedback loop since more data will increase SHM applications in turn increasing the amount of data available. I see this as the most viable long term path to scale the technology and make it more accessible.

5 Conclusion and Future Work

This analysis only considers scale models in a controlled environment and does not account for all sources of ambient noise. Furthermore, while the structures being evaluated are different in terms of materials and construction, they are similar in geometry. More research is needed to investigate the effectiveness of TL-based SHM in the context of heterogeneous buildings with topological variability, and where additional sources of noise, such as varying soil conditions are present. Additionally since the experimental models used in this research were not constructed for the purpose of this report or for compatibility in a transfer learning framework, allot of data was discarded on damage cases that were not mutual between the structures. Future research can be conducted where damage scenarios across structures are consistent, and this would allow for a much larger range of classes to be accounted for in a model. A natural extension to this work is to investigate cases where multiple physical source buildings are used to inform the model. This can potentially shrink the bias introduced by using a single source structure. Furthermore, the results of this experiment have shown that in the presence of sufficient data, the target-only model performs best by eliminating bias all together. This suggests the potential benefit of an ensemble combining both the target-only and transfer learning model. A model using such a framework can leverage data at the expense of bias during the initial phase of operation when a relatively small amount of data is available on the target structure. The network can then dynamically adjust the weighting of the two models to favour the target-only model as training data increase so that bias can be removed at this phase.

References

1. Anaissi, A., Khoa, N.L.D., Rakotoarivelo, T., Alamdari, M.M., Wang, Y.: Adaptive online one-class support vector machines with applications in structural health monitoring. ACM Trans. Intell. Syst. Technol. (TIST) **9**(6), 1–20 (2018)
2. Anaissi, A., Lee, Y., Naji, M.: Regularized tensor learning with adaptive one-class support vector machines. In: Cheng, L., Leung, A.C.S., Ozawa, S. (eds.) ICONIP 2018. LNCS, vol. 11303, pp. 612–624. Springer, Cham (2018). https://doi.org/10.1007/978-3-030-04182-3_54
3. Anaissi, A., Makki Alamdari, M., Rakotoarivelo, T., Khoa, N.L.D.: A tensor-based structural damage identification and severity assessment. Sensors **18**(1), 111 (2018)
4. Anaissi, A., Zandavi, S.M., Suleiman, B., Naji, M., Braytee, A.: Multi-objective variational autoencoder: an application for smart infrastructure maintenance. Appl. Intell. 1–16 (2022)
5. Bull, L., et al.: Foundations of population-based SHM, part I: homogeneous populations and forms. Mech. Syst. Sig. Process. **148**, 107141 (2021)

6. Dyke, S.: Report on the building structural health monitoring problem phase 2 analytical (2011)
7. Frangopol, D.M., Messervey, T.B.: Maintenance principles for civil structures. Encyclopedia of Structural Health Monitoring (2009)
8. Gardner, P., Bull, L., Dervilis, N., Worden, K.: On the application of kernelised Bayesian transfer learning to population-based structural health monitoring. Mech. Syst. Sig. Process. **167**, 108519 (2022)
9. Gardner, P., Bull, L., Gosliga, J., Dervilis, N., Worden, K.: Foundations of population-based SHM, part III: heterogeneous populations-mapping and transfer. Mech. Syst. Sign. Process. **149**, 107142 (2021)
10. Gardner, P., Liu, X., Worden, K.: On the application of domain adaptation in structural health monitoring. Mech. Syst. Sig. Process. **138**, 106550 (2020)
11. Goodfellow, I., et al.: Generative adversarial networks. Commun. ACM **63**(11), 139–144 (2020)
12. Gosliga, J., Gardner, P., Bull, L., Dervilis, N., Worden, K.: Foundations of population-based SHM, part II: heterogeneous populations-graphs, networks, and communities. Mech. Syst. Sig. Process. **148**, 107144 (2021)
13. He, Y., Chen, H., Liu, D., Zhang, L.: A framework of structural damage detection for civil structures using fast Fourier transform and deep convolutional neural networks. Appl. Sci. **11**(19), 9345 (2021)
14. Ierimonti, L., Cavalagli, N., Venanzi, I., García-Macías, E., Ubertini, F.: A transfer Bayesian learning methodology for structural health monitoring of monumental structures. Eng. Struct. **247**, 113089 (2021)
15. Kavitha, S., Daniel, R.J., Sumangala, K.: High performance mems accelerometers for concrete SHM applications and comparison with cots accelerometers. Mech. Syst. Sig. Process. **66**, 410–424 (2016)
16. Khoa, N.L.D., Anaissi, A., Wang, Y.: Smart infrastructure maintenance using incremental tensor analysis. In: Proceedings of the 2017 ACM on Conference on Information and Knowledge Management, pp. 959–967 (2017)
17. Khoa, N.L.D., Makki Alamdari, M., Rakotoarivelo, T., Anaissi, A., Wang, Y.: Structural health monitoring using machine learning techniques and domain knowledge based features. In: Zhou, J., Chen, F. (eds.) Human and Machine Learning. HIS, pp. 409–435. Springer, Cham (2018). https://doi.org/10.1007/978-3-319-90403-0_20
18. Makki Alamdari, M., Anaissi, A., Khoa, N.L., Mustapha, S.: Frequency domain decomposition-based multisensor data fusion for assessment of progressive damage in structures. Struct. Control. Health Monit. **26**(2), e2299 (2019)
19. Michael, J.B., Robert, E.l., Long beach, C.: Los Alamos Los Alamos national laboratory Los Alamos, New Mexico 87545 (2000)
20. Puruncajas, B., Vidal, Y., Tutivén, C.: Vibration-response-only structural health monitoring for offshore wind turbine jacket foundations via convolutional neural networks. Sensors **20**(12), 3429 (2020)
21. Xu, S., Noh, H.Y.: Knowledge transfer between buildings for seismic damage diagnosis through adversarial learning. arXiv preprint arXiv:2002.09513 (2020)

Subscriber Matching in Energy Internet Using the Firefly Algorithm

Lina Benchikh[1](✉), Lemia Louail[2], and Djamila Mechta[1]

[1] LRSD Laboratory, Faculty of Sciences, University Ferhat Abbas Setif 1, Setif, Algeria
{lina.benchikh,mechtadjamila}@univ-setif.dz

[2] Université de Lorraine, CNRS, CRAN, 54000 Nancy, France
lemia.louail@univ-lorraine.fr

Abstract. The Energy Internet (EI) distribution paradigm is a fundamental shift from the traditional centralized energy system towards a decentralized and localized one. This distribution promotes the use of renewable energy sources, which can be harnessed locally and distributed efficiently through microgrids or smart grids, leading to increased energy efficiency, lower operational costs, and improved reliability and resilience. EI involves routing energy from producers to consumers through a complex network. One of the challenges in energy routing is to find the best path for transferring energy between producers and consumers. However, achieving this goal is not an easy task, as it requires finding the best producer for a consumer to ensure efficient and effective energy distribution. In this paper, we propose a new subscriber-matching approach based on the firefly's behavior. This approach helps a consumer find the best set of producers with the best energy price. Furthermore, the proposed method considers the case of multiple sources for one consumer, unlike previous works.

Keywords: Energy Internet · energy routing · energy-efficient path · subscriber matching · Firefly algorithm · bio-inspired algorithm

1 Introduction

Energy Internet (EI) refers to a new paradigm in the global energy system, aimed at creating a highly decentralized, integrated, and intelligent energy network. This concept seeks to optimize the production, distribution, and consumption of energy by incorporating advanced technologies such as the Internet of Things (IoT), artificial intelligence, big data analytics, and blockchain. The main goal of EI is to create a more efficient, reliable, and sustainable energy system that is better able to meet the growing demand for energy, particularly in developing countries, and reduce greenhouse gas emissions. In this system, energy can be produced from a variety of sources, including renewable sources like solar and wind, and then distributed over a smart grid to consumers in real-time.

K. Daimi and A. Al Sadoon (Eds.): ICR 2023, LNNS 721, pp. 418–432, 2023.
https://doi.org/10.1007/978-3-031-35308-6_35

Additionally, energy storage solutions such as batteries and hydrogen fuel cells play a critical role in this concept, allowing excess energy to be stored and used when needed. Overall, the Energy Internet represents a major shift in the way energy is produced, distributed, and consumed, and has the potential to transform the global energy system into one that is more efficient, cost-effective, and environmentally sustainable [1,2].

Energy routing refers to the process of directing the flow of energy in an energy network or grid to optimize its distribution and consumption. The goal of energy routing is to minimize energy loss and improve the overall efficiency of the energy system. In a traditional energy grid, energy is typically generated at large centralized power plants and then distributed to consumers through a network of transmission and distribution lines. Energy routing takes this one step further by using advanced technologies such as artificial intelligence, machine learning, and the IoT to dynamically direct the flow of energy based on real-time demand and supply data. For example, in a smart grid, energy routing algorithms can be used to optimize the distribution of energy from renewable sources such as wind and solar, taking into account factors such as the availability of energy from these sources, the current demand for energy, and the availability of energy storage solutions such as batteries. Energy routing has the potential to greatly improve the efficiency and sustainability of the energy system, reducing energy waste and helping to meet the growing demand for energy in an environmentally responsible way [2–4].

Energy Efficient Path refers to the most optimal way of transferring energy from a producer to a consumer while minimizing energy losses and costs. The goal of finding an energy-efficient path is to ensure that energy is distributed effectively and efficiently, taking into account the available energy resources, the energy demands of consumers, and the overall network infrastructure [5].

Subscriber matching in the Energy Internet refers to the process of connecting energy producers (such as individuals or businesses with their own renewable energy systems) with energy consumers in real-time. This process is facilitated through the use of advanced technologies such as blockchain, the Internet of Things (IoT), and smart grid systems. The idea behind subscriber matching is to create a more decentralized and flexible energy system where excess energy generated by one producer can be sold directly to a nearby consumer, rather than being fed back into the traditional energy grid. This can help to reduce energy waste and improve the overall efficiency of the energy system. In a subscriber matching system, energy producers and consumers can be matched based on their real-time energy needs and availability. For example, a homeowner with a rooftop solar system may have excess energy that they can sell to a nearby business during the day when the business has higher energy demand. The transaction can be recorded on a blockchain-based platform, allowing for a secure, transparent, and tamper-proof record of the transaction. Subscriber matching has the potential to revolutionize the energy industry by enabling a more decentralized and efficient energy system, where energy can be produced and consumed locally and in real-time [6,7].

In this paper, we propose to solve the subscriber matching problem in EI by applying a bio-inspired approach based on the Firefly's behavior.

The remainder of the paper is organized as follows: in the next section, we present the state of the art. Section 3 presents the proposed approach. Section 4 shows the performance evaluation of our approach. Finally, Sect. 5 concludes this paper.

2 Related Works

In order to balance the supply/demand and solve energy-efficient path problems, the authors of [8] proposed a bio-inspired Energy Routing Protocol based on Ant Colony Optimization (ACO). This protocol runs through 3 steps: Collecting information, subscriber matching, and determining the best energy path. The graph of the network is modeled as follows: the producer represents the ant nest, the consumer represents the source of food and the output energy of each producing node represents the ForwardAnt. This model supports the transport of energy to the consumer. Each node has the link state information of all connected nodes in order to build the neighbor's list. Each node chooses the next hop among its neighbors until it reaches the consumer. When the consumer is distinguished, the producer will construct the ForwardAnt with the requested energy. Then the procedure of determining the efficient path by choosing the best next-hop for the consumer among its neighbors starts. As a result, they identify for each consumer a producer that can supply the required energy and determine the optimal path between them. This can be done in a way that minimizes the overall cost while ensuring that the energy demand of each consumer is met. There are some limitations to consider in this work; for instance, only the case of one source load was taken into account.

The energy routing method described in [9] was inspired by the foraging behavior of bees and builds upon the BCO (Bee Colony Optimization) algorithm. The bee colony is represented as follows: the bee hive is the consumer, the flower patch is the producer, the nectar is the energy packet, the scouts represent the energy request message and its response according to its direction and the foragers are the output energy of the producer. Two types of bee agents are implemented: Scout Agents and Forager Agents. Scout Agents travel in the network from one node to another to find the requested energy. After obtaining the objective, the scout constructs and saves the selected path from the consumer to the found producer. Then, it goes back to the consumer following the same path, trying to recruit the foragers using a dance. The dance is abstracted in the quality (Cost) of its founded path. Forager Agents are the main bee agent workers and have two roles. The first role is to notify producers that their corresponding consumers have accepted the energy supply within a predetermined period of time. The second role consists of transporting the energy from the producer to the hive through a specific path. The consumer follows the chosen path in order to reduce costs in terms of power consumption and traveled distance. The same as the previous technique, BCO permits the transfer of energy in an efficient manner with the minimum latency and transmission cost, but, it does not consider the multi-source scenario.

Based on the collective behavior of autonomous agents that interact to find a global solution. Authors in [10] proposed an optimized energy routing method using Particle Swarm Optimization (PSO) to solve the shortest path problem. This method runs in three phases similar to the previous one. Each node constructs its neighbors' list. Then, the producer constructs the packets with the requested energy after receiving the identity of the consumer and its energy demand. After that, the procedure of determining the efficient path by PSO starts. It first generates random particles i.e, a suggested path from the producer to the consumer composed of random nodes which represent the total length of the path. After that, the fitness value is calculated to get the best particles by taking into account latency, distance, and the quality of the link (cost).

In [11] a discrete Artificial Bee Colony (ABC) algorithm for energy routing is introduced. This method runs through 5 steps: Food source representation where the food source in ABC describes a solution i.e, the solution is a path composed of a set of nodes between a consumer and a producer. After that, Discrete ABC initialization phase to provide a better exploration of the search space and to only get feasible solutions. Then, Discrete ABC employed bee phase starts after calculating the fitness value. Next, Discrete ABC Onlooker bee phase begins in which the food source selection process starts, i.e. when the food source information is transmitted by the employed to the onlooker bees, the onlooker bee uses the roulette wheel mechanism and selects a food source to exploit. After that the scout bees take their information from the best solution that they got so far and cross it with the corresponding solution. Finally, to solve the congestion problem a congestion control phase starts. Two congestion management strategies have been used in energy routing protocols. The first one helps to remove all power energy routers and lines that do not meet the transferring power. The second consists of using the energy datagram mode. With this method, the optimal non-congestion path is found.

In [6], the authors implemented various bio-inspired algorithms to find the best load set, the optimal source, and the optimal non-congestion paths with minimum loss. The authors proposed a centralized peer-to-peer energy trading architecture. Then, to assign the best producer for each consumer in terms of minimal cost and power loss, the subscriber matching mechanism starts. In the case of multi-source consumer (heavy load), the particle swarm optimization algorithm was used to determine the amount of power for a group of producers and to achieve minimum power transmission loss and cost. To avoid congestion, an Improved Ant Colony Optimization (IACO) energy routing protocol was implemented.

The authors of [12] proposed a routing approach inspired by bees' colony foraging behavior in order to address routing issues. The bees' colony-inspired energy routing approach was developed to define a non-congestion minimum energy loss path and the best set of producers in terms of energy cost and power transmission losses, to satisfy the consumers' requests at the time by solving three main problems: subscriber matching, efficient energy routing, and scheduling energy transmissions to face congestion. Similarly to [9], the authors used two types of bees (scouts and foragers). Here, the method used to solve the shortest path problem is similar to that used in [6]. Instead of removing all power lines and Energy Routers that do not support the transmitted power to solve congestion and overflow; the authors employed the power packets concept (sending power packets via multiple paths). The search process starts from the consumer node (source node). A central controller is used to enable the peer-to-peer energy trading process. This algorithm generates a list of producers for each consumer who can provide the consumer's energy demand in the corresponding period. Multiple scenarios are available: multiple sources and one consumer demand, multiple sources, and one big consumer (heavy load), and multiple available sources with multiple consumers' demand.

Because of the centralized architecture used in [6,11,12], and the absence of multiple sources of energy in [8–10], we propose a new decentralized approach in the following section to resolve the subscriber matching problem in Energy Internet.

3 Research Proposal

To improve the energy efficiency of the EI by selecting the best producers for the consumers, it is essential to have a method that balances the energy supply and the energy demand. With this goal in mind, we have developed a new subscriber matching scheme based on the Firefly algorithm. This proposed scheme operates as follows.

3.1 Firefly Algorithm

The Firefly Algorithm [13] is a meta-heuristic optimization algorithm inspired by the flashing behavior of fireflies. The algorithm is used to find the optimal solution for optimization problems that involve finding the optimum of a function. The Firefly Algorithm is based on the behavior of fireflies, where they use bio-luminescence to communicate with each other and attract mates. The first rule is that fireflies are unisex. The algorithm uses the intensity of the light emitted by fireflies to represent the fitness of the solution, and the attractiveness between fireflies is used to represent the optimization process. In the Firefly Algorithm, the position of each firefly in the search space corresponds to a potential solution to the optimization problem. The algorithm iteratively updates the position of each firefly in the search space, based on the attractiveness of neighboring fireflies, until a satisfactory solution is found. The Firefly Algorithm has been successfully applied to a variety of optimization problems in various fields such as engineering, finance, and medicine [14–16].

The firefly algorithm works as follows [17]:

- Initializing the population of fireflies with randomly generated positions and light intensities.
- Defining a fitness function that calculates the fitness value of each firefly based on its position in the search space.
- Specifying the maximum number of iterations and setting the iteration counter to zero.
- While the iteration counter is less than the maximum number of iterations:
  - For each firefly in the population, calculate the attractiveness of neighboring fireflies based on their light intensities and distances from the current firefly.
  - Move the firefly towards the more attractive neighboring fireflies, with a step size that is proportional to the attractiveness and inversely proportional to the distance between fireflies.
  - Update the light intensity of the firefly based on its new position.
  - Evaluate the fitness value of the firefly based on its new position, and update the population of fireflies with the best solution found so far.
  - Increment the iteration counter.
- Return the best solution found by the algorithm.

Algorithm 1 describes the work of the firefly algorithm.

Algorithm 1. Pseudo-code of basic Firefly algorithm [18]

Input: objective function $f(x)$
Output: the best solution
Initialize the fireflies population $X = f(x_1, x_2, ..., x_n)$
Evaluate each firefly x_i in the initial population by $f(x_i)$
Light intensity I_i at x_i is determined by $f(x_i)$

while termination criterion not reached **do**
    for $i \leftarrow 1, n$ **do**
        for $j \leftarrow 1, n$ **do**
            if $I_i > I_j$ **then**
                Compute the attractiveness
                Move firefly i toward j
            end if
        end for
    end for
    Evaluate the population
    Rank the fireflies, find the current best
end while
Return the global best solution x^*

3.2 Energy Internet Network Architecture

EI comprises several components:

- Energy Generator: renewable energy sources such as wind turbines, solar panels, and hydroelectric power plants that provide clean and sustainable energy.
- Energy Storage devices: systems used to store excess energy produced by the energy generation systems and to release it when needed such as batteries, fuel cells, and thermal storage.
- Energy Transmission and Distribution system: Power lines and transformers are used to transmit and distribute energy from the energy generators and storage systems to the end-users.
- Energy Management system: Energy Routers (ERs) are the hardware that manages and optimizes the Energy Internet network. It collects and analyzes data from the energy generation, storage, and distribution systems, and uses advanced algorithms to optimize the energy flow and minimize energy waste.
- Smart meters: used to determine the nature of users and represent the main components of advanced energy systems.
- Producers: nodes that only produce energy and sell it to other nodes.
- Consumers: nodes that need energy. Therefore, they buy it from producers or prosumers.
- Prosumers: nodes that generate energy from Distributed Renewable Energy Sources, consume it and sell their own surplus to other consumers.

Figure 1 shows an example of an Energy Internet network with its different components.

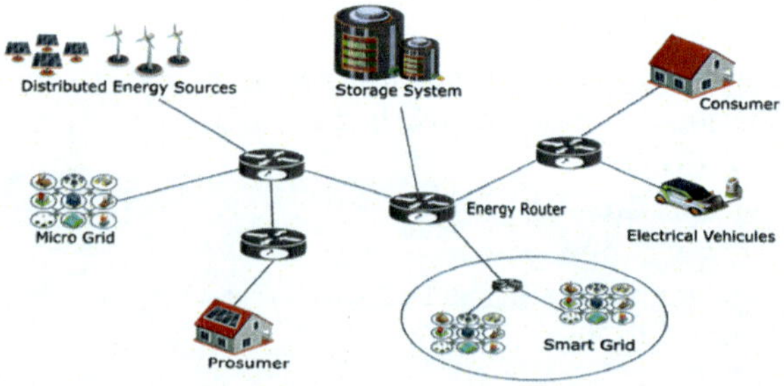

Fig. 1. Energy Internet model

The components of Energy Internet are interconnected and work together to create an integrated and efficient energy system. Users are furnished with Distributed Renewable Energy Sources (DRESs) and/or Distributed Storage Devices (DSDs), connected to the energy routers. These routers manage both communication and power flow in the network. The power and communication flow are bidirectional. Peer-to-peer energy trading allows both prosumers and consumers to exchange energy directly without the need for the utility grid. This made the transmission of energy through power links more complex. To handle the power flow in EI, Energy Routers (ERs) need to be equipped with efficient energy routing algorithms that allow an efficient energy transmission from one or multiple sources to the destination.

In order to simulate the network, the EI is represented as a connected graph G. Where, the vertices $V = (v_1, v_2...v_n)$ represent the network nodes. Each node represents an Energy Router (ER) directly connected to producers, consumers, and/or prosumers. The edges E represent the power links that link the nodes, where e_{ij} is the power link that connects router v_i to router v_j.

3.3 Firefly-Based Energy Routing for Energy Internet (FER-EI)

In this section, we describe our proposed approach called FER-EI (Firefly-based Energy Routing for Energy Internet). This approach helps to solves the subscriber matching problem in Energy Internet. The objective of the subscriber matching process is to combine a group of subscribers (Energy producers) in a way that maximizes the overall satisfaction of consumer demand, subject to certain constraints. These constraints may include cost, quantity offered by each subscriber, power loss, and distance. Our approach determines the best set of subscribers.

According to the decentralized architecture, each node possesses all the necessary information about other nodes. As a result, each consumer can generate all possible combinations of subscribers that can fulfill their required energy demand.

In order to represent the behavior of fireflies in our network we assume that:

- Each firefly represents a prosumer x_i in the network.
- The brightness of a firefly depends on the objective function $f(x)$.
- Three roles are defined. Fireflies that demand energy are consumers. Those who have energy are producers. Fireflies that don't have energy are neither consumers nor producers
- Fireflies are attracted to each other regardless of their roles.
- The consumer chooses the less bright producer.
- In case of the same brightness, the consumer chooses randomly.

To simulate the fireflies' behaviors the FER-EI approach runs in the following steps:

- Step1: Initialization phase
  1. Initializing parameters.
  2. Generate fireflies' swarm population with their positions.

3. Generate the number of subscribers n in the network, the quantity of energy Qnt_i, and the position Pos_i for each participant i,

$$Qnt = \{Qnt_1, Qnt_2, Qnt_3, ..., Qnt_n\})$$

$$Qnt\_i = rand(MinQnt, MaxQnt)$$

where $MaxQnt$ represents the capacity of the DSD and $MinQnt$ represents the needed energy.

$$Pos = (PosX, PosY)$$

$$PosX = \{PosX_1, PosX_2, PosX_3, ..., PosX_n\}$$

$$PosY = \{PosY_1, PosY_2, PosY_3, ..., PosY_n\}$$

$$PosX_i = rand(0, S)$$

$$PosY_i = rand(0, S)$$

where S represents the search space.

- Step2: Computing the fitness value
  1. Get the Energy Demand ED_i from first firefly x_i that has $Qnt_i < 0$. As a reminder, $Qnt_i < 0$ means that the participant has no energy and therefore is considered a consumer.
  2. Calculate the objective function of participants x_j that have a quantity of energy $Qnt_j > 0$. A peer-to-peer energy trading system is applied. Each node operates independently, with the ability to make decisions locally based on its own network requirements.

$$f(x_j) = \alpha * \frac{price_{x_j}}{MaxPrice} + \beta * \frac{Distance_{x_i/x_j}}{MaxDistance}$$

α and β are factors that indicate the relative significance of the price and the distance.

$$price_{x_j} = (Qnt_{xj} * cost_{xj})$$

$cost_{x_j}$ represents the energy unit price of the producer x_j.
The power loss is related to two main factors: the distance between nodes, and the capacity of both power lines losses and ER losses that build the path. Here, we consider that all path links have the same capacity in the network. The same as all energy routers. The distance, on the other hand,

is calculated as follows:

$$Distance_{x_i/x_j} = \sqrt{(posX_{x_i} - posX_{x_j})^2 + (posY_{x_i} - posY_{x_j})^2}$$

- Consumer x_i starts searching for energy from fireflies (producers) who have $f(x_j) > 0$.
- Choose the firefly (producer) x_j with the lowest $f(x_j) > 0$.

– Step3: Update the energy quantity of consumer x_i and the chosen producer x_j:
  - if producer x_j has the exact amount of energy needed by consumer x_i ($Qnt_j = ED_i$), the updates to apply are:

$$Qnt_i = Qnt_i + Qnt_j$$

$$ED_i = 0$$

$$Qnt_j = 0$$

  x_j is added to the group of subscribers and is deleted (temporarily) from the search space.
  - Otherwise
    * if producer x_j has less energy than the amount needed by x_i ($Qnt_j < ED_i$), the updates to apply are:

$$Qnt_i = Qnt_i + Qnt_j$$

$$ED_i = ED_i - Qnt_j$$

$$Qnt_j = 0$$

    * if the producer x_j has more than the energy needed by the consumer x_i (($Qnt_j > ED_i$), the updates will be:

$$Qnt_i = Qnt_i + ED_i$$

$$Qnt_j = Qnt_j - ED_i$$

$$ED_i = 0$$

Here, the consumer got the needed energy; it leaves the group of consumers. The next consumer starts running the same procedure until all the consumers are satisfied.

The instructions are condensed into the subsequent FER-EI Algorithm 2:

Algorithm 2. FER-EI algorithm

```
Input: ED_i, Qnt_i = Qnt_1, Qnt_2, ...., Qnt_n, Pos_i = Pos_1, Pos_2, ...., Pos_n
Output: Best set of producers
Initialize the prosumers population X_i = (x_1, x_2, ...., x_n)
while x_i exist do /*consumers exist*/
    get x_i /*get the consumer*/
    calculate the objective function F(x_j) of each producer x_j
    while ED_i ≠ 0 do /*The demand energy no reached*/
        choose producer x_j such as {x_j ∈ X_i, F(x_j) > 0, min(F(X_i))}
        if ED_i == Qnt_j then
            Qnt_i = Qnt_i + Qnt_j
            ED_i = 0
            Qnt_j = 0
        else if ED_i < Qnt_j then
            Qnt_i = Qnt_i + Qnt_j
            ED_i = ED_i − Qnt_j
            Qnt_j = 0
        else
            Qnt_i = Qnt_i + ED_i
            Qnt_j = Qnt_j − ED_i
            ED_i = 0
        end if
        x_j /* leaves the search space*/
        j = j + 1 /* next producer*/
    end while/* best producers found for current consumer*/
    i=i+1 /* next consumer*/
end while
Return the global best group of producers for each consumer
```

4 Performance Evaluation

The proposed algorithm was implemented in MATLAB r2019a version 9.6. The simulation code was run on a laptop with an 11th Gen Intel(R), Core(TM), i7-11370H @ 3.30 GHz, 8.00 GB RAM, 64-bit operating system. In the following, experiments were performed to verify the efficiency of the proposed approach. Figure 2 shows an example of an Energy Internet network with 17 nodes represented as a graph.

4.1 Multiple Energy Sources and One Consumer Demand

In this section, we consider the case where many producers can provide the energy needed by the same consumer. To find the best set of these producers, in terms of price and distance, the FER-EI approach starts running. Each firefly

Table 1. Energy information of the producers and the consumer

Producer	*energy (kw)*	*cost (usd/kw)*	*Pos(x,y)*	*Compared to*	*Distance*	*price (usd)*	*ED (kw)*	*Compared to*	*Distance*	*price (usd)*	*ED (kw)*
N1	15	0.068	(5,3)	***N4***	5.5902	0.4080	−9	***N16***	2.8284	0.2040	−12
N2	25	0.043	(6.5,5.5)	***N4***	2.6926	0.6880	−9	***N16***	5.7009	0.5590	−12

Table 2. α variation in multiple energy sources and one consumer demand

Producer		*0.1*	*0.2*	*0.3*	*0.4*	*0.5*	*0.6*	*0.7*	*0.8*	*0.9*
N4	**fitness of N1**	5.0720	*4.5537*	4.0355	3.51	2.9991	2.4809	***1.96***	1.4444	0.9262
	fitness of N2	2.4921	2.2917	2.0912	1.98	1.6903	1.4898	1.28	1.0889	0.8885
N16	**fitness of N1**	2.56660	*2.3035*	2.0411	1.7787	1.5162	1.2538	*0.9913*	0.7289	0.4664
	fitness of N2	5.1867	4.6725	4.1583	3.6441	3.1299	2.6158	2.1016	1.5874	1.0732

travels the network to find a solution presented by a producer (firefly). The fitness value of each solution is computed. Then, the solution (the best producer) with the minimum fitness value will be selected by respecting all constraints.

In this example: N1, and N2 are considered producers. N4 and N16 are considered consumers. The rest of the nodes are considered relay points (routers).

Table 1 represents the information of each participant in the system, where consumers are listed with their distance and price compared to N1 and N2, position, and energy demand. The producers are listed along with their respective energy production capacities, cost, and position. This information is essential for identifying the optimal energy distribution strategy in the system, which involves determining how much energy should be allocated to each source and the most efficient way to transfer the energy to the consumer while minimizing energy losses and costs.

N4 can get the needed energy from both N1 and N2. The same for N16. To select the best producer for each consumer, the FER-EI algorithm calculates the fitness value of each producer and then chooses the best one for each consumer according to these values. The optimization results of the proposed approach with different values of α are illustrated in Table 2. Figure 2 shows the best producer for each consumer. Where the best producer for consumer 16 is N1 and for consumer 4 is N2.

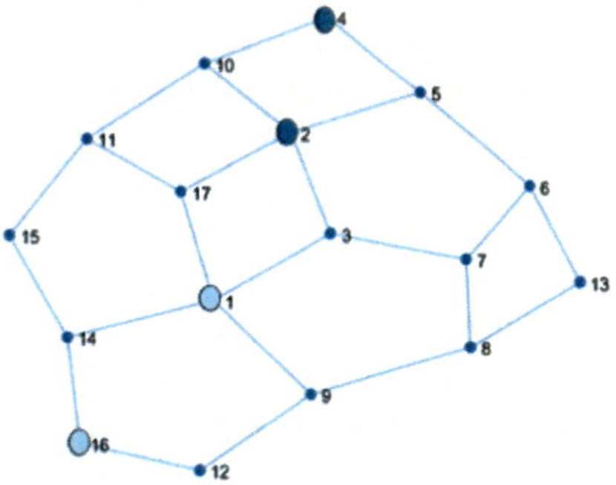

Fig. 2. Best producer for the consumer N1 and N2

4.2 Multiple Available Sources and One Big Consumer

In this case, according to Table 3, there are two consumers (N4 and N16) with five producers (N1, N2, N6, N7 and N15). Here, to satisfy the consumer energy demand, the FER-EI algorithm selects the solution that has the best fitness value by getting the maximum power and the minimum price value to maximize the stability of the network. Then, to get the rest of the power, the same procedure will be generated. Finally, energy information is updated. In case of not having energy, the consumer load cannot be provided.

Table 3. Energy information of the participants

Participant	*Pos(x,y)*	*energy (kw)*	*cost (usd/kw)*
N1	(5, 3)	15	0.068
N2	(6.5, 5.5)	25	0.043
N6	(9.5, 6.5)	10	0.041
N7	(8, 3)	10	0.023
N15	(1, 4)	17	0.053
N4	(7.5, 8)	−40	/
N16	(3, 1)	−30	/

Table 4. α variation in multiple energy sources and one consumer demand

Producer		*0.1*	*0.2*	*0.3*	*0.4*	*0.5*	*0.6*	*0.7*	*0.8*	*0.9*
N4	**fitness of N1**	4.1551	5.0161	4.7291	4.4421	4.1551	3.8681	3.5811	3.2940	3.0070
	fitness of N2	2.2063	2.4981	2.4008	2.3035	2.2063	2.1090	2.0118	1.9145	1.8173
	fitness of N6	2.0700	2.3280	2.2420	2.1560	2.0700	1.9840	1.8980	1.8120	1.7260
	fitness of N7	2.9725	4.2040	3.7935	3.3830	2.9725	2.5620	2.1515	1.7410	1.3305
	fitness of N15	4.8761	6.5297	5.9785	5.4273	4.8761	4.3249	3.7737	3.2224	2.6712
N16	**fitness of N1**	2.7496	2.6707	2.5919	2.5131	2.4342	2.3554	2.2765	2.1977	2.1188
	fitness of N2	5.2598	4.8187	4.3776	3.9365	3.4954	3.0544	2.6133	2.1722	1.7311
	fitness of N6	7.7862	7.0578	6.3293	5.6008	4.8723	4.1439	3.4154	2.6869	1.9585
	fitness of N7	4.9156	4.4461	3.9766	3.5071	3.0376	2.5681	2.0985	1.6290	1.1595
	fitness of N15	3.4040	3.2024	3.0009	2.7993	2.5978	2.3962	2.1947	1.9931	1.7916

As illustrated in Table 3, N4 and N16 can buy energy from multiple sources (N1, N2, N6, N7 and N15). Many groups are possible to provide the needed energy. To get the best set, the FER-EI algorithm will choose for each consumer the best producers in terms of their fitness value. The optimization results of the proposed approach with different values of α are shown in Table 4. Figures 3 and 4 summarize the best set of producers for the consumers N4 and N16 respectively.

The analysis reveals that the ideal producers for satisfying the energy demands of consumer N4 are N2, N6, and N7. Among them, N6 is the most efficient one, but it is unable to fulfill the required energy demand. N5 is included in the group, but it also falls short of the desired quantity. Eventually, N2 is selected to join the group, leading to the fulfillment of the energy requirements of the consumer. As a result, the updated quantity values are as follows: $Qnt_{N6} = 0$, $Qnt_{N7} = 0$ and $Qnt_{N2} = 5$.

For consumer N16, if the value of α is between 0.1 and 0.6, the best producers for fulfilling its energy needs are N1 and N15. However, N1, although the most efficient, is not able to satisfy the energy demand. Therefore, N15 is selected to

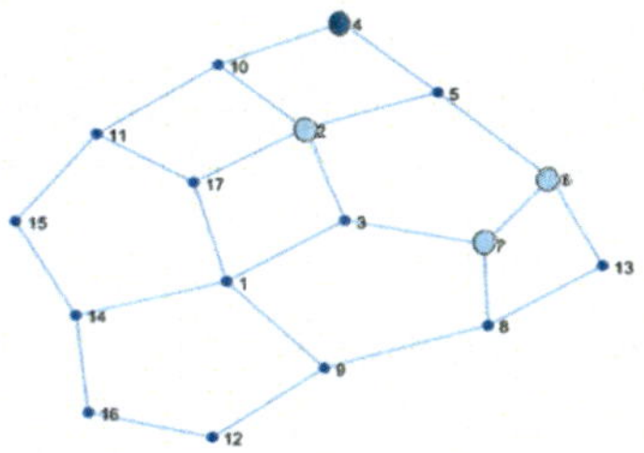

Fig. 3. Best set of producers for the consumer N4

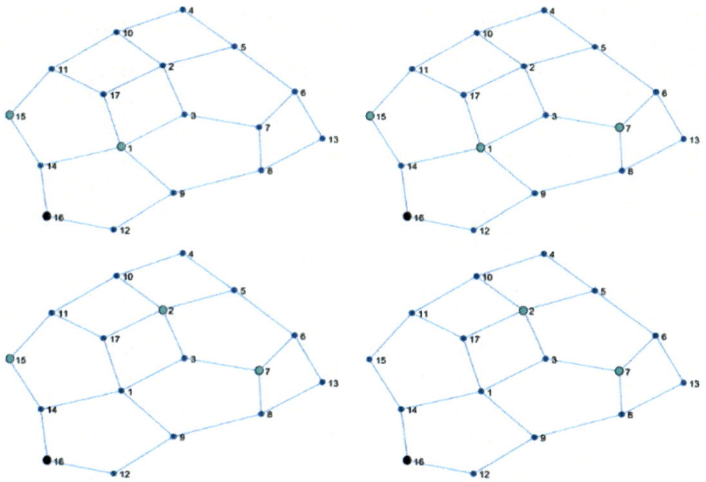

Fig. 4. Best set of producers for the consumer N16 with $0.1 \leq \alpha \leq 0.6$ (top left), $\alpha = 0.7$ (top right), $\alpha = 0.8$ (bottom left) and $\alpha = 0.9$ (bottom right)

join the group and meets the energy requirements of the consumer. Consequently, the new quantity values are updated to $Qnt_{N1} = 0$ and $Qnt_{N15} = 2$.

In the case where $\alpha = 0.7$, the most suitable producers to meet the energy requirements of consumer N16 are N1, N7, and N15. Despite being the most efficient one, N7 cannot supply the required energy demand, and N15 falls short of the desired quantity even when added to the group. Ultimately, N1 is selected, and the energy requirements of the consumer are met. Thus, the updated quantity values are as follows: $Qnt_{N7} = 0$, $Qnt_{N15} = 0$, and $Qnt_{N1} = 12$. The same is true for $\alpha = 0.8$, but N2 is selected instead of N1, resulting in $Qnt_{N2} = 22$. Finally, with $\alpha = 0.9$ the best producers are N7 and N2, the updated quantity values are as follows: $Qnt_{N7} = 0$, $Qnt_{N2} = 5$.

5 Conclusion

The Energy Internet distribution paradigm is a trans-formative concept that has the potential to revolutionize the way we produce, distribute and consume energy. This paper addresses the energy routing problem by solving the subscriber matching issue. We proposed a new approach, FER-EI, based on the Firefly algorithm. With this bio-inspired technique, our approach finds the best set of producers for an energy consumer at an optimal price. The simulation results have proven the efficiency of the proposed approach. As future work, we plan on trying our approach on much bigger networks and analyzing its performance in such a context.

References

1. Zhou, K., Yang, S., Shao, Z.: Energy internet: the business perspective. Appl. Energy **178**, 212–222 (2016)
2. Hebal, S., Harous, S., Mechta, D.: Energy routing challenges and protocols in energy internet: a survey. J. Electr. Eng. Technol. **16**(6), 3197–3212 (2021)
3. Wang, K., et al.: A survey on energy internet communications for sustainability. IEEE Trans. Sustain. Comput. **2**(3), 231–254 (2017)
4. Hussain, S.M.S., et al.: The emerging energy internet: architecture, benefits, challenges, and future prospects. Electronics **8**(9), 1037 (2019)
5. Hussain, H.M., et al.: What is energy internet? Concepts, technologies, and future directions. IEEE Access **8**, 183127–183145 (2020)
6. Hebal, S., et al.: Hybrid energy routing approach for energy internet. Energies **14**(9), 2579 (2021)
7. Abdella, J., Shuaib, K., Harous, S.: Energy routing algorithms for the energy internet. In: 2018 International Conference on Intelligent Systems (IS). IEEE (2018)
8. Hebal, S., Mechta, D., Harous, S.: Aco-based distributed energy routing protocol in smart grid. In: 2019 IEEE 10th Annual Ubiquitous Computing, Electronics and Mobile Communication Conference (UEMCON) (2019)
9. Hebal, S., Harous, S., Mechta, D.: Latency and energy transmission cost optimization using BCO-aware energy routing for smart grid. In: 2020 IEEE IWCMC (2020)
10. Mechta, D., Harous, S., Hebal, S.: Energy-efficient path-aware routing Protocol based on PSO for Smart Grids. In: 2020 IEEE International Conference on Electro Information Technology (EIT) (2020)
11. Hebal, S., Harous, S., Mechta, D.: Solving energy routing problem in energy internet using a discrete artificial bee colony algorithm. In: 2022 IEEE IWCMC (2022)
12. Fawaz, A., Mougharbel, I., Kanaan, H.Y.: New routing application using bees colony for energy internet. In: 2022 3rd International Conference on Smart Grid and Renewable Energy (SGRE). IEEE (2022)
13. Yang, X.-S., Slowik, A.: Firefly algorithm. In: Swarm Intelligence Algorithms, pp. 163–174. CRC Press (2020)
14. Choudhury, A., et al.: Segmentation of brain MR images using quantum inspired firefly algorithm with mutation. In: IWBBIO, Maspalomas, Gran Canaria, Spain, 27–30 June 2022
15. Thepphakorn, T., Pongcharoen, P.: Modified and hybridised bi-objective firefly algorithms for university course scheduling. Soft Comput. 1–38 (2023)
16. Tilahun, S.L., Ngnotchouye, J.M.T.: Firefly algorithm for discrete optimization problems: a survey. KSCE J. Civ. Eng. **21**(2), 535–545 (2017). https://doi.org/10.1007/s12205-017-1501-1
17. Li, J., et al.: A survey on firefly algorithms. Neurocomputing **500**, 662–678 (2022)
18. Yang, X.-S.: Nature-Inspired Metaheuristic Algorithms. Luniver Press (2010)

Posters

Training Problem-Solvers by Using Real World Problems as Case Studies

Martin Q. Zhao(✉) and Robert Allen

Department of Computer Science, Mercer University, Macon, GA, USA
{zhao_mq,allen_r}@mercer.edu

Abstract. Employers of software engineers seek to hire who are not only excellent software developers but also possess three important skills: interpersonal communication, team collaboration, and problem solving. Mercer University's Computer Science Department has a history of using real world problems for projects to motivate students and provides a rich environment for them to develop their problem solving and interpersonal skills. High-profile events like the Super Bowl can draw interests from students in a variety of courses. This poster will present the plan for using a project centered on Super Bowl to attract student's interest, tailor teaching materials and hands-on exercises around this popular topic, and make appropriate assignments to students in two ongoing courses. The resultant software product can be extended in future courses to help train our students into problem solvers.

Keywords: Case-based learning · Collaborative learning · Innovative teaching · CS Education · Problem Solving Skills

1 Introduction

Employers of software engineers tell us that they seek to hire students who are not only excellent software developers but also possess three important skills: interpersonal communication, team collaboration, and problem solving. It is imperative that software engineering educators incorporate the development and nurturing of these important skills into their curriculum. Additionally, programs need to find ways to attract cohorts of students who will quickly embrace the practice of these skills.

Mercer University's Computer Science Department has a history of using real world problems for projects to motivate our students. Recently, we made curricular changes to further address this growing need of employers seeking to hire software engineers. We have seen how using real world problems motivates students and provides a rich environment for them to develop their interpersonal communication skills, team collaboration, and problem-solving skills.

A highly motivational, real-world case study could be related to the Super Bowl, or similarly popular events. The high-profile nature of such an annual event will draw a variety of student interests. A project centered on such a popular event could be designed which blends student talents from multiple computer science courses. We are forming a virtual software development "company" that uses students from a variety of courses

K. Daimi and A. Al Sadoon (Eds.): ICR 2023, LNNS 721, pp. 435–440, 2023.
https://doi.org/10.1007/978-3-031-35308-6_36

to build the case study project. Every student will need to collaborate with all the other students, using their interpersonal communication skills to solve an interesting problem.

In this poster, we focus on using one real world problem, Super Bowl, to attract student's interest, tailor teaching materials and hands-on exercises around this topic, and make appropriate assignments to students in intermediate programming (CSC 205 – Programming II) and Database Systems (CSC 312).

2 Methods/Innovative Teaching Pedagogies

Object-oriented programming (OOP) is still the predominant program design paradigm and taught in college courses to train software engineers. The very term object points directly to entities, concepts, and transactions in real world business processes, and prescribes a design logic focusing on organizing program modules to reflect the semantics (properties and operations) of and relationships amongst these objects. Software applications with a sound OO design tends to be easier to accommodate user requirements and to evolve with changing business situations.

It is also beneficial to using real world scenarios in teaching the concepts and principles of OOP. One general theme used in CSC 205 can help relate objects and their collaborations to real world scenarios as follows:

- Objects vs. (sub-)system: employees vs. company (with departments); each focuses on a set of responsibilities;
- Class vs. object: job descriptions vs. people fill in the jobs;
- Object responsibilities: know + do something = identify and specify the job, in terms of knowledge and skills;
- Collaboration = message passing: objects interact with one another in the process of fulfilling the goal in business;
- Cohesion and Coupling: organize employees in functional departments and set up communication protocols.

Problems: how to train "good" programmers? It is similar to training good "writers". Write about everything you see in the world with (Java) code: identifying the objects; specify their responsibilities; and provide a solution using them to write your (Java) code.

Various case studies have been used in classes taught in the CSC department, including Programming II, Database Systems, and Software Engineering. The topics evolved from "classroom samples" [5] extended from textbooks [1] to units from real world R&D projects [3]. Lately, the case studies used include the following:

- Super Bowl: It all started from drawing a bowling alley to "visualize" OO concepts as designed into GUI components and containers, layout managers, and event handling mechanisms; and then gradually extended to animating a Curling game in a Winter Olympics year, or American football after a Super Bowl game, since MQZ usually teaches Programming II in the spring.
- CSViewer for a Rhesus Monkey Knowledge Model (supported through a NSF grant) [7]: Teams of students in several database, software engineering, and data science courses have been involved in DB and GUI development, and related data preparation

and analytics tasks. When the Programming II class saw the recently released v1.0.2 [6], some students were intrigued and commented, "I want to do that." (Fig. 1b)

- Chinese Learning App: with Oracle Bone Script parsing (from a PDF and recognition using OCR); image and text data management with DB; GUIs supporting searching and learning (through animation, TTS) [on going]

3 Methods/Case-Based Collaborative Learning

In general, teaching and learning is not the same as filling human brain with knowledge like filling up a gas tank. Knowledge acquired through lectures and class examples need to be practices in hands-on exercises. What one learned from other courses and/or real life experiences need to be integrated into this learning-practice process. The related principles have been put forward and evolved through out human civilization. Analects [2] starts with quoting *Kongzi* (孔子, known as Confucius), a great teacher: "Is it not pleasant to learn with a constant perseverance and application?" How to develop effective curricular materials and leverage latest technological advancements to engage students in enjoyable learning and practicing activities remains a challenge to CS educators.

Our strategies include developing and updating courses (especially during recent curriculum reforms), promoting collaboration between classes, adopting assignments with real world applications, using knowledge from courses in other CS programs (IST, CYS, etc.). Essentially, we employ the "learning by doing" principle.

In this paper, we will use a Super Bowl theme/collaborative case currently adopted in spring 2023 as an example. The focus is on a Programming II section, while (teams of) students in another (database) class will collaborate.

- Concepts and skills in Programming II: design a class, levels of abstraction; GUI, collections, IO; recursion; etc.
- Case-based learning: identify cases = aspects of the problem that can be handled by the skills practiced;
- Collaborative learning: teacher guides the plan and design; provides templates/codebase, and
  - Assigns specific tasks to students: as labs and projects, with samples fed in through lectures.
  - Students become curriculum developers, and produce useable software products.
- Collaborative learning: use the same topic across several classes (subjects/semesters), on different aspects
  - Programming II: this spring, learning and practicing GUI, data structures, algorithms (like recursion);
  - Database DB design and implementation, content creation and management, and DB connectivity;
  - Software Engineering I & II, in 2023–24 academic year: for an enjoyable app for Super Bowl fans.
- Collaborative learning: potentially involving students from other schools/departments on graphics design, business, or even legal aspects.

4 Results/Super Bowl Project Collaborated in Programming and Database Classes

Again, the presentation here is mostly based on the Programming II class, for which a more detailed plan is available.

- After a review on Java (covered in Programming I) and two projects on (using and) Designing a Class, the Super Bowl theme will be used for the remaining 4 projects {scoreboard; historical highlights; auto-play; stats for fun} as follows:
- A game window: setting up the stage with a provided 2D game mini-framework, which includes

  - Interfaces: Drawable, Movable, Controllable, which specify WHAT objects in the type can do (like move);
  - Abstract classes: SceneEntity, Sprite, Avatar, which provide base data structures and functions for subclasses to access and/or inherit, yet forbid direct instantiation of these generic types;
  - Base/Utility classes: GameWindow with menu and hosting a GamePanel with a tabbed structure for various use cases (such as point-by-point replay), and a ShapeTransform class for moving ColoredShape objects (which combines a Color and a Shape, both standard Java types) for making SceneEntity objects.
  - Suggested implementing classes: specifying HOW objects in types QuarterBack, RunningBack, Field, and Scoreboard (, and even Referee, Artist, CheerLeader, Audience, if needed) will behave.

- Historical highlights: practicing data management with types in the Java Collections Framework (JCF).

  - Linear types (e.g., Lists and Queues): for Games, Teams, star Players; Artists; Cities (queue), etc. [#]
  - Set and map: distinct teams and the games they attended.
  - Custom types/types used in combination: game score recording with score time stamps, etc. [#]

- Auto-play: employing recursion/backtracking algorithms (often used in a maze app) to guide the running back to maneuver through defenders and get touchdown.
- Stats for fun: try to expose the students with using a third-part API (like JFreeChart[8]) to visualize results (such as with a bar chart). [#]

Note: Entries with # could use help from the DB class. While JDBC (as introduced in [4]) and Java is the default programming language in the database class, one team is assigned to explore the ways to use WebSwing [9] to show the Java GUIs in a web browser.

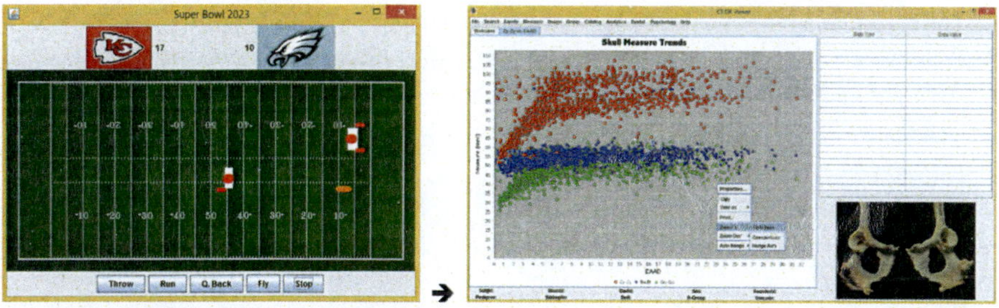

Fig. 1. a) Super Bowl Scoreboard under development b) A Screenshot of CSViewer v1.0.2

5 Conclusions and Future Works

The courses are ongoing, with students deeply engaged (in Programming II) and/or voted for the project topic (in Database Systems). Now in the programming class, we have a quarterback and a running back on the field, about to throw and catch a football (Fig. 1a). The quarterback can swing his arm and throw a ball; the ball flying is driven with a timer; and the running back carries a "catch-box" and can be moved by button press trying to receive the ball. Teams to build a database and related GUIs are formed in the database class, and the teams kicked off the process with a planning phase. The poster that will be presented at the conference will have complete diagrams and screenshots for demonstration and discussions.

This project can be extended into other courses, such as Software Engineering, and future offerings of the programming and database classes. Skills built up through this project can be applied in R&D projects like CSViewer and future employment.

References

1. Horstmann, C.: Object-Oriented Design and Patterns, 2nd edn. Wiley (2005)
2. Confucius. The Analects (论语 *lunyu,* as available on the Chinese Text Project's website. The Chinese Text Project is an online open-access digital library that makes pre-modern Chinese texts available to readers and researchers all around the world.). https://ctext.org/analects/xue-er. Accessed 1 Mar 2023
3. Zhao, M.Q.: Knowledge Models for SA Applications and User Interface Development for the SITA System. Final Report, ARFL/RI, Rome, NY, 15 July 2011
4. Zhao, M.Q.: A First Course in Database Systems. Linus Learning, Ronkonkoma, NY (2018)
5. Zhao, M.Q., White, L.: Engaging software engineering students using a series of OOAD workshops. In: Proceeding of ASEE 2006, Chicago, IL, 18–21 June 2006
6. Zhao, M.Q., Widener, E.R., Francis, G., Wang, Q.: Building a Knowledge Model of Cayo Santiago Rhesus Macaques: Engaging Undergraduate Students in Developing Graphical User Interfaces for a NSF Funded Research Project. Paper accepted by ICR 2023, Madrid, Spain (2023)
7. Zhao, M.Q., Maldonado, M., Kensler, T.B., Kohn, L.A.P., Guatelli-Steinburg, D., Wang, Q.: Conceptual design and prototyping for a primate health history model. In: Arabnia, H.R., Deligiannidis, L., Tinetti, F.G., Tran, Q.-N. (eds.) Advances in Computer Vision and Computational Biology, pp. 511–522. Springer, New York (2021). https://doi.org/10.1007/978-3-030-71051-4_40

8. The JFreeChart Project.https://www.jfree.org/jfreechart/. Accessed 16 Feb 2023
9. WebSwing | Run your Java Application in a web browser. https://www.webswing.org/. Accessed 22 Mar 2023

User Friendly Indoor Navigation Application for Visually Impaired Users in Museums Using 3D Sound

Nusaiba Al Sulaimani(✉), Ali Al-Humairi, and Sharifa Al Khanjari

Department of Computer Science, GUtech, Halban, Muscat, Sultanate of Oman
{nusaiba.alsulaimani,ali.alhumairi,
sharifa.alkhanjari}@gutech.edu.om

Abstract. As we move towards smart cities, it is important to consider the accessibility for people with disabilities. We consider visually impaired individuals by designing a mobile application that they can use to navigate autonomously around a museum. We propose combining current traditional non-technical accessibility methods with the use of 3D sounds technology.

Keywords: Visual Impairments · Human Computer Interaction · Indoor Navigation · 3D Sounds · BLE Beacons

1 Introduction

It is estimated that 2.2 billion people suffer from some form of visual impairment globally [1]. This means it is important to consider them when designing applications for a smart city. There are several studies that were done to support the autonomous mobility of the visually impaired. They all conclude the need for research in the area of indoor navigation [2–5].

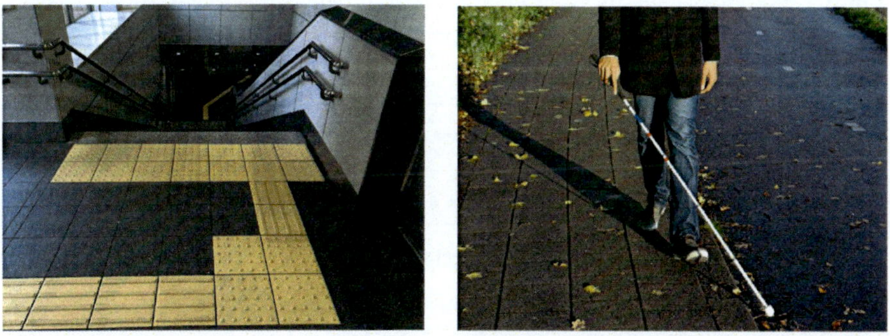

Fig. 1. Tactile tiles on the floor (LEFT)[9] and visually impaired individual using cane (RIGHT) [10]

K. Daimi and A. Al Sadoon (Eds.): ICR 2023, LNNS 721, pp. 441–444, 2023.
https://doi.org/10.1007/978-3-031-35308-6_37

Some traditional methods visually impaired individuals rely on to get around include using a cane to feel their surroundings, a guide dog and floor tactile. However, today there are many applications and technologies they can use to support their mobility. There are a number of applications that were researched specifically with the aim to help with navigation. An example is the app FIND, which is an application that was designed specifically to help people with disabilities navigate indoors [3]. Their approach included a heuristic analysis, a focus group and usability experts early in the development phase to come up with a product that would provide a positive user experience to their users [3]. Other solutions include the use of "Smart-canes", which are canes that help detect possible obstacles that a person may encounter while moving around. Smart glasses were also used for purpose of object detection [2, 6].

We are currently implementing an indoor navigation solution for a museum to enhance the experience of the visually impaired guest using BLE beacons, to help them achieve depth perception using 3D sounds combined with floor tactile for path finding and safety (Fig. 1).

2 Methodology

Several researchers have been studying indoor navigation techniques specifically for the visually impaired. However, not many focus on the user experience. It is important to consider the usability of the app in the early stages when developing a software [3].

We started our research by conducting qualitative interviews with 3 people who suffer from visual impairment to get an understanding of the kind of apps that they use in their daily life to help them with accessibility and mobility. Our focus is understanding their preferences and general experience using mobile applications. We asked about the accuracy, user-friendliness, and usefulness of the apps they use.

We found that despite a very high inaccuracy in some apps, the visually impaired users continue to use them. They depend on voiceover screen readers which makes following the accessibility guidelines for app building important to consider. The usability guidelines we found relevant to us was conducting a user test once the application is built. Additionally, including content descriptions to support the voiceover by labeling textboxes and buttons are also important because visually impaired users rely on the voiceover screen reader and voice over commands to use the applications [8] (Fig. 2).

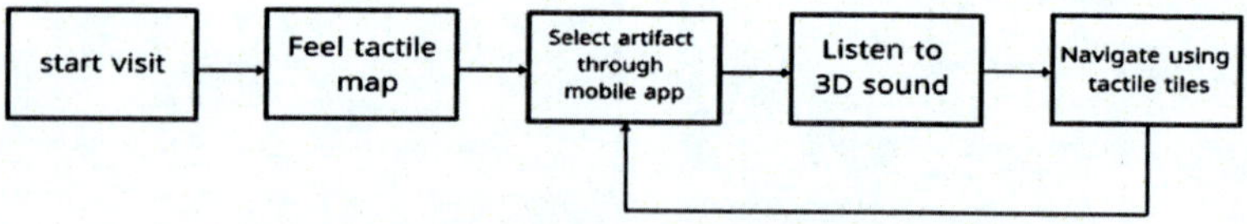

Fig. 2. Map to user experience through museum

We are currently researching a solution using BLE beacons to locate where the 3D sounds is coming from to provide depth perception. BLE beacons have been used for indoor navigation combined with other technologies such as computer vision in many researchers [7]. There are several researches that used the 3D sounds to provide depth perception in museums, however, our solution is unique because we are combining the use of technology with the traditional physical floor tactiles to provide a path for the user. This is because visually impaired individuals need their sense of hearing to avoid moving obstacles.

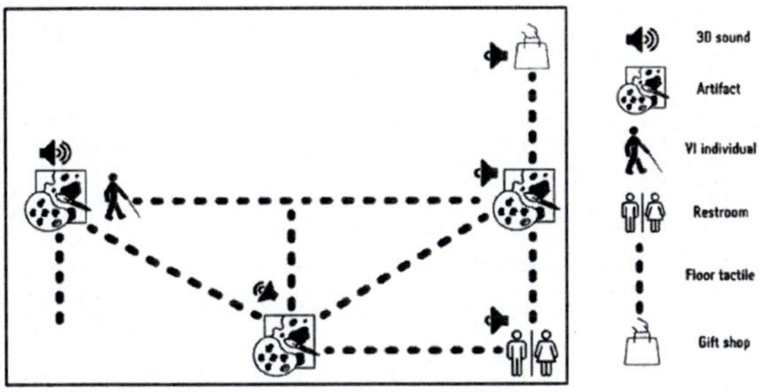

Fig. 3. Illustrative example explaining how 3d sounds can guide the VI user to the artifact

Upon entering the museum, the visually impaired user can feel a tactile map to understand the floor plan. The application can be used by the user for navigating through the museum, relying on the floor tactiles as a guiding path. For the app to locate the position of the user, a 2D map is embedded in the application that contains the exact position of each BLE beacon. Using trilateration, the positions of the beacons can be used to estimate the precise position of the user. Additionally, gyroscope sensors can find user's direction in relation to the beacons, which can then generate 3D sounds from that direction [11].

In Fig. 3, an illustration is provided on how the app can be used by someone with visual impairment to navigate through a museum. As the user gets closer to an artifact, the volume of the 3D sound will increase, while it will decrease as they move further away. The sound will originate from the direction of the artifact, serving as a helpful guide for visually impaired individuals to independently reach their desired destination.

3 Conclusion and Future Works

Implementing Indoor Navigation Solutions is very likely to change the lives of visually impaired individuals. Our research is still in its early stages; however, we discuss how we can provide a visually impaired user an auditory perception of their surroundings to eliminate the need for audio instructions to reach to a position. We are currently developing this app, and our main challenge is finding an accurate estimation for the users' position.

Future works include conducting a user study to study the efficiency of the solution and evaluating the accessibility of the application in terms of accuracy and comfort for the visually impaired user.

References

1. World Health Organization. (2022, January). Blindness and visual impairment. Fact Sheet. Retrieved March 27, 2023. https://www.who.int/news-room/fact-sheets/detail/blindness-and-visual-impairment
2. Mantoro, T., Zamzami, M.: Realtime indoor navigation system for visually impaired person using direct-based navigation. In: 2022 5th International Conference of Computer and Informatics Engineering (IC2IE), Jakarta, Indonesia, 2022, pp. 320–324 (2022). https://doi.org/10.1109/IC2IE56416.2022.9970063
3. Shahini, F., Nasr, V., Zahabi, M.: A Friendly Indoor Navigation App for People with Disabilities (FIND) (2022)
4. Ou, W., Zhang, J., Peng, K., Yang, K., Jaworek, G., Mueller, K., Stiefelhagen, R.: Indoor Navigation Assistance for Visually Impaired People via Dynamic SLAM and Panoptic Segmentation with an RGB-D Sensor (2022). https://doi.org/10.1007/978-3-031-08648-9_19
5. Aakash Krishna, G.S., Pon, V.N., Rai, S., Baskar, A.: Vision system with 3D audio feedback to assist navigation for visually impaired. Procedia Comput. Sci. **167**, 235–243 (2020). ISSN 1877-0509. https://doi.org/10.1016/j.procs.2020.03.216
6. Idrees, A., Iqbal, Z., Ishfaq, M.: An Efficient Indoor Navigation Technique To Find Optimal Route For Blinds Using QR Codes (2020)
7. Gang, H.-S., Pyun, J.-Y.: A smartphone indoor positioning system using hybrid localization technology. Energies **12**, 3702 (2019). https://doi.org/10.3390/en12193702
8. Apple Inc. (n.d.). Inclusion. Human Interface Guidelines. Retrieved March 28, 2023. https://developer.apple.com/design/human-interface-guidelines/foundations/inclusion/
9. Samurai Tours. (2018, May 17). Japan's tactile paving blocks. Retrieved March 31, 2023. https://www.samuraitours.com/japans-tactile-paving-blocks/
10. Lighthouse for the Blind and Low Vision. (n.d.). Everything you need to know about white canes. Retrieved March 31, 2023. https://lhblind.org/everything-you-need-to-know-about-white-canes/
11. Cantón Paterna, V., Calveras Augé, A., Paradells Aspas, J., Pérez Bullones, M.A.: A Bluetooth low energy indoor positioning system with channel diversity, weighted trilateration and Kalman filtering. Sensors **17**, 2927 (2017). https://doi.org/10.3390/s17122927

Using AI to Capture Class Attendance

Fatmah Alantali[1], Adhari Almemari[1], Maryam Alyammahi[1], Benson Raj[1], Mohsin Iftikhar[1](✉), Muhammad Aaqib[2], and Hanif Ullah[2]

[1] Higher College of Technology, Fujairah, UAE
{H00386666,H00415297,H00415326,braj,miftikhar}@hct.ac.ae
[2] Ulster University, Northern BT15 1ED, UK
{Aaqib-m,h.ullah}@ulster.ac.uk

Abstract. The primary goal of this work is to provide an overview of the project's design and, equally important, its implementation. Face Recognition is a computer application implemented for identifying or verifying human faces from a digital camera image or video. Our system employed a face recognition system to register the attendance of students upon entry and exit from Higher College of Technology (HCT) premises. The proposed system involves capturing and analyzing the facial features of individuals and comparing them to a database of the registered students. The experimental analysis of the proposed system shows that our method for facial recognition systems is quite accurate, effective, and reliable. Moreover, it would be used as an automated attendance management system in real-world scenarios. Furthermore, we performed manual testing to evaluate the application's input and output, as well as the conformance of our programming and coding to the project's specifications.

Keywords: Artificial Intelligence · Face Recognition · Histogram of Gradient · Higher Colleges of Technology · Haar Cascade classifier

1 Introduction

Since the number of students in the HCT is increasing, it will get more crowded when people are entering and leaving. HCT is a large academic institution that offers an extensive variety of courses and programs. One of the main difficulties faced by HCT is maintaining proper students' attendance logs. Currently, the tutor takes attendance manually; however, this approach has proven unreliable due to several reasons, including an increasing number of students and students arriving late.

Face recognition technology was used to track attendance, which was an innovative approach to handling attendance procedures. Facial recognition was a more precise and fast procedure than other systems, which reduced the possibility of faking attendance [1]. Facial recognition had the advantage of enabling passive authentication, which meant that the individual being identified did not need to authenticate their identity [2]. While installing a face recognition system at a college's entrance gate can be a useful option for various reasons, such as improving the accuracy, speed, convenience, and security of the college's student attendance system.

K. Daimi and A. Al Sadoon (Eds.): ICR 2023, LNNS 721, pp. 445–449, 2023.
https://doi.org/10.1007/978-3-031-35308-6_38

As a team, we discussed the problem and came up with a great idea that will effectively achieve the goal of the problem. As much as possible, we attempt to develop a system that would be novel and contemporary and assist us in resolving this issue. Therefore, we came up with the concept and idea of smart gates. These smart gates would significantly reduce congestion.

Furthermore, these gates make it simple to identify a person based on their facial print. Therefore, we suggested a system for taking attendance that uses face recognition to help students get to class on time. To build our system, we used the Python programming language and artificial intelligence (AI) to recognize the faces of the students. The reason behind this choice is that Python provides a variety of libraries for AI and machine learning (ML) [3]. Moreover, Python is more prevalent in AI than other languages. Face recognition uses AI systems to recognize human faces in the background. Additionally, the algorithm often searches for human eyes first, followed by the brows, nose, mouth, nostrils, and iris. This project's aim is to design and integrate all facial recognition requirements because this solution reduces scanning times and enhances HCT input operations.

2 Literature Review

As we mentioned in the introduction section, the number of students at HCT and all universities is drastically increasing. Also, we know that with the increase in the number of students, crowding occurs when entering and leaving the HCT; for example, overcrowding in entering the HCT causes delays in attending lectures, so the student is registered as being late, and there are many other problems as well.

Solving this problem required us to produce solutions, which we were able to do. However, we have brainstormed solutions that will help us solve the mentioned problem. While implementing these solutions, it would lead to a significant reduction in congestion.

In the literature, we have observed that several companies have utilized this technology to simplify processes; these technologies are found in airports [4], the Tahaluf Company [5], and other organizations. However, upon examining the technology employed by these companies, we have noticed that they only have mechanisms that recognize facial imprints with ease but do not address congestion effectively. Because these companies have implemented gates that require individuals to stand still for their face prints to be scanned, this fails to tackle the issue of overcrowding during entry and exit at HCT.

Our proposed system aims to address the problems of registration and delays experienced by the HCT when students enter or leave the campus. Therefore, we developed a system that makes it easy for students to go through the scanning point without having to wait in line at any gate. Finally, with our system, the students can walk through the designated area as cameras scan their faces and register their details in the system.

3 Libraries Used

- Cmake: An object library compiles source files but does not archive or link their object files into a library. Actually, this library is used for managing the dependencies of face detection techniques such as Dlib, OpenCV.

- Dlib: We used the Dlib library to detect faces based on HOG features. There are several reasons for choosing the library [6]; including its high accuracy during face detection and its capability to detect faces in challenging conditions.
- OpenCV-python: A library of Python bindings designed to solve computer vision problems. Initially, we used this library for image analysis using the HAAR Cascade to identify faces in the images [7].
- We employed the above libraries in our system because they facilitate pre-built techniques and schemes that are optimized for face recognition tasks.

4 Proposed System

The proposed system is equipped with cameras that can effortlessly scan the features of the image. To begin with, we need to obtain the facial prints of each student and attach them to the system. Once the system saves the face print, it will be simple to enter and exit the HCT. When a student, teacher, or any member of staff passes in front of these cameras, the cameras will take a scan of the person's face and then connect it to the system. The camera will not recognize them, and after recognizing the face, a box will appear on the student's face with his information, and if the face print is not recognized, a box will appear with (unknown) (Fig. 1).

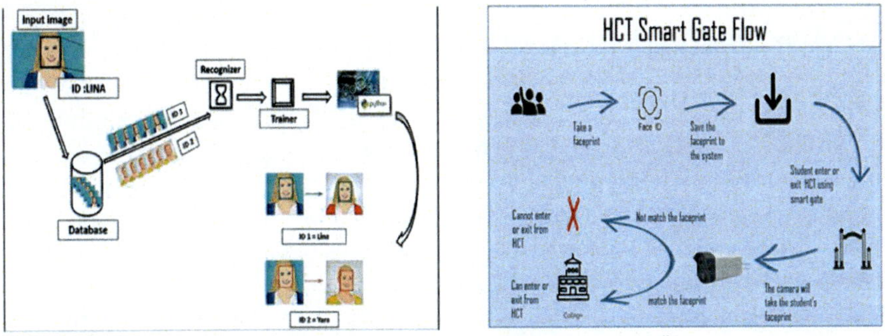

(a) (b)

Fig. 1. (a) Database (b) System architecture.

The following steps were deployed.

1. Image acquisition: Initially, we captured the image using a camera placed in the entrance gate.
2. Detect faces: Here we used histogram of oriented gradients (HOG) to detect the students' faces.
3. Encoding features: The next step was to extract the unique face characteristic for each image, as faces are found in the sample image. In general, whenever we obtain face localization, the extremely precise 128-d facial features are retrieved for each image input and kept in records files for face recognition system.
4. Face-recognition: finally, we used a face recognition system for identification. Therefore, we performed feature comparisons against the features recorded in the data [8]. The investigation image is shown beside the associated verified face, and the matched face's name is recognized and used to register or mark attendance successfully [9].

5 Preliminary Testing Results

To test the capabilities of the system, the IDs of multiple users were used, as shown in Fig. 2 (a). It is evident from Fig. 2 (b) that 98.7% accuracy was detected when the person stood in front of the image capturing module.

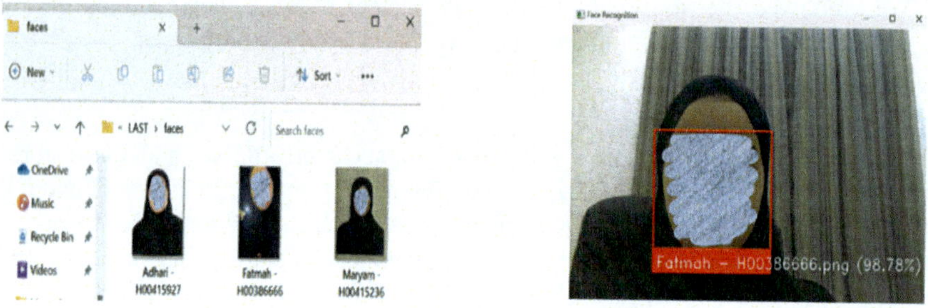

(a) (b)

Fig. 2. (a) Data file (b) Face Recognition.

6 Conclusion and Future Work

As mentioned earlier, the proposed system is based on a camera that captures the face print and then connects it to the system to see if it has been recognized. Therefore, in this system, we used a webcam initially to show the idea in general and how it works. The webcam provides a simple and quick way on how the mechanism of our developed system works. However, in the future, it will be more essential to incorporate a real camera and connect it to the system for the purposes of attendance and facial recognition. The system first needs the database of students' images so that it can compare the faceprint it will take with the image in the database. Moreover, in the future, the proposed method will deal with noisy images, observe the effect on accuracy by increasing the number of samples and cases, and also check the behavior of the person from their facial features using the face recognition system. A real camera would do this job perfectly and would give a full overview of our work.

References

1. Bhatti, K., Mughal, L., Khuhawar, F., Memon, S.: Smart attendance management system using face recognition. EAI Endorsed Transactions on Creative Technologies, 5(17) (2018)
2. Quraishi, N., Naimi, M.E., Ghousi, S., Kumar, S.: Smart attendance using real-time recognition (2021)
3. Top 9 Python Libraries for Machine Learning in 2023. upGrad Blog. https://www.upgrad.com/blog/top-python-libraries-for-machine-learning/ upGrad. (2022)
4. Air Canada trials facial recognition technology – Business Traveller. (2023, February 22). Business Traveller. https://www.businesstraveller.com/business-travel/2023/02/22/air-canada-trials-facial-recognition-technology/

5. تحالف. (n.d.). Takeleap. https://takeleap.com/ar/services/computer-vision/tahaluf-smart-vending-machine
6. Dlib C++ library. (n.d.). Retrieved March 15, 2023. http://dlib.net
7. Introduction (n.d.). Retrieved March 15, 2023. https://docs.opencv.org/3.4/da/d60/tutorial_face_main.html team, O. (2023). From OpenCV: https://opencv.org/about/
8. Face Recognition: recent advancements and research challenges (2023). From IEEE: https://ieeexplore.ieee.org/document/9984308
9. An improved face recognition algorithm and its application in attendance management system (2020). Array. https://www.sciencedirect.com/science/article/pii/S2590005619300141

Author Index

K. Daimi and A. Al Sadoon (Eds.): ICR 2023, LNNS 721, pp. 451–452, 2023.
https://doi.org/10.1007/978-3-031-35308-6